LUNG VOLUME REDUCTION SURGERY

LUNG VOLUME REDUCTION SURGERY

Edited by

MICHAEL ARGENZIANO, MD
MARK E. GINSBURG, MD

Columbia University College of Physicians and Surgeons; The New York Presbyterian Hospital–Columbia Presbyterian Center, New York, NY

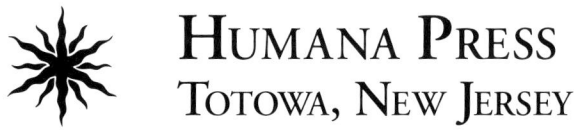

HUMANA PRESS
TOTOWA, NEW JERSEY

© 2002 Humana Press Inc.
999 Riverview Drive, Suite 208
Totowa, New Jersey 07512
humanapress.com

For additional copies, pricing for bulk purchases, and/or information about other Humana titles, contact Humana at the above address or at any of the following numbers: Tel.: 973-256-1699; Fax: 973-256-8341, E-mail: humana@humanapr.com; or visit our Website: http://humanapr.com

Cover Illustration: Diffuse severe pulmonary emphysema in a 66-year-old man. *See* Fig. 3 on p. 68.

Cover design by Patricia F. Cleary.

Production Editor: Mark J. Breaugh.

This publication is printed on acid-free paper. ∞
ANSI Z39.48-1984 (American National Standards Institute) Permanence of Paper for Printed Library Materials.

Printed in the United States of America. 10 9 8 7 6 5 4 3 2 1

Library of Congress Cataloging-in-Publication Data

Lung volume reduction surgery / [edited by] Michael Argenziano, Mark E. Ginsburg
     p. ; cm.
   Includes bibliographical references and index.
   ISBN 0-89603-848-3 (alk. paper)
   1. Pneumonectomy. 2. Lungs--Surgery. 3. Emphysema, Pulmonary--Treatment. I.
Argenziano, Michael. II. Ginsburg, Mark E.
   [DNLM: 1. Pneumonectomy. WF 668 L9637 2001]
   RD539 .L867 2001
   617.5'42--dc21
                                                                2001024308

DEDICATIONS

To my parents, Anna and Gaetano,
who set me upon my current path;
and to my wife, Maria,
and our sons, Michael, Anthony, and Nicholas,
who have made it worth traveling.
—Michael Argenziano, MD

To honor my parents Jeanne and Ben;
and for my wife, Gail,
and my children, Adam, Allison, Kerry, and Rebecca:
may all your dreams come true.
—Mark E. Ginsburg, MD

PREFACE

In a landmark paper published in 1995, Dr. Joel Cooper reported the initial results of a procedure that he termed "bilateral pneumectomy." A modern reincarnation of an operation conceived nearly a half century earlier by Otto Brantigan, Dr. Cooper's technique involved bilateral resection of significant amounts of diseased lung tissue in emphysema patients, in an effort to improve respiratory function by decompressing the thoracic cavity and increasing pulmonary elastic recoil. Almost instantaneously, worldwide interest and enthusiasm were directed toward this potential panacea for the millions of patients suffering and dying from end-stage emphysema. Lung volume reduction surgery (LVRS), as the new procedure soon came to be known, became the subject of numerous articles in the lay media, if not in scientific journals, gaining the attention of patients, physicians, and the general public. Despite a paucity of objective data, surgeons willing to perform the procedure were inundated by hundreds of self-referring patients desperate for a new lease on life.

Dozens of centers began to perform LVRS, in the manner described by Cooper, and a trickle of scientific reports eventually ensued. According to these early reports, short-term results were promising, although outcomes had not been positive in all patients. Nonetheless, before long, the operation was being performed across the country, fueled by positive reports from centers operating on highly selected patient cohorts, and more importantly, by patient and physician enthusiasm.

This enthusiasm for LVRS had several effects. Almost suddenly, questions about how our society should implement new surgical technology and about the role of insurers in determining coverage, and thereby access, to new procedures became central issues. The ethics of randomized trials for the study of apparently beneficial surgical treatments became hotly debated. Fundamental questions were raised concerning the long-term efficacy, cost-effectiveness, selection criteria, timing, and optimal surgical approaches for LVRS. The previously quiescent field of pulmonary physiology was reinvigorated.

In 1996, after a review of preliminary data failed to provide conclusive evidence of a clear benefit of LVRS for emphysema, the Health Care Financing Administration (HCFA) imposed a moratorium on Medicare reimbursement for the new procedure until a properly designed, randomized trial could be performed. Thus, through the collaboration of HCFA and the NHLBI, the multicenter National Emphysema Treatment Trial (NETT) was conceived. As of the writing of this book, the trial is underway, with results still several years away. It is the hope of the physicians and patients involved in this trial that valuable information is gained, with the ultimate goal of determining if (and for whom) the operation is in fact beneficial.

Lung Volume Reduction Surgery was conceived in response to the enthusiasm, controversy, confusion, and disappointment that, in the experience of the editors, have variously (and often simultaneously) characterized the attitudes of clinicians and scientists toward this novel and potentially revolutionary operation. In the chapters that follow, we attempt to elucidate the current state of knowledge surrounding LVRS, in order to define the clinical and scientific landscape for those interested in this field. In Part One, experts in clinical medicine and the basic sciences review the diagnosis, pathophysiology, and medical management of emphysema, in order to ground the reader in the disciplines that form the basis of our current knowledge. In Part Two, the technical aspects and clinical results of LVRS are reviewed, with additional emphasis on organizational issues important for those involved or planning to be involved in LVRS programs. This book is intended for readers of diverse backgrounds, including surgeons, pulmonologists, primary care physicians, physiologists, radiologists, basic scientists, physical and occupational therapists, and nurses. It is the hope of the editors that the information contained in this book will be of help to these professionals and to all those who share the mission of providing the best possible care to patients with emphysema.

The question of whether LVRS will have a future role in the treatment of emphysema is currently unanswered. A clear and complete answer to this question will likely require years of clinical experience, careful analysis of properly designed randomized trials, and perhaps most importantly, a redefinition by society of the importance of palliation in the treatment of incurable diseases. Despite the controversy that is certain to surround LVRS in the coming years, the debate that has been generated has already had positive effects. The enthusiasm generated by this novel operation has brought a fresh perspective and a new generation of researchers into the fields of pulmonary physiology and end-stage lung disease. In this environment, a unique opportunity exists for both clinicians and researchers to uncover the physiologic and molecular determinants of this devastating disease. Although LVRS may one day be shown to improve (and perhaps prolong) the lives of patients suffering from emphysema, it is far more exciting to think that the research initiated in these early LVRS years might one day lead to an actual cure of the disease.

Michael Argenziano, MD
Mark E. Ginsburg, MD

CONTENTS

CONTRIBUTORS

MICHAEL ARGENZIANO, MD • *Division of Cardiothoracic Surgery, New York Presbyterian Hospital–Columbia Presbyterian Center, New York, NY*

JOHN H.M. AUSTIN, MD • *Department of Radiology, New York Presbyterian Hospital, New York, NY*

DAVID BALFE, MBBCH, FCP, SA • *Division of Pulmonary/Critical Care Medicine, Cedars Sinai Medical Center, Los Angeles, CA*

MATTHEW N. BARTELS, MD, MPH • *Division of Rehabilitation Medicine, Columbia University College of Physicians and Surgeons, New York, NY*

YAHYA M. BERKMEN, MD • *Department of Radiology, New York Presbyterian Hospital, New York, NY*

FRANCES BROGAN, MSN, RN • *Lung Volume Reduction Program, New York Presbyterian Hospital, New York, NY*

JEANINE D'ARMIENTO, MD • *Division of Pulmonary, Allergy, and Critical Care Medicine, Columbia University College of Physicians and Surgeons, New York, NY*

JOSEPH J. DEROSE, JR., MD • *Division of Cardiothoracic Surgery, New York Presbyterian Hospital–Columbia Presbyterian Center, New York, NY*

ELLISE S. DELPIIIN, MD, MPH • *Department of Anesthesiology, New York University School of Medicine, New York, NY*

CLAUDE DESCHAMPS, MD • *Division of General Thoracic Surgery, Mayo Clinic, Rochester, MN*

MARK E. GINSBURG, MD • *Division of Cardiothoracic Surgery, New York Presbyterian Hospital–Columbia Presbyterian Center, New York, NY*

LYALL A. GORENSTEIN, MD • *Division of Cardiothoracic Surgery, New York Presbyterian Hospital–Columbia Presbyterian Center, New York, NY*

CHARLES W. HOOPES, MD • *Section of General Thoracic Surgery, University of Michigan Medical Center, Ann Arbor, MI*

MARK D. IANNETTONI, MD • *Section of General Thoracic Surgery, University of Michigan Medical Center, Ann Arbor, MI*

PATRICIA A. JELLEN, MD • *Lung Volume Reduction Program, New York Presbyterian Hospital, New York, NY*

MARK J. KRASNA, MD • *Division of Thoracic Surgery, University of Maryland, Baltimore, MD*

ZAB MOHSENIFAR, MD, FCCP • *Division of Pulmonary/Critical Care Medicine, Cedars Sinai Medical Center, Los Angeles, CA*

GREGORY D. N. PEARSON, MD • *Department of Radiology, New York Presbyterian Hospital, New York, NY*

STEVEN M. SCHARF, MD, PhD • *Division of Pulmonary and Critical Care Medicine, Long Island Jewish Medical Center, New Hyde Park, NY*

NEIL W. SCHLUGER, MD • *Division of Pulmonary, Allergy, and Critical Care Medicine, Columbia University College of Physicians and Surgeons, New York, NY*

LARRY L. SCHULMAN, MD • *Division of Pulmonary Medicine, Columbia University College of Physicians and Surgeons, New York, NY*

MARIA C. SHIAU, MD • *Department of Radiology, New York Presbyterian Hospital, New York, NY*

JOSHUA R. SONETT, MD • *Division of Thoracic Surgery, University of Maryland, Baltimore, MD*

KENNETH M. STEINGLASS, MD • *Division of Cardiothoracic Surgery, New York Presbyterian Hospital–Columbia Presbyterian Center, New York, NY*

BYRON THOMASHOW, MD • *Division of Pulmonary Medicine, Columbia University College of Physicians and Surgeons, New York, NY*

JAMES P. UTZ, MD • *Division of Pulmonary and Critical Care Medicine, Mayo Clinic, Rochester, MN*

ANTONIO L. VISBAL, MD • *Division of General Thoracic Surgery, Mayo Clinic, Rochester, MN*

CHUN K. YIP, MD • *Division of Pulmonary, Allergy, and Critical Care Medicine, Columbia University College of Physicians and Surgeons, New York, NY*

I

DIAGNOSIS, PATHOPHYSIOLOGY, AND MEDICAL MANAGEMENT OF EMPHYSEMA

1 The Pathogenesis and Pathophysiology of Emphysema

Neil W. Schluger, MD
and Jeanine D'Armiento, MD

CONTENTS

CURRENT CONCEPTS IN THE MOLECULAR PATHOGENESIS OF EMPHYSEMA

Emphysema, the "abnormal permanent enlargement of the airspaces distal to the terminal bronchioles, accompanied by destruction of their walls and without obvious fibrosis," is the result of a complex pathophysiologic process that occurs in the setting of one or more of several risk factors, of which by far the most important is cigarette smoking. Other risk factors for the development of emphysema include exposure to environmental tobacco smoke and/or high levels of ambient air pollution, sex, and race. Socioeconomic factors and occupational exposures may also contribute to or form part of the stimulus, which sets in motion the chain of events, which lead ultimately to destruction of lung tissue.

The prevailing hypothesis explaining the pathogenesis of emphysema, the "proteinase-antiproteinase theory," holds that the natural defenses of the lung are overwhelmed by the ongoing secretion and activation of tissue proteases in the lung which are secreted mainly by neutrophils and perhaps alveolar macrophages as well. Under normal conditions, there is both constituitive and sporadic release of proteolytic

From: *Lung Volume Reduction Surgery*
Edited by: M. Argenziano and M. E. Ginsburg © Humana Press Inc., Totowa, NJ

enzymes into the lung. These enzymes fall into several categories, including serine proteinases (secreted mainly by neutrophils), cysteine proteinases (secreted mostly by macrophages), and matrix metalloproteinases (secreted by both neutrophils and macrophages). Inhibitors of these proteinases, such as α-1-antitrypsin, prevent destruction of the lung's extracellular matrix under normal circumstances. In the proteinase-antiproteinase theory, emphysema may result when there is an imbalance in the system, such that proteinase release or activity is augmented, or antiproteinase release or activity is diminished, or some combination of the two occurs in an unequal manner such that there is a net excess of proteolytic activity.

Matrix Proteins and Proteinases in the Pathogenesis of Emphysema

The first target of proteolytic enzymes to be identified (and linked to the development of emphysema) within the extracellular matrix (ECM) of the lung appears was elastin. Indeed, a careful morphologic study of lung specimens resected from patients undergoing surgery for lung cancers has demonstrated decreased elastin content in areas of centriacinar, distal acinar, and irregular air-space enlargement (1). Elastin is at the core of the elastic fibers, which form the structural matrix of the lung, and can be cleaved by a number of enzymes present in lung parenchyma, including neutrophil elastase, proteinase 3, cathepsin G, gelatinase, metalloelastase, cathepsin L, and cathepsin S. Normally, elastin synthesis in the lung begins during the late fetal period and continues throughout lung development, which continues through adolescence, although the peak synthesis occurs during the early post-natal period (2). The exact source of elastin production in the lung is unclear, although myofibroblasts, chondroblasts, and smooth muscle cells are all capable of production. Interestingly, alveolar epithelial cells have not been shown to be sources of elastin synthesis.

Recent evidence suggests that elastin synthesis in the lung and else-where may be regulated to a significant degree by retinoids. Elastin synthesis by rat pulmonary interstitial fibroblasts is increased by retinoic acid. In a study by McGowan et al., pulmonary interstitial fibroblasts were isolated from fetal and postnatal rat lungs and the retinoid levels (retinoic acid, retinoic acid receptors, and cellular retinol binding protein) in the cells quantitated and correlated with timing of elastin production (3). Levels of all of these retinoids were highest just before maximal elastin synthesis, consistent with the hypothesis that endogenous retinoic acid could contribute to the postnatal increase in elastin synthesis by lung fibroblasts. Further work by the same group demonstrated that when inhibitors of retinoid metabolism were used to reduce the flux of retinyl esters to retinoic acid, gene expression of elastin was reduced in lung tissue of rats *(4)*. The magnitude of the effect of inhibitors was retinol dependent and was significantly reduced in lung tissue that was vitamin A-deficient, lending further support to the notion that stores of retinoids may increase elastin gene expression during fetal and early postnatal life. Most recently, fetal lung morphology in normal and vitamin A-deficient rats was studied by Antipatis et al. who demonstrated that elastin was expressed in normal rats from day 19 of gestation until the second postnatal day, whereas offspring of vitamin A-deficient maternal rats had altered lung development, with underdeveloped bronchial passages containing less elastin. Fetal lung elastin gene expression was reduced by nearly half in these animals *(5)*.

The degradation of elastin readily explains the early development of the disease in the rare human disorder of α-1-antitrypsin deficiency *(6)*. However, as noted above, this represents only 1% of all human patients who suffer from emphysema *(7)* and the relationship of α-1-antitrypsin to the major form of human emphysema induced by cigarette smoking remains unclear. In fact, studies over the past 20 yr have failed to demonstrate elastase excess or inhibitor deficiency in the development of other forms of human emphysema *(8,9)*. Even in α-antitrypsin-deficient human patients, there is no direct biochemical evidence for actual proteolysis of elastin in vivo *(10)*. Finally, it has been shown that the elastin gene is disrupted in the human disease of supravalvular aortic stenosis, which causes the narrowing of arteries *(11)*. Despite the apparent lack of elastin in these human patients, there are no abnormalities observed in the lung.

Most significantly perhaps, there are a number of discrepancies between the emphysema observed in the elastase-induced animal model and human emphysema. First, there are differences in the morphological phenotype that have been identified at the ultrastructural level *(12)*. Second, the elastase-induced animals suffer from an acute (within 4 h) severe hemorrhagic and inflammatory response *(12)*, which could induce a variety of nonspecific initiators of the emphysematous process *(13)*. Third, this acute form of emphysema induced after a single intratracheal instillation of enzyme is in direct contrast to human emphysema, which develops only after chronic insult to the tissue over a period of years. Overall, the lack of direct evidence has led a number of investigators to question the exact role of elastase in human emphysema *(8,13)*.

As incomplete as our understanding is about the exact role of elastase in emphysema, the picture is even more unclear for the role of other degradative enzymes and their substrates. There has also been considerable investigation into the role and importance of collagen and other matrix proteins important in emphysema pathogenesis. Wright and Churg have demonstrated that smoke-induced emphysema in guinea pigs is associated with collagen breakdown and repair, as evidenced by careful morphometric analysis *(14)*. This interesting study revealed that after 1 mo of smoke exposure there was a significant decrease in the volume proportion of collagen in the lungs, whereas after 6–12 mo of smoke exposure, there was actually an increase in the volume proportion of collagen. This study suggests that smoke-induced emphysema reflects breakdown and resynthesis of a variety of connective tissue proteins, in addition to elastin. The hypothesis that turnover of collagen is important in the development of emphysema is also supported by studies of Selman, who also used a guinea pig model to demonstrate increased expression of collagenase mRNA in alveolar macrophages in response to smoke exposure *(15)*. This increased gene expression was associated with increased enzyme activity and supports the conclusion that interstitial collagen degradation plays a role in the development of lung emphysema.

Other work in animals lends support to a potential role of collagen and collagenase in emphysema. On the one hand, when bacterial collagenase was injected into the lungs of hamsters, no emphysematous lesions developed *(16)*. However, there are some correlative studies that suggest that collagenase, a matrix metalloproteinase that degrades the fibrillar collagens, may be involved in a number of lung diseases including respiratory disorders *(17–20)*. Furthermore, there are a number of observations that suggest that collagen is degraded or damaged in pulmonary emphysema. For example, antibodies to collagen have been found in the serum of patients with emphysema *(21)*. In the inherited disorder type-VI Ehlers-Danlos syndrome, there is a decreased structural integrity of collagen fibrils and emphysematous changes were reported in these patients *(22)*. It has also been shown that collagen is affected in the various emphysema animal models. In papain-induced emphysema, dissolution of collagen fibrils is seen shortly after instillation of the enzyme *(23)*. Similarly, collagen is rapidly degraded in elastase-induced emphysema *(24)*. Finally, short exposure to toxic amounts of oxygen in rats will lead to emphysematous changes and collagen degradation with no changes in elastin *(25)*.

In emphysema, the complex interactions between the various components of the ECM are perturbed *(26)*. Such a disturbance can only be examined within the framework of the whole tissue and any resulting disease state is only evident in the whole organism. A number of animal model systems have, therefore, been employed to analyze the pathophysiology of emphysema. The first involves the intratracheal instillation of a number of proteinases into various animal species. Although valuable information has been gained through these experiments, their usefulness is limited because of the nonphysiological conditions created by the introduction of large quantities of enzymes into the lungs of animals (see also aforementioned for further disadvantages of the various animal models using this methodology). The second approach has taken advantage of a number of genetic animal models of emphysema including the blotchy *(25)* and the tight skin (Tsk) mouse *(27)*. Unfortunately, the use of these mutants is limited because they have a pleiotropic phenotype.

Recently, apparent support for the involvement of elastolytic enzymes in emphysema came from studies performed on a metalloelastase knockout mouse (MME -/-). These mice do not express the metalloelastase gene and are normal at baseline *(28)*. When the animals are exposed to cigarette smoke, at the human equivalent of 2000 cigarettes/d, they do not develop emphysematous changes in the lung as do wild-type animals. Although the data are novel and highly suggestive that the lack of the metalloelastase enzyme is protecting the animals from emphysema, there is no direct evidence demonstrating that excess elastolytic activity of metalloelastase is critically involved in emphysema formation. Furthermore, the investigators demonstrate that the macrophage is abnormal in the MME-/- mice. When the MME -/- mice are exposed to cigarette smoke, there is no increase in macrophage infiltration into the lung as is seen with wild-type mice.

Further evidence in support of the role of matrix metalloproteinases, including collagenase, is provided by the work of both D'Armiento and Ohnishi *(29,30)*. D'Armiento created a transgenic mouse that overexpresses collagenase, and histological analysis of the lungs revealed disruption of the alveolar walls and coalescence of the alveolar spaces with no evidence of fibrosis or inflammation *(29)*. These findings were strikingly similar to the changes in the lungs of humans with emphysema. Ohnishi et al. observed that membrane-type metalloproteinase-1 (MT1-MMP) and matrix metalloproteinase-2 (MMP-2) were present in elevated levels in pneumocytes, fibroblasts, and alveolar macrophages from emphysematous lungs as compared to normal lung tissue *(30)*. Interestingly, in this study, neutrophil elastase (as measured by enzyme immunoassay [EIA]) and α-1-antitrypsin (assayed by laser nephelometric immunoassay) were not present in elevated amounts in the emphysematous lungs.

Most recently, investigators have examined alveolar macrophages from 10 emphysema patients and 10 normal volunteers and measured protease activity and mRNA levels *(31)*. In this study, Finlay et al. demonstrated that there were elevated levels of gelatinase B and interstitial collagenase mRNA in the macrophages of smokers. In contrast, the mRNA for metalloelastase was not detected. In addition, the investigators demonstrated an increase in collagenase activity in the macrophages from the emphysema patients as compared to the normal patients. In conjunction with the transgenic mouse data, the results of this study strongly suggest a significant role for collagen-digesting MMPs in matrix degradation in emphysema.

The studies aforementioned provide evidence for a role of a variety of connective tissue proteins in the pathogenesis of emphysema. This is perhaps not surprising given the heterogeneous nature of damage in emphysematous lungs in humans. It may well be that at different time-points in the disease process, different matrix proteins are degraded and/or synthesized, with the ultimate result being that destruction of lung tissue eventually becomes widespread, but not uniform.

PATHOPHYSIOLOGY OF EMPHYSEMA

The molecular events described above lead to destruction of lung tissue, and as a result abnormalities in pulmonary function develop *(32)*. The abnormalities manifest themselves in four related, but distinct, areas: limitation to airflow (obstructive physiologic defect), abnormalities of gas exchange, abnormalities in lung mechanics, and dyspnea. These abnormalities are certainly interrelated, but the pathogenesis of each has its own unique features such that a separate discussion of each on its own is warranted.

Limitation of Airflow

The hallmark finding on a pulmonary spirogram (flow-volume loop) in patients with emphysema is a marked reduction in the forced expiratory volume/forced vital capacity (FEV_1/FVC) ratio, and a marked absolute decrease in the FEV_1 itself. These findings are illustrated in the typical flattened or scooped-out appearance of the flow volume loop as illustrated in Fig. 1. Other abnormalities of pulmonary function that accompany the reduced FEV_1/FVC ratio in patients with emphysema include an increased residual volume (RV) and total lung capacity (TLC), which result from the air trapping and hyperinflation that are characteristic of this disease.

In general, reductions in or limitations to expiratory airflow arise from one of two mechanisms: increased airways resistance or decreased elastic recoil (decreased driving pressure). In obstructive airways diseases such as asthma and chronic bronchitis, there is clearly increased resistance to airflow that occurs because the airway lumen is narrowed

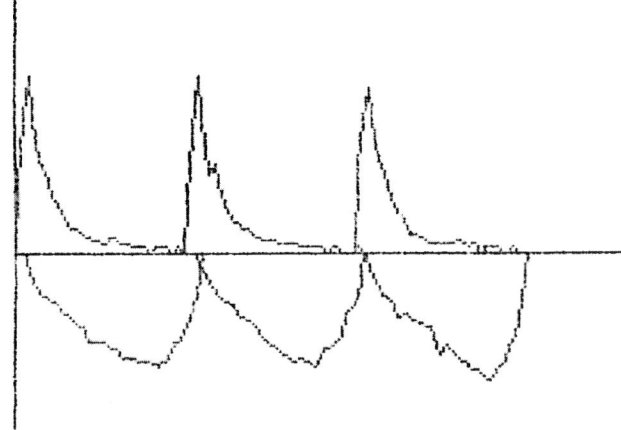

Fig. 1. A series of flow-volume loops from a patient with severe emphysema. Note the typical scooped-out appearance of the expiratory limb of the curve.

by bronchospasm and inflammation. In emphysema, however, there is typically little ongoing airway inflammation or bronchospasm, and it is likely that the majority of the airflow limitation arises from diminished elastic recoil. However, air trapping caused by early closure of overly compliant lung units also contributes to limitation of airflow and may represent a component of increased resistance to flow in these patients. At the level of the small airways, the loss of elastic recoil leads to increased collapsibility characteristic of emphysema, and this can cause increased airflow resistance. This is a fundamentally different mechanism from the increased resistance seen in patients with asthma.

Overinflation of the Lungs

Typically, RV, TLC, and functional residual capacity (FRC) are increased in patients with emphysema. The RV/RCL ratio is increased as well. The reasons for these increases in lung volume are fairly straightforward, and relate mainly to air trapping caused by early airway closure in patients with very collapsable lung units. As the so-called equal pressure point of the airways (the point at which the transpulmonary pressure equals or overcomes the distending pressure of the small airways) moves more distally because of the loss of elastic tissue in the lungs, early airway closure upon expiration, and hence air trapping, occurs.

As a result of the hyperinflation of the lungs seen in emphysema, remodeling of the thoracic cage results. The ribs are repositioned upward and outward, and the diaphragm is flattened. This results in the familiar barrel-chested appearance seen in emphysema. Radiographically, these changes are best appreciated on a lateral chest film where the flattened diaphragm and the increased retrosternal airspace are apparent.

Although hyperinflation of the chest may, in fact, be a partially compensatory mechanism in emphysema (airways enlarge and therefore resistance to airflow decreases at higher lung volumes) it is likely that the major effect of hyperinflation on respiratory mechanics is a negative one because of the significant mechanical disadvantage imposed on the muscles of respiration by the distension associated with hyperinflation. Most of the negative effects of hyperinflation appear to be focused on the diaphragm. This occurs in several ways, which have been well summarized by Senior and Shapiro *(33)*. First, with flattening of the diaphragm, muscle fiber length is shortened, and less force is generated for any given contraction. Second, the geometry of the reconfigured chest wall is such that force generated by the contraction of the diaphragm is less effectively applied than in a person with a normally shaped chest wall. This is because the zone of apposition between the chest wall and the flattened diaphragm is less than in normals. Third, the increased radius of curvature of the diaphragm decreases the transpulmonary pressure generated by contraction. Fourth, the thoracic cage itself operates at a mechanical disadvantage (there is resistance to inspiration because the thoracic cage is inflated over its usual resting position) and the respiratory muscles have to perform additional work to achieve inspiration.

The mechanical disadvantage imposed on the respiratory musculature results in a significantly higher cost of breathing in emphysema patients than that observed in normal individuals. Both in the resting state and in situations of acute respiratory failure, the oxygen cost of breathing in patients with emphysema is considerably higher than in normals. In a study by Sridhar, oxygen cost of breathing was correlated inversely with lung function, and in some patients with emphysema, overall resting energy expenditure was higher than in controls. Certainly in patients with respiratory failure and possibly in stable patients at rest, the increased oxygen cost of breathing caused by emphysema may be responsible for the overall hypermetabolic state and malnutrition that is commonly seen.

Abnormalities of Gas Exchange

A hallmark of pure emphysema is that arterial blood Po_2 and Pco_2 levels are maintained to a greater degree than in patients with chronic bronchitis and a similar degree of pulmonary impairment. However, gas exchange is by no means normal in patients with emphysema. There are at least two mechanisms of hypoxemia at play in such patients. One is reduction in diffusing capacity (DL_{CO}), which occurs because of the loss of alveolar surface area, which is part and parcel of the process of emphysema in the lungs. Although the reduction in diffusing capacity is straightforward to understand, isolated reductions in diffusion do not play a significant role in resting hypoxia. The second, and more clinically significant determinant of abnormal gas exchange, is ventilation-perfusion mismatching. This was established in a seminal experiment by Wagner et al. more than 20 yr ago and has been noted even in the early stages of disease *(34,35)*. Using the multiple inert gas-elimination technique (MIGET) to assess the distribution of ventilation and perfusion in the lungs, these investigators demonstrated that in patients with so-called type-A chronic obstructive pulmonary disease (COPD) (i.e., emphysema), a large portion of ventilation goes to lung regions with very high V_A/Q ratios *(35)*. There is very little ventilation to regions of low V_A/Q ratio (Fig. 2). In contrast, patients with type-B COPD (chronic bronchitis) have a high proportion of their blood flow distributed to regions with low V_A/Q ratios (Fig. 3), resulting in a significant physiologic shunt. Thus, even in patients with severe emphysema, the low level of shunting explains the usually good response to supplemental oxygen that is observed.

Whereas considering gas-exchange abnormalities in patients with emphysema, it is worth commenting on the observation that in response to supplemental oxygen administration, PCO_2 levels often rise to dangerous levels, thus worsening respiratory acidosis. Generations of medical students and house officers have been taught that this occurs because a hypoxic drive to breathe has been extinguished. However, Aubier et al. from the Meakins-Christie Laboratory in Montreal, Canada, demonstrated 20 yr ago that the main contributor to the development of hypercarbia in such cases was a worsening of V_A/Q mismatch, with a blunted hypoxic stimulus and the Haldane effect (an effect related to the interaction between the transport mechanisms for oxygen and carbon dioxide) playing a less-significant role *(36)*.

Dyspnea

The final result of all of the derangements seen in patients with emphysema is dyspnea, the sensation that breathing has become difficult. Dyspnea is an extremely complicated phenomenon, and is certainly multifactorial in its etiology *(37,38)*. Several tools have been developed to quantify dyspnea, and some of the treatments used in patients with emphysema, such as pulmonary rehabilitation, improve dyspnea without significantly improving pulmonary function. Understanding the mechanisms underlying dyspnea may lead to new treatments for this disorder.

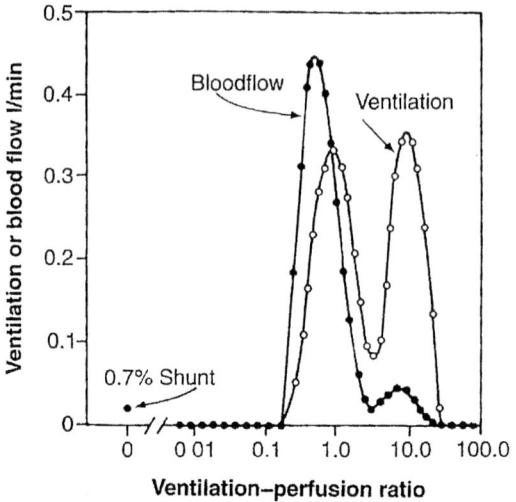

Fig. 2. Ventilation–perfusion relationships in a patient with emphysema. There is a high degree of ventilation in regions of the lung with high V_A/Q ratios. Figure from *(35)*.

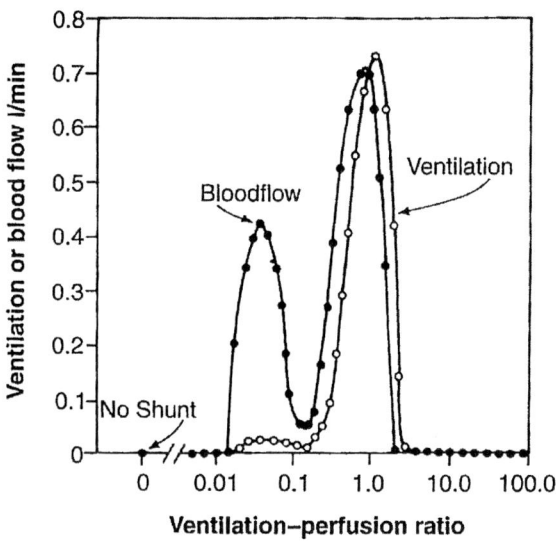

Fig. 3. Ventilation–perfusion relationships in a patient with chronic bronchitis. There is a high degree of blood flow in the lung directed at regions that have very low V_A/Q ratios. Figure from *(35)*.

REFERENCES

1. Cardoso WV, Sekhon HS, Hyde DM, Thurlbeck WM (1993) Collagen and elastin in human pulmonary emphysema [see comments]. *Am Rev Respir Dis* 147(4):975–981.
2. Swee MH, Parks WC, Pierce RA (1995) Developmental regulation of elastin production. Expression of tropoelastin pre-mRNA persists after down-regulation of steady-state mRNA levels. *J Biol Chem* 270(25):14 899–14 906.
3. McGowan SE, Harvey CS, Jackson SK (1995) Retinoids, retinoic acid receptors, and cytoplasmic retinoid binding proteins in perinatal rat lung fibroblasts. *Am J Physiol* 269(4 Pt 1):L463–472.
4. McGowan SE, Doro MM, Jackson SK (1997) Endogenous retinoids increase perinatal elastin gene expression in rat lung fibroblasts and fetal explants. *Am J Physiol* 273(2 Pt 1):L410–416.
5. Antipatis C, Ashworth CJ, Grant G, Lea RG, Hay SM, Rees WD (1998) Effects of maternal vitamin A status on fetal heart and lung: changes in expression of key developmental genes. *Am J Physiol* 275(6 Pt 1):L1184–1191.
6. Laurell C, Erickson S (1963) The electrophoretic alpha-1-globulin pattern of serum in alpha-1-antitrypsin deficiency. *Scand J Clin Lab Investigat* 15:132–140.
7. Snider GL (1989) Chronic obstructive pulmonary disease: risk factors, pathophysiology and pathogenesis. *Annu Rev Med* 40:411–429.
8. Hance AJ, Crystal RG (1975) The connective tissue of lung. *Am Rev Respir Dis* 112(5):657–711.
9. Laros CD, Kuyper CM (1976) The pathogenesis of pulmonary emphysema (II). *Respiration* 33(5):325–348.
10. Curran ME, Atkinson DL, Ewart AK, Morris CA, Leppert MF, Keating MT (1993) The elastin gene is disrupted by a translocation associated with supravalvular aortic stenosis. *Cell* 73(1):159–168.
11. Kuhn C, Tavassoli F (1976) The scanning electron microscopy of elastase-induced emphysema. A comparison with emphysema in man. *Lab Invest* 34(1):2–9.
12. Johanson WJ, Pierce AK (1972) Effects of elastase, collagenase, and papain on structure and function of rat lungs in vitro. *J Clin Invest* 51(2):288–293.
13. Hoidal JR, Niewoehner DE (1983) Pathogenesis of emphysema. *Chest* 83(4):679–685.
14. Wright JL, Churg A (1995) Smoke-induced emphysema in guinea pigs is associated with morphometric evidence of collagen breakdown and repair. *Am J Physiol* 268(1 Pt 1):L17–20.
15. Selman M, Montano M, Ramos C, et al (1996) Tobacco smoke-induced lung emphysema in guinea pigs is associated with increased interstitial collagenase. *Am J Physiol* 271(5 Pt 1):L734–743.
16. Crystal RG, Gadek JE, Ferrans VJ, Fulmer JD, Line BR, Hunninghake GW (1981) Interstitial lung disease: current concepts of pathogenesis, staging and therapy. *Am J Med* 70(3):542–568.
17. Bruce MC, Poncz L, Klinger JD, Stern RC, Tomashefski JF, Jr, Dearborn DG (1984) Biochemical and pathologic evidence for proteolytic destruction of lung connective tissue in cystic fibrosis. *Am Rev Respir Dis* 132(3):529–535.
18. Christner P, Fein A, Goldberg S, Lippmann M, Abrams W, Weinbaum G (1985) Collagenase in the lower respiratory tract of patients with adult respiratory distress syndrome. *Am Rev Respir Dis* 131(5):690–695.
19. Gadek JE, Kelman JA, Fells G, et al (1979) Collagenase in the lower respiratory tract of patients with idiopathic pulmonary fibrosis. *N Engl J Med* 301(14):737–742.

20. Michaeli D, Fudenberg HH (1974) Antibodies to collagen in patients with emphysema. *Clin Immunol Immunopathol* 3(2):187–192.
21. Pinnell SR, Krane SM, Kenzora JE, Glimcher MJ (1972) A heritable disorder of connective tissue. Hydroxylysine-deficient collagen disease. *N Engl J Med* 286(19):1013–1020.
22. Kilburn KH, Dowell AR, Pratt PC (1971) Morphological and biochemical assessment of papain-induced emphysema. *Arch Intern Med* 127(5):884–890.
23. Yu SY, Keller NR (1978) Synthesis of lung collagen in hamsters with elastase-induced emphysema. *Exp Mol Pathol* 29(1):37–43.
24. Riley DJ, Kramer MJ, Kerr JS, Chae CU, Yu SY, Berg RA (1987) Damage and repair of lung connective tissue in rats exposed to toxic levels of oxygen. *Am Rev Respir Dis* 135(2):441–447.
25. Fisk DE, Kuhn C (1976) Emphysema-like changes in the lungs of the blotchy mouse. *Am Rev Respir Dis* 113(6):787–797.
26. Pierce J, Hocott J, Ebert R (1961) The collagen and elastin content of the lungs in emphsyema. *Ann Intern Med* 55:210–222.
27. Green MC, Sweet HO, Bunker LE (1976) Tight-skin, a new mutation of the mouse causing excessive growth of connective tissue and skeleton. *Am J Pathol* 82(3):493–512.
28. Hautamaki RD, Kobayashi DK, Senior RM, Shapiro SD (1997) Requirement for macrophage elastase for cigarette smoke-induced emphysema in mice. *Science* 277(5334):2002–2004.
29. D'Armiento J, Dalal SS, Okada Y, Berg RA, Chada K (1992) Collagenase expression in the lungs of transgenic mice causes pulmonary emphysema. *Cell* 71(6):955–961.
30. Ohnishi K, Takagi M, Kurokawa Y, Satomi S, Konttinen YT (1998) Matrix metalloproteinase-mediated extracellular matrix protein degradation in human pulmonary emphysema. *Lab Invest* 78(9):1077–1087.
31. Finlay GA, O'Driscoll LR, Russell KJ, et al (1997) Matrix metalloproteinase expression and production by alveolar macrophages in emphysema. *Am J Respir Crit Care Med* 156(1):240–247.
32. Celli BR (1995) Pathophysiology of chronic obstructive pulmonary disease. *Chest Surg Clin N Am* 5(4):623–634.
33. Senior RM, Shapiro S (1998) Chronic Obstructive Pulmonary Disease: epidemiology, pathophysiology, and pathogenesis. In: *Pulmonary Diseases and Disorders*. Fishman, A.P., ed. New York: McGraw-Hill.
34. Barbera JA, Ramirez J, Roca J, Wagner PD, Sanchez-Lloret J, Rodriguez-Roisin R (1990) Lung structure and gas exchange in mild chronic obstructive pulmonary disease. *Am Rev Respir Dis* 141(4 Pt 1):895–901.
35. Wagner PD, Dantzker DR, Dueck R, Clausen JL, West JB (1977) Ventilation-perfusion inequality in chronic obstructive pulmonary disease. *J Clin Invest* 59(2):203–216.
36. Aubier M, Murciano D, Milic-Emili J, et al (1980) Effects of the administration of O2 on ventilation and blood gases in patients with chronic obstructive pulmonary disease during acute respiratory failure. *Am Rev Respir Dis* 122(5):747–754.
37. Manning HL, Schwartzstein RM (1995) Pathophysiology of dyspnea. *N Engl J Med* 333(23):1547–1553.
38. Mahler DA, Jones PW (1997) Measurement of dyspnea and quality of life in advanced lung disease. *Clin Chest Med* 18(3):457–469.

2 Cardiopulmonary Exercise Testing in the Evaluation of the Patient with Emphysema

David Balfe, MBBCH, FCP (SA)
and Zab Mohsenifar, MD, FCCP

INTRODUCTION

Comprehensive exercise testing offers an opportunity to study the cellular, cardiovascular, and ventilatory systems' responses simultaneously under controlled conditions *(1)*. Physical exercise requires the interaction of physiologic mechanisms that enable the cardiovascular and respiratory systems to supply exercising muscles with the fuel

From: *Lung Volume Reduction Surgery*
Edited by: M. Argenziano and M. E. Ginsburg © Humana Press Inc., Totowa, NJ

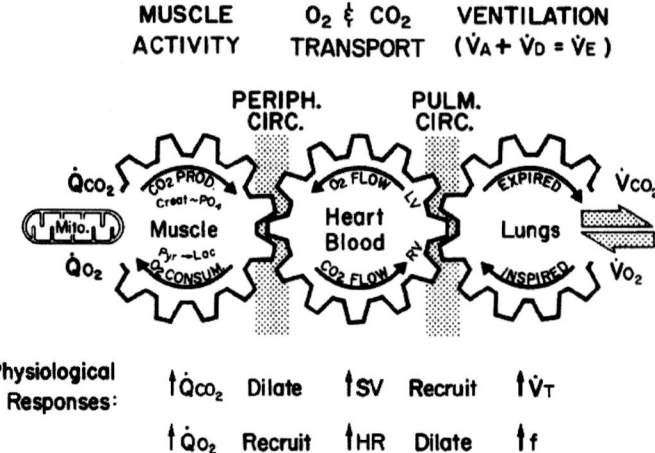

Fig. 1. Gas transport mechanisms for coupling cellular to pulmonary respiration. The gears represent functional interdependence of the physiological components of the system. (Printed with permission from Wasserman K, Hansen JE, Sue DY, Casaburi R, Whipp BJ, Principles of Exercise Testing and Interpretation 1999, 3rd ed., Lipincott, Williams & Wilkins.)

required to meet increased oxygen demand (VO_2) and remove excess carbon dioxide production (VCO_2). This coupling of respiratory, cardiovascular, and muscle gas transport systems is illustrated in Fig. 1 *(1)*. The physiologic reserve capacity of the cardiovascular and respiratory systems is significantly high enough that even if much of this capacity is lost, demands of daily living will be met adequately *(2)*. Abnormalities of exercise performance may be influenced by diseases of the heart, lungs, pulmonary and peripheral circulation, hemoglobin, muscles and/or cytochrome systems *(3)*. In this chapter, we will initially discuss various methods of cardiopulmonary testing, and later we will discuss its applications in patients undergoing lung volume reduction surgery.

BROAD OVERVIEW OF METHODS
OF CARDIOPULMONARY EXERCISE TESTING

Exercise testing allows the objective measurement of exercise capacity that can be compared with the ideal exercise capacity corrected for age, gender, height, and weight. In addition, symptoms that limit exercise can be elucidated and the physiologic responses to exercise can be analyzed in order to highlight patterns suggesting underlying organ dysfunction. Unfortunately, there is a lack of standardization concerning the performance of clinical exercise testing *(2)*. This applies to the methods used, variables being measured, and interpretive techniques. There are a number of predicted formulas that can be used to calculate the maximum VO_2, work rate, heart rate, and minute ventilation *(1,2,4)*. Exercise tests can be noninvasive, symptom limited, steady state, performed with arterial blood sampling, or with the presence of a pulmonary artery catheter *(2)*. In addition, the tests can be conducted on various types of equipment: treadmill, cycle ergometer, step testing, or using an arm ergometer. The tests can be performed on room air or on supplemental oxygen. Using an electrically braked cycle ergometer leads to a more predictable increase in oxygen uptake than with a treadmill *(2)*, using a treadmill results in an approx 7 % higher oxygen consumption than a cycle *(5)*, increases in ventilation and blood lactate levels tend to be higher in cycling *(6)*. The work performed on a treadmill is dependent on the weight of the subject, but this is not as significant with the cycle ergometer *(7)*.

SAFETY ISSUES IN CARDIOPULMONARY EXERCISE TESTING

The safety of exercise testing has been well established and the risks to the patient are very small as long as simple precautions are observed. The risk of a myocardial infarction (MI) or serious arrythmia is estimated at 1/10 000 submaximal tests *(8)*, increasing to 1/2500 maximal tests if the patient has a history of MI *(9)*. We feel that the test should be supervised by an experienced physician who is familiar with the patient's history and physical examination, and who is knowledgeable in resuscitative techniques. Before 1980, exercise tests were supervised by physicians 90% of the time. However, over the past 15 yr, cost containment initiatives have encouraged more extensive use of specially trained health professionals (nurses, exercise physiologists, physician assistants, and physical therapists) *(10–12)*.

Absolute contraindications to exercise testing

1. The presence of an acute febrile illness.
2. EKG features of myocardial ischemia.
3. Uncontrolled heart failure.
4. Pulmonary edema.
5. Unstable angina.
6. Acute myocarditis.
7. Uncontrolled hypertension (> 250 mm systolic, 120 mm diastolic).
8. Uncontrolled asthma *(2)*.

Relative contraindications to exercise testing

1. Recent (less than 4 wk previously) MI.
2. Aortic valve disease.
3. Resting tachycardia (HR >120/min).
4. Resting EKG abnormalities.
5. Poorly controlled diabetes.
6. Poorly controlled epilepsy.
7. Cerebrovascular disease.
8. Respiratory failure *(2)*.

SPECIFIC ISSUES RELATING TO CHRONIC OBSTRUCTIVE PULMONARY DISEASE AND EMPHYSEMA

Chronic obstructive pulmonary diseases (COPD) are characterized by reduced maximal expiratory flow and include various disease entities such as chronic obstructive bronchitis, asthmatic bronchitis, and emphysema. At least 14 million people in the United States suffer from COPD, and the prevalence of this disease seems to be increasing *(13–16)*. As many as 2 million people suffer from emphysema, and the overall death rate for emphysema in the United States has been estimated at 20 000/yr, the fifth leading cause of death in North America *(13,16–18)*. Exercise testing in patients with COPD has been stimulated by the increasing numbers of patients entering pulmonary rehabilitation programs *(19)*, in addition to the availability of specific treatments for this condition, i.e., pulmonary transplantation and lung volume reduction surgery (LVRS).

TYPES OF CARDIOPULMONARY EXERCISE TESTING FOR PATIENTS WITH COPD

The simplest validated exercise test is the 6-min walk test performed either on or off oxygen. The inability to walk at least 200 m during this test has been shown to correlate with increased postoperative mortality *(20)*. Patients with severe COPD present a number of difficulties when an incremental exercise test is performed. Their exercise capacity is frequently extremely limited *(21)*, it is therefore difficult to obtain sufficient physiologic data. The exercise duration can be improved, however, by using small increments in the exercise load *(21)* and by using supplemental oxygen. Currently, the National Emphysema and Treatment Trial (NETT) is comparing the efficacy of LVRS and maximal medical therapy. Exercise tolerance is an important outcome measure in the study and the exercise techniques used in the NETT trial could serve as a standardized way of performing an incremental exercise test in patients with severe COPD.

Patients are exercised on an electrically braked cycle ergometer, which has the capability for electronic computer control to provide ramp workloads as low as 5 W/ min. The test is initially performed with arterial blood sampling, whereas subsequent tests during the trial may or may not use arterial sampling. The exercise tests are performed on an FIO_2 of 30%, the patients breathing in the O_2 and air mixture delivered from a high-flow blender to a large Douglas bag (>30 L). After being connected to the exercise equipment and getting on the cycle ergometer, the patient is observed for 5 min at rest, 3 min at 0 W cycling, and subsequently during a symptom-limited incremental exercise test (5 W/ min increments) *(22)*. Exercise is considered maximal if one or more of the following criteria are met:

1. The patient's predicted maximal VO_2 is reached.
2. A clinically significant EKG abnormality develops.
3. Serum lactate increases to greater than 8 mmol/L.
4. Breathing reserve is less than 15 L /min.
5. The heart rate reserve is less than 10 beats/min.
6. The arterial PO_2 falls below 50 mmHg or the oxygen saturation falls below 84%.

The following parameters are measured:

1. Level of work (WR).
2. Heart rate (and the difference between heart rate and maximal predicted heart rate—the heart rate reserve).
3. EKG.
4. Blood pressure.
5. Respiratory rate.
6. Tidal volume (and the tidal volume to inspiratory capacity ratio).
7. Minute ventilation (VE) (and the difference between VE and maximal voluntary ventilation—the breathing reserve).
8. Oxygen consumption (VO_2), carbon dioxide production (VCO_2), and the relationship of these measures to the minute ventilation (VE/VO_2 and VE/VCO_2).
9. The VO_2/WR relationship.
10. The VO_2/heart rate response—the oxygen pulse.

RESPONSES TO EXERCISE IN CHRONIC OBSTRUCTIVE LUNG DISEASE

The two main factors reducing exercise capacity in COPD/emphysema are the reduced ventilatory capacity and the increased ventilatory requirement *(1)*. Other factors include exercise-induced hypoxemia, cardiac dysfunction, and deconditioning *(23)*. Both airway obstruction

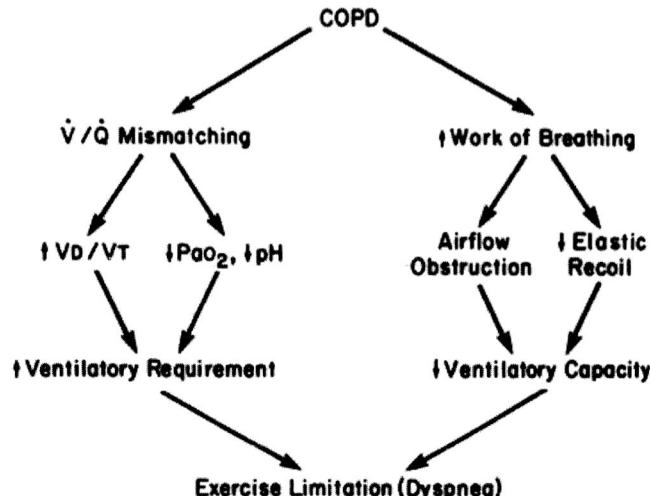

Fig. 2. Factors that play a role in exercise limitation and dyspnea in patients with chronic obstructive pulmonary disease. (Printed with permission from Wasserman K, Hansen JE, Sue DY, Casaburi R, Whipp BJ, Principles of Exercise Testing and Interpretation 1999, 3rd ed., Lipincott, Williams & Wilkins.)

and a reduction in lung elastic recoil are responsible for the decreased ventilatory capacity; the increased ventilatory requirements are a result of inefficient ventilation of the lungs because of mismatching of ventilation to perfusion *(1)* (Fig. 2). There is often a reduction in work that can be performed as a consequence of oxygen demand exceeding the maximal oxygen carrying capacity of the oxygen transport chain *(21)*, and this is largely because of the failure of the available ventilatory reserve to meet the increasing ventilatory demands *(24,25)*. The VO_2/WR response is often normal in patients with COPD, the oxygen cost of breathing, however, is much higher in COPD as compared to normal *(21)*. There is a greater time constant for CO_2 excretion than O_2 consumption (50–60 s vs 30–40 s). Patients with COPD have increased numbers of lung units with high ventilation/perfusion ratios, these regions receiving up to 50% of blood flow, further exacerbating the delay in CO_2 output. The ventilatory response to exercise is dependent on the metabolic rate, the "set point level of arterial CO_2" and the wasted ventilation fraction *(VD/Vt)*. The required minute ventilation at any given time may be calculated using the following equation:

$$VE = (863 \times VCO_2)/(PACO_2 \times (1\text{-}VD/Vt))$$

with the arterial $_pCO_2$ ($PaCO_2$) generally being substituted for the alveolar CO_2 ($PACO_2$) *(21,26)*. Patients with stable COPD regulate

$PaCO_2$ at a reasonably constant level despite increasing work rates, in patients with severe COPD, however, the $PaCO_2$ may increase with exercise, worsening exercise-associated acidosis *(1)*. Minute ventilation is frequently increased at rest in addition to being increased for a given level of exercise *(1,21)*. This is frequently a result of the increased *VD/Vt* ratio, requiring an abnormal level of ventilation to maintain a normal $PaCO_2$ *(27)*.

Many patients with COPD are hypoxemic, either at rest and/or during exercise. The degree of widening of the alveolar-arterial oxygen gradient with exercise is related to the degree of ventilation perfusion mismatching, particularly in regions of low ventilation/perfusion ratios (21).

DYNAMIC HYPERINFLATION AND ITS CONSEQUENCES

In patients with chronic lung diseases, the tidal volume tends to be lower and the respiratory rate tends to be higher at a given level of VE. A close relationship has been noted between measured vital capacity and maximal tidal volume during exercise *(1,21)*. In patients with COPD, flow rates can be shown to reach the envelope of the resting maximal flow volume curve, which may contribute to exercise limitation *(28,29)*. Normal subjects increase respiratory rate by decreasing inspiratory time *(Ti)* fractionally less than expiratory time *(Te)*—as a consequence, the inspiratory duty cycle (*Ti*/total respiratory time) increases. In contrast, patients with COPD often show no increase in the inspiratory duty cycle, preserving greater time for exhalation. This is achieved by increasing inspiratory flow rates. There is, however, an associated increase in intrathoracic gas volume as a consequence of airflow limitation and increased respiratory frequency, eventually leading to a point on the thoracic cage pressure/volume relationship where inspiratory muscles function inefficiently, eventually leading to a large increase in thoracic gas volume with resultant fall in inspiratory flow *(21,30)*. During exercise, the development of dynamic hyperinflation with a progressive increase in end-expiratory lung volume (EELV) imposes an additional elastic load on the ventilatory system, resulting in a reduction in inspiratory capacity, and is closely related to exertional dyspnea *(31–33)*. This is in contrast to normal subjects in whom the EELV decreases with exercise *(33)*. Traditionally, the maximal voluntary minute ventilation (MVV) (or multiple of the FEV1) has been compared to the maximal VE as an estimate of ventilatory capacity. Measuring the MVV in patients with COPD has shortcomings, however. Significant differences exist in the breathing patterns during the 12–15 s MVV maneuver and the breathing patterns during heavy exercise *(33)*.

Ventilatory capacity can vary during exercise because of bronchodilation or bronchoconstriction, and is dependent on the lung volume where the tidal breathing occurs relative to the total lung capacity (TLC) and residual volume (RV). Measurements of the resting inspiratory capacity have been shown to closely correlate with maximal work in COPD patients *(34)*. Breathing at higher lung volumes increases the inspiratory elastic load and, consequently, the work of breathing. Breathing at low lung volumes limits the available ventilatory reserve because of encroachment on the flow volume envelope. Reducing the total lung volume and residual volume, either medically by the use of bronchodilators (medical volume reduction) or surgically (surgical volume reduction), may indeed offer significant benefits by reducing EELV and subsequently availing more inspiratory capacity.

The technique of measuring the exercise inspiratory capacity, which allows superimposition of the exercise tidal volume loop on the maximal flow volume loop allows measurement of the EELV and the end inspiratory lung volume during exercise. This analysis provides more useful information about the cause of ventilatory limitation than analysis of the breathing reserve and breathing pattern (tidal volume and respiratory rate relationship) alone *(33)*. Fig. 3 represents flow volume loops during exercise and compares the pattern in a healthy young male to that in a patient with emphysema.

CARDIOVASCULAR RESPONSE TO EXERCISE IN COPD PATIENTS

Patients with COPD can have coexisting cardiovascular diseases, because smoking is a risk factor for both COPD and ischemic heart disease and hypoxia can exacerbate ischemic heart disease. In patients with COPD, increases in cardiac output with exercise is less in comparison with normal subjects *(35)*. Possible explanations for this phenomenon include cardiac dysfunction and elevations in pulmonary artery pressure with exercise due as a result hypoxia and or capillary destruction or obstruction, even in the absence of cor pulmonale *(21,35,36)*.

EFFICACY OF LVRS

LVRS has been shown to significantly improve forced vital capacity (FVC), forced expiratory volume in 1 s (FEV1), and MVV, in addition to RV and TLC *(37)*. Furthermore, lung elastic recoil has been shown to increase significantly after LVRS *(38)*. The exercise capacity of patients with emphysema is thought to be determined by the mechanical constraints placed on maximal ventilation *(39)*. Therefore, improvements in lung

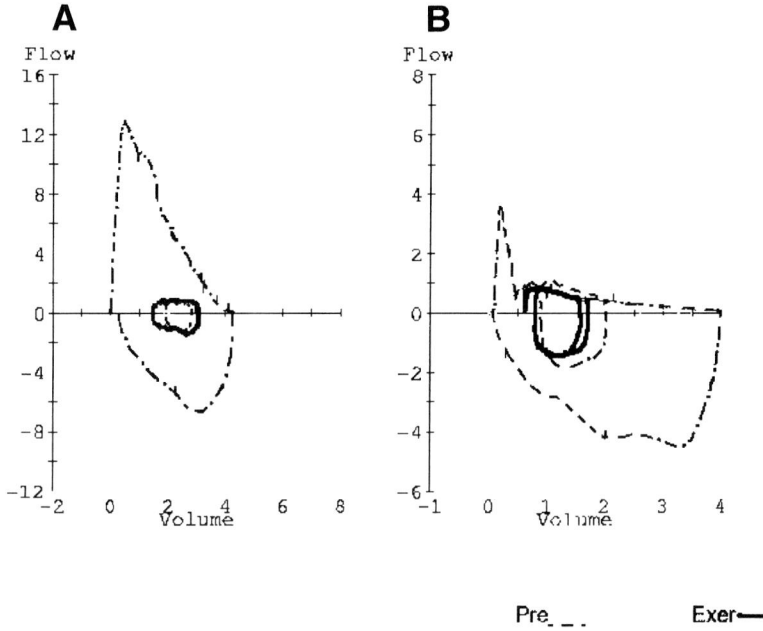

Pre __ .   Exer—

Fig. 3. Exercise flow volumes pre- and during exercise. Graph A represents the normal increase in tidal volume with exercise associated with a reduction in the end expiratory lung volume accompanied by an increase in the end inspiratory lung volume and no encroachment on the maximal resting flow volume loop. Graph B represents a patient with COPD, with an exercise-associated increase in the EELV. In addition, there is encroachment on the expiratory component of the maximal pre-exercise flow volume loop.

mechanics may explain the improvements noted following LVRS, specifically, the combination of the reduction in pulmonary hyperinflation, reduction in breathing frequency, reduction in mechanical constraints on tidal volume and reduction in functional residual capacity (FRC) *(40)*. Improvements in exercise tolerance following LVRS include longer 6-min walk distances, increased maximal workloads, higher maximal VO_2, and improved indices of gas exchange *(41)*. Currently in the NETT trial, the 6-min walk test, maximal VO_2, and maximum work rate are measured, with the maximum work rate as one of two primary outcomes to be analyzed *(13,23,42–45)*.

Significant increases in the 6-min walk test have been noted following LVRS, from 300 to 370 m in normocapnic patients, and from 197 to 274 m in hypercapnic patients. The maximal VO_2 has also been shown to significantly increase in both normocapnic and hypercapnic patients following LVRS, from 14.6 to 17.02 mL/Kg/min and

11.7 to 14.7 mL/Kg/min, respectively *(37)*. The same study also noted significant increases in the maximal Vt (0.85 to 1.05 L and 0.8 to1.2 L, respectively, in normocapnic and hypercapnic patients); similarly, maximal minute ventilation increased from 29.2 to 33.5 L/min in normocapnic and 22.5 to 31 L/min, respectively, in hypercapnic patients *(37)*.

The role of cardiovascular adaptations and altered heart–lung inter-actions in the improvements noted following LVRS is unclear. Most patients with severe emphysema have mild to moderate pulmonary hypertension, which may contribute to their exercise limitation *(46)*. The consequences of LVRS on the pulmonary circulation are felt to be twofold: 1) resection of emphysematous lung tissue could reduce the vascular bed and increase pulmonary vascular resistance; and 2) better mechanical properties of the respiratory system with improved elastic recoil and less dynamic hyperinflation might counteract this effect and lead to a decrease in pulmonary vascular resistance *(43,47)*. Strong correlations have been noted between improvements in gas exchange (the alveolar-arterial gradient) and reductions in mean exercise pulmo-nary artery pressure following ARDS, although these associations were not evident at rest *(47,48)*. Other investigators have shown a trend to improvement in the VD/Vt ratio following LVRS *(44)*. It is of interest that close correlations have been previously noted between the cardiac output and maximal VO_2 at maximal exercise in patients with predomi-nant cardiac dysfunction or pulmonary vascular disease. It is a possibil-ity, therefore, that the increased VO_2 noted following LVRS could, in part, represent an improvement in cardiac output *(48,49)*. A strong association has been noted between the increases in FEV1 and the improvements in VO_2 following LVRS *(47,48)*. Thus it appears that there is a dichotomy between improvement in maximal VO_2 and PaO_2 follow-ing LVRS. The former depends on improvements in FEV1, whereas the latter depends on improvement in pulmonary artery pressure.

LVRS has been shown to produce significant improvement in relief of dyspnea in many patients *(44)* in addition to improved quality-of-life scores *(50)*. These improvements are generally associated with improve-ments in pulmonary function and exercise tolerance. However, the exact mechanism for the improvement in dyspnea is not precisely defined *(50)*. Exercise testing before and after LVRS, including the use of the exercise flow volume loop and, in selected circumstances, invasive hemodynamic exercise testing will continue to improve our knowledge and help to ascertain the nature and duration of improvement in these patients. Moreover, as additional information is obtained from ongoing clinical trials, the exercise test will help to define which patients are suitable candidates for the procedure *(37)*.

REFERENCES

1. Wasserman K, Hansen JE, Sue DY, Casaburi R, Whipp BJ (1999) In: *Principles of Exercise Testing and Interpretation* 3rd ed. Lipincott, Williams & Wilkins, Baltimore, Maryland.
2. Jones NL, Moran Campbell EJ (1982) *Clinical Exercise Testing*, 2nd ed. Philadelphia, Pennsylvania: W. B. Saunders Co.
3. Goldring RM (1984) Specific defects in cardiopulmonary gas transport, *Am Rev Respir Dis* 129 (Suppl): S57–S59.
4. Blackie SP, Fairburn MS, McElvaney GN, Morrison NJ, Wilcox PG, Pardy RL (1989) Prediction of maximal oxygen uptake and power during cycle ergometry in subjects older than 55 years of age. *Am Rev Respir Dis* 139: 1424–1429.
5. Shephard RJ (1971) Standard tests of aerobic power, In: Shephard RJ, ed, *Frontiers of Fitness*. Springfield, IL: Charles C Thomas.
6. Shephard RJ (1966) The relative merits of the step test, bicycle and treadmill in the assessment of cardiorespiratory fitness. *Int Z Angew Physiol* 23: 219–230.
7. Wasserman K, Whipp BJ (1975) Exercise physiology in health and disease. *Am Rev Respir Dis* 112: 219–249.
8. Rochmis P, Blackburn H (1971) Exercise tests, a survey of procedures, safety and litigation experience in approximately 170,000 tests. *JAMA* 17: 1061–1066.
9. Shephard RJ (1970) For exercise testing - a review of procedures available to the clinician. *Bull Physiopathol Resp* 6: 425–474.
10. Franklin, BA, Gordon S, Timmis GC, O'Neill W (1997) Is direct physician supervision of exercise stress testing routinely necessary. *Chest* 111: 262–265.
11. Stuart RJ Jr, Ellestad MH (1980) National survey of exercise testing facilities. *Chest* 77: 94–97.
12. Cahalin LP, Blessey, RL, Kummer D, et al (1987) The safety of exercise testing performed independently by physical therapists. *J Cardiopulm Rehabil* 7: 269–276.
13. Utz JP, Hubmayr RD, Deschamps C (1998) Lung volume reduction surgery for emphysema: out on a limb without a NETT (Review). *Mayo Clinic Proc* 3: 552–566.
14. Higgins MW, Thom T (1989) Incidence, prevalence, and mortality: intra and inter country differences. *Lung Biol Health Dis* 43: 23–43.
15. Petty TL (1997) A new national stategy for COPD. *J Respir Dis* 18:363–369.
16. Feinleib M, Rosenberg HM, Collins JG, Delozier JE, Pokras R, Chevarley FM (1989) Trends in COPD morbidity and mortality in the United States. *Am Rev Respir Dis* 140 (Suppl): S9–S18.
17. American Thoracic Society (1995) Standards for the diagnosis and care of patients with chronic obstructive lung disease. *Am J Respir Crit Care Med* 152(Suppl): S77–S120.
18. American Lung Society (1993) Lung disease data. New York : American Lung Association.
19. Lacasee Y, Wong E, Guyatt GH, King D, Cook DJ, Goldstein RS (1996) Meta-analysis of respiratory rehabilitation in chronic obstructive pulmonary disease. *Lancet* 348: 1115–1119.
20. Szekely, LA et al. (1997) Preoperative predictors of operative morbidity and mortality in COPD patients undergoing bilateral lung volume reduction surgery. *Chest* 111: 550–558.

21. ERS Task Force (1997) Clinical exercise testing with reference to lung diseases: indications, standardization and interpretation strategies. *Eur Respir J* 10: 2662–2689.
22. The National Emphyema Treatment Trial Research research protocol.
23. Benditt, JO, Lewis S, Wood DE, Klima L, Albert RK (1997) Lung volume reduction surgery improves maximal O_2 consumption, maximal minute ventilation, O_2 pulse, and dead-space-to-tidal volume ratio during leg cycle ergometry. *Am J Respir Crit Care Med* 156: 561–566.
24. Cooper JD, Patterson AG (1996) Lung volume reduction surgery for severe emphysema. *Semin Thorac Cardiovasc* Surg 8(1): 52–60.
25. Yusen, RD, Trulock EP, Pohl MS, Biggar DG, et al. (1996) Results of lung volume reduction surgery in emphysema. *Semin Thorac Cardiovasc* Surg 8(1): 99–1090.
26. Weisman IM, Zeballos RJ, eds. (1994) An integrated approach to the interpretation of the CPET, Clinical exercise testing in Clinics in Chest Medicine Philadelphia: W.B. Saunders.
27. Wagner PD, Gale GE. Ventilation perfusion relationships. In: Whipp BJ, Wasserman K, eds. Pulmonary physiology and pathophysiology of exercise. New York: Dekker, 1991; 121–142.
28. Potter WA, Olafsson S, Hyat RE (1971) Ventilatory mechanics and expiratory flow limitation during exercise in patients with obstructive lung disease. *J Clin Invest* 50: 910–919.
29. Gallagher C (1990) Exercise and chronic obstructive pulmonary disease. *Med Clin N Am* 74: 619–641.
30. Jones NL, Berman LB (1984) Gas exchange in chronic air-flow obstruction. *Am Rev Respir Dis* 129 (Suppl): S81–S83.
31. Dodd DS, Brancatisano T, Engel LA (1988) Chest wall mechanics during exercise in patients with severe chronic air flow obstruction. *ARRD* 129: 33–38.
32. O'Donnell DE, Webb KA (1993) Exertional breathlessness in patients with chronic airflow limitation. *ARRD* 148:1351–1357.
33. Johnson BD, Weisman IM, Zeballos RJ, Beck KC (1999) Emerging concepts in the evaluation of ventilatory limitation during exercise - the exercise flow volume loop. *Chest* 116: 488–503.
34. Murariu C, Ghezzo H, Milic-Emili J, Gautier H (1998) Exercise limitation in obstructive lung disease. *Chest* 114: 965–968.
35. Stewart RI, Lewis CM (1986) Cardiac output during exercise in patients with COPD. *Chest* 89: 199–205.
36. Agusti AG, Barbera JA, Roca J, Rodriguez-Roisin R, Wagner PD, Agust-Vidal A (1990) Hypoxic vasoconstriction and gas exchange during exercise in chronic obstructive pulmonary disease. *Chest* 97: 268–275.
37. O'Brien GM, Furukawa S, Kuzma, AM, Cordova F, Criner GJ (1999) Improvements in lung function, exercise and quality of life in hypercapnic COPD patients after lung volume reduction surgery. *Chest* 115: 75–84.
38. Gelb AF, Brenner M, McKenna R, Fischel R, Zamel N, Schein MJ (1998) Serial lung function and elastic recoil 2 years after lung volume reduction surgery for emphysema. *Chest* 113: 1497–1506.
39. Potter WA, Olafsson S, Hyatt RE (1971) Ventilatory mechanics and expiratory flow limitation during exercise in patients with obstructive lung disease. *J Clin Invest* 50: 910–919.
40. O'Donnell DE, Webb KA, Bertley JC, et al. (1996) Mechanisms of relief of exertional breathlessness following unilateral bullectomy and lung volume reduction surgery in emphysema. *Chest* 110: 18–27.

41. Gelb AF, McKenna RJ, Brenner M, Schein MJ, Zamel N, Fischel R (1999) Lung function 4 years after lung volume reduction surgery for emphysema. *Chest* 116: 1608–1615.
42. The National Emphysema Treatment Trial Research Group (1999) Rationale and Design of the National Emphysema Treatment Trial, A Prospective Randomized Trial of Lung Volume Reduction Surgery. *Chest* 116: 1750–1761.
43. Sciurba FIC, Rogers RM, Keenan RJ, Silvka WA, Gorcsan J III, Ferson PF, et al (1996) Improvement in pulmonary function and elastic recoil after lung volume reduction surgery for diffuse emphysema. *N Engl J Med* 334: 1096–1099.
44. Keller CA, Ruppel G, Hibbett A, Osterloh J, Naunheim KS (1997) Thoracoscopic lung volume reduction surgery reduces dyspnea and improves exercise capacity in patients with emphysema. *Am J Respir Crit Care Med* 156: 60–67.
45. The National Emphyema Treatment Trial Research Group (1999) Rationale and design of the national emphysema treatment trial (NETT): a prospective randomized trial of lung volume reduction surgery. *J Thorac Cardiovasc Surg* 118: 518–528.
46. Light RW, Mintz HM, Linden GS, Brown SE (1984) Hemodynamics of patients with severe chronic obstructive pulmonary disease during progressive upright exercise. *Am Rev Respir Dis* 130: 391–395.
47. Oswald-Mammosser M, Kessler R, Massard G, Wihlm J, Weitzenblum E, Lonsdorfer J (1998) Effect of lung volume reduction surgery on gas exchange and pulmonary hemodynamics at rest and during exercise. *Am J Respir Crit Care Med* 158: 1020–1025.
48. Wagner PD (1998) Functional consequences of lung volume reduction surgery for COPD (Editorial). *Am J Respir Crit Care Med* 158: 1017–1019.
49. Balfe DL, Nathanson A, Wasserman K, Mohsenifar Z. Does pulmonary artery catheterization add to traditional cardiopulmonary exercise testing in diagnosing dyspnea? submitted for publication.
50. Cooper JD, Trulock EP, Triantafillou AN, Patterson GA, Pohl MS, Deloney PA, Sundaresan RS, Poper CL (1995) Bilateral pneumonectomy (volume reduction) for chronic obstructive pulmonary disease. *J Thorac Cardiovasc Surg* 109:106–119.

3   Cardiovascular Effects of Emphysema

Steven M. Scharf, MD, PhD

CONTENTS

INTRODUCTION
THEORETICAL EFFECTS OF EMPHYSEMA
  ON CARDIOVASCULAR FUNCTION
EFFECTS OF EMPHYSEMA ON CARDIOVASCULAR FUNCTION
CARDIOVASCULAR FUNCTION IN SEVERE EMPHYSEMA
CONCLUSIONS
REFERENCES

INTRODUCTION

The recent reintroduction of lung volume reduction surgery (LVRS) for the treatment of severe emphysema has led to a renewed interest in the pathophysiology of this debilitating condition. Severe shortness of breath is generally the most distressing symptom of the emphysematous form of the chronic obstructive pulmonary disease (COPD) spectrum. The origin of this symptom is likely to be multifactorial and, hence, the mechanisms by which LVRS may alleviate symptoms is also likely to be multifactorial. Given the interactions between respiratory and cardiovascular systems, it is not surprising that there is interest in the effects of LVRS on cardiovascular function and how these effects are integrated into the overall response. Whereas the cardiovascular effects of COPD have been the subject of hundreds of scientific studies, the majority of these studies do not distinguish between the major subgroups of COPD, chronic bronchitis, and emphysema. Because most patients have significant symptoms of chronic bronchitis, these studies, by design, do not give a comprehensive view of the cardiovascular effects of relatively "pure" emphysema. One problem regarding this is how to

From: *Lung Volume Reduction Surgery*
Edited by: M. Argenziano and M. E. Ginsburg © Humana Press Inc., Totowa, NJ

define emphysema, on clinical, pathological, or physiological grounds and distinguish this from chronic bronchitis. Some of these issues influence the interpretation of studies purporting to assess the hemodynamic effects of emphysema.

In this chapter we will address a number of issues. We will describe the pathophysiologic effects of emphysema which could, in theory, affect cardiovascular function. We will review some studies of the cardiovascular effects of emphysema in animal models and in human disease. We will address the issue of whether or not there is a cardiovascular limitation to exercise tolerance in patients with emphysema. We will review what few data are available in patients undergoing LVRS. Finally, we will review directions for current and possibly future research in cardiovascular effects of emphysema.

THEORETICAL EFFECTS OF EMPHYSEMA ON CARDIOVASCULAR FUNCTION

Increased Pulmonary Vascular Resistance and Ventricular Interdependence

Table 1 lists some of the theoretical mechanisms by which emphysema could adversely affect cardiovascular function. Emphysema leads to increased pulmonary vascular resistance (PVR) and hyperinflation. Theoretically, hyperinflation could have a number of possible cardiovascular effects independent of effects on PVR, which will be reviewed later. Anything that increases PVR, by increasing right ventricular (RV) afterload, can lead to structural changes in the RV (i.e., cor pulmonale) (1). Increased PVR, if severe enough, could theoretically limit cardiac output, especially during exercise. By limiting the increase in cardiac output, oxygen delivery to the periphery, and hence, exercise capacity is limited. Further, because myocardial fibers are a syncitium, it is possible that the biochemical events leading to structural changes in the RV as a result of chronic RV overload could affect fibers around the left ventricle (LV) and change LV function. Indeed, following pulmonary hypertension caused by experimental banding of the pulmonary artery (PA) in animals (2,3) Laks et al. found remodeling of LV, as well as RV myocardium. Theoretically, this could affect LV systolic performance. In addition, there are parallel interactions between the ventricles acting both in diastole (4) and systole (5). The importance of these interactions, often referred to as ventricular interdependence, is increasingly recognized in diseases as diverse as sleep apnea and COPD. During diastole, RV overload stiffens the LV. This works by decreasing the radius of curvature of the LV septum and decreasing LV preload. In addition, the

Table 1
Theoretic Mechanisms by Which Emphysema Could Adversely Affect Cardiovascular Function

Increased Pulmonary Vascular Resistance
Hypoxia-induced vasospasm (acute)   Hypoxia-induced vascular remodeling (chronic)   Loss of cross-sectional area because of tissue (precapillary) destruction   Compression of pulmonary capillaries (intra-alveolar vessels) by regional   hyperinflation   Sympathetic vasoconstriction

Hyperinflation

Compression of IVC because of flattening and configurational change in the
     diaphragm
 Compression of the intrathoracic portion of the IVC
 Increased pleural pressure, especially at end-expiration: could raise right atrial
     pressure atrial pressure.
 Increased cardiac fossa pressure, inhibiting RV and LV diastolic ventricular
     filling

Effects on Cardiac Function
Increased load on the RV, leading to inhibition of LV diastolic filling (diastolic   interdependence)   Adverse affect of RV overload on LV myocardial fibers (whole heart   hypothesis, of chronic RV overload) - systolic function   Effects of chronic hypoxia on cardiac function - systolic and diastolic

presence of the pericardium acts as an "amplifier" for these effects *(4)*. RV contraction against an increased afterload actually aids LV systolic function *(5)*. This is because both ventricles contract against a common center of gravity. The importance of "systolic positive interdependence" has been well documented for LV to RV interaction. Whereas RV to LV effects are less, in the presence of pulmonary hypertension, these could be greater *(5)*.

Hyperinflation

The hyperinflation associated with positive end-expiratory pressure (PEEP) may be one good model to study the cardiovascular effects of emphysema. Due compression of intra-alveolar pulmonary vessels hyperinflation is associated with increased PVR *(6,7)*. In the presence of co-existing pulmonary hypertension, high levels of PEEP can even lead to acute cor pulmonale and circulatory collapse *(8)*. Hyperinflation could also affect return of venous blood to the right atrium via the inferior vena cava (IVC). This could occur at the level of either the diaphragm or the intrathoracic IVC. Consistent with this notion, Nakhjavan et al. *(9)* demonstrated inspiratory collapse of the IVC at the level of the diaphragm in patients with emphysema, but not in normals. This is illustrated in Fig. 1. This has implications for control of cardiac output in exercise. Normally, during exercise, decreasing inspiratory intrathoracic pressure aids venous return to the right heart and increases cardiac output (thoracic pump). As a result of inspiratory IVC collapse, this mechanism may be unavailable to patients with emphysema. Hence, cardiac output may be limited during exercise not only because of increased RV afterload, but because of decreased RV preload as well. In supine dogs, Fessler et al. *(10)* demonstrated collapse of the IVC during PEEP induced hyperinflation. This led to a rightward shift of the point of flow limitation in the venous return curve. This means that venous return into the right atrium, normally increasing with decreasing right atrial pressure, becomes limited at higher than normal right atrial pressures with PEEP *(11,12)*. In humans, the IVC is relatively short and it is possible that IVC collapse is less likely to occur than in dogs with relatively longer IVCs. However, closure of the IVC at the level of the diaphragm could have much the same effect as collapse of the intrathoracic portion of the IVC. Finally, hyperinflation would be expected to lead to mechanical interactions between the heart and lungs. Not only does increased lung volume increase end-expiratory pleural pressure, but by directly compressing the mediastinum, pressures in the cardiac fossa may even increase more than those measured at the pleural surface of the lung *(13,14)*. In patients with COPD, during exercise or voluntary hyperventilation, parallel increases in right atrial and PA wedge pressure *(Pw)* have been attributed to hyperinflation of the lower lobes (intrinsic PEEP) with concomitant increases in cardiac fossa pressures *(15,16)*. By "compressing" the heart, especially during exercise, the lungs would thus inhibit ventricular diastolic filling. This could further decrease LV stroke volume and cardiac output. We next consider what is known about the effects of emphysema (as opposed to chronic bronchitis) on cardiovascular function in experimental animals and in patients.

EFFECTS OF EMPHYSEMA ON CARDIOVASCULAR FUNCTION

Emphysema is defined as "a condition of the lung characterized by abnormal, permanent enlargement of airspaces distal to the terminal bronchiole, accompanied by the destruction of their walls, and with

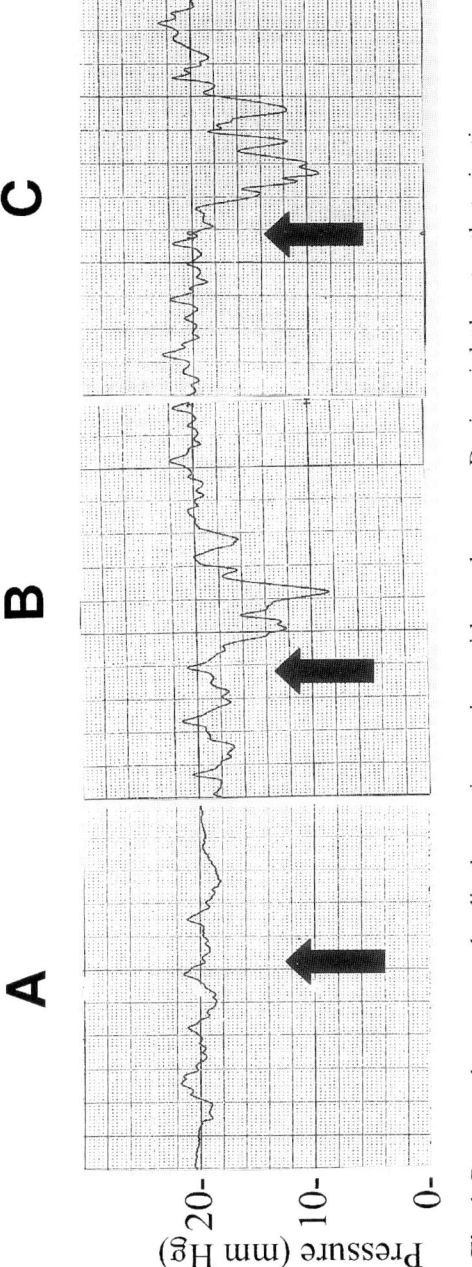

Fig. 1. Pressure drop across the diaphragm in a patient with emphysema. During right heart catheterization pressures in the IVC were recorded from three positions: A = 1 cm below the dome of the diaphragm; B = 1 cm above the dome of the diaphragm; C = right atrium. The arrows mark the onset of inspiration. Note as the catheter advances across the diaphragm (A to B) there is the appearance of inspiratory swings in venous pressures. This figure indicates that during the inspiration there is closure of the IVC with failure to transmit the decreases in intrathoracic pressure in this patient.

33

fibrosis" (17). There is an association between the development of cor pulmonale and emphysema. Approximately 6% of patients with emphysema have been reported to develop cor pulmonale each year (18). This is important because, given equal severities of airflow obstruction, the presence of cor pulmonale is the best predictor of mortality (19). Further, mortality rate is inversely related to PVR (20,21), with PVR values greater than 600 dyne-s/cm^5 (see Fig. 2) or signs of RV hypertrophy being associated with poor prognosis. There are several purported mechanisms for the development of pulmonary hypertension in emphysema (see Table 1). Because in humans there are often multiple confounding factors present leading to the development of pulmonary hypertension, such as concomitant cardiac disease, bronchitis, or thromboembolic disease, the study of relatively "pure" animal models of emphysema offers some advantages for dissecting out those factors responsible for pulmonary hypertension in emphysema. Many studies have centered around deciding whether chronic hypoxia or obliteration of pulmonary vasculature is primarily responsible for the development of pulmonary hypertension and cor pulmonale in emphysema.

Effects of Emphysema on Cardiovascular Function— Experimental Animal Models

In order to study the effects of emphysema on pulmonary mechanics, respiratory muscle function, and hemodynamics, animal models of emphysema have been developed, often in which a protease (elastase or papain) is instilled into the trachea of an animal (22). An animal model of emphysema has been defined similarly to emphysema in humans as "an abnormal state of the lungs in which there is enlargement of the airspaces distal to the terminal bronchiole" (23). Generally, experimental models study panlobular emphysema and may, in fact, be most analogous to the human condition α-1 antitrypsin deficiency. On the other hand, most smoking-related emphysema, the most common clinically relevant situation, is centrilobular and is associated with some degree of chronic bronchitis. Similar to human disease, animal models of emphysema are associated with increased lung volumes and decreased in diffusion capacity, flow rates, and elastic recoil. Thus, hemodynamic changes with animal models of emphysema are relevant to human disease.

Wright et al. (24) investigated the effects of chronic exposure to cigarette smoke on the structure and function of pulmonary vasculature in guinea pigs. They found an increase in PA pressure after 1-mo exposure, even though at this time there were no parenchymal structural changes. With the progression of time, pulmonary vascular pressures remained elevated, but did not progressively increase increase even in

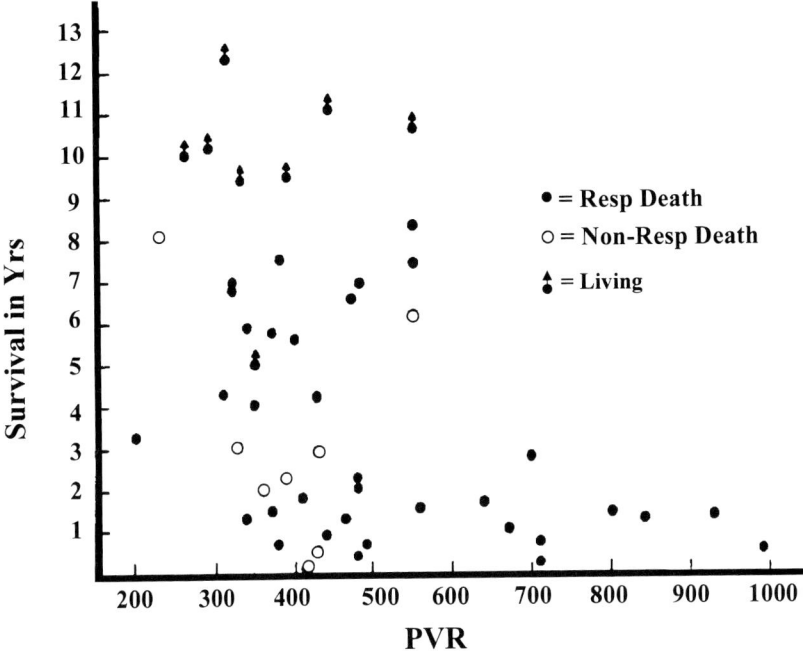

Fig. 2. Plot of survival in years as a function of initial PVR in COPD patients. From *(20)*, with permission.

the face of progressive destruction of lung parenchyma. There was neither hypoxia nor hypercapnia. Given the dissociation between parenchymal and vascular abnormalities, these workers concluded that neither vascular obliteration nor hypoxia was necessary for producing pulmonary hypertension with smoking. Pulmonary hypertension appeared to be a result of smoking-induced inflammation in the pulmonary capillary bed, possibly because of the release of proteolytic enzymes or vasoactive substances.

Sato et al. *(25)* studied pulmonary hemodynamics over 4 wk in normoxic awake rats with elastase-induced emphysema. There was a nonsignificant increase in pulmonary vascular pressures in the elastase group. Inhalation of a hypoxic gas mixture produced greater pulmonary vascular pressure increases in the elastase group; however, this was related to greater increases in cardiac output, not PVR. This finding suggested that, with emphysema, there may greater sympathadrenal tone leading to greater venous return and cardiac output. This indirect evidence that pulmonary vascular reactivity is increased in emphysma led to the suggestion that this was one mechanism leading to the development of cor pulmonale. On the other hand, in a similar model, Tseng et al. *(26)* found that hemodynamic changes with emphysema were in fact correlated with the development of parenchymal morphologic changes and heightened vascular reactivity did not appear to play a role in the development of pulmonary hypertension. These authors concluded that hypoxia is not necessary for the development of cor pulmonale, but rather that in emphysema pulmonary hypertension resulted from "direct destruction of connective tissue and pulmonary vessels" *(26)*.

Martorana et al. *(27)* studied the relationship between parenchymal morphometry and pulmonary hemodynamics in a normoxic, normocapnic dog model of papain-induced emphysema. They did find a correlation between indices of tissue destruction and both PA pressure and PVR. They also observed an inotropic effect with increased cardiac output and decreased Pw in emphysematous compared to control animals. Thus, early in the course of emphysema, both tissue destruction, as well as sympathetic activation *(28)* contribute to increased PVR. On the other hand, it is possible that chronic sympathetic activation could lead to vasoconstriction, myocardial necrosis, depletion of myocardial-receptors and decreased myocardial catecholamine stores *(29,30)*, thus diminishing cardiac function in the long run with emphysema. Conceivably, this could account for some of the clinical studies reporting decreased LV function in emphysema.

Using plots of stroke volume against transmural filling pressure to characterize cardiac function (modified Starling curves), Mink et al. *(31)*, observed pulmonary hypertension and decreased RV, but normal LV, function in acutely emphysematous dogs. These findings suggested that RV function deteriorated because of increased RV afterload, but that there was no change in overall myocardial contractile function. However, in a chronic dog model of emphysema, this group *(32)* demonstrated decreased LV systolic function, with a parallel rightward shift in the LV end-systolic pressure-volume curve and increased diastolic LV stiffness *(33,34)*. Chronically increased RV stress with emphysema could have led to increased LV diastolic stiffness. Alternatively, because LV and RV myocytes are not separate, but rather a syncitium, remodeling of myocardium because of stress on one ventricle could trigger remodeling in myocardium of the opposite ventricle *(2,3)*. Finally, the measured alterations in LV stress-strain relations could have resulted from mechanical interactions between the heart and lungs *(13–15)*. Either pleural or esophageal pressures were used by by this group *(31,32,34)* to calculate transmural pressures (the stress). This may have resulted in the underestimation of cardiac surface pressure with emphysema-associated pulmonary hyperinflation because cardiac surface pressure may increase more with lung inflation than esophageal pressure *(13–16,35)*. Thus, the true transmural pressure would have been overestimated at any given cardiac volume, leading to the conclusion that stiffness was increased with emphysema. These possibilities remain speculative and we agree with Gomez et al. that the mechanisms changing LV function in emphysema "must await future studies *(34)*."

Effects of Emphysema on Cardiovascular Function—Human Disease

There have been many studies on the hemodynamics of patients with COPD. However, there are several problems interpreting this vast clinical literature regarding the understanding the hemodynamic effects of emphysema. First, many studies of COPD do not distinguish between emphysema and, the more common, chronic bronchitis. Another is that the definition of emphysema may not be the same in all studies. Emphysema may be defined physiologically and clinically as normal oxygenation and minimal hypercapnia (pink and puffing), hyperinflation, decreased diffusion capacity, and perhaps, decreased elastic recoil. Newer studies often incorporate radiologic findings, especially with high-resolution computed tomography (HRCT), in the definition of emphysema in individual patients. Finally, emphysema may be defined pathologically on the basis of tissue destruction. Because most patients with COPD have, in fact, both emphysema and chronic bronchitis, the distinctions are often illusory.

Filley et al. *(36)* described two clinical types of COPD. "Pink puffers" were defined as patients with airflow limitation who were thin, had a narrow cardiac silhouette, no history of heart failure, and had a normal hematocrit. These patients tended to be normoxic and normocapnic at rest. "Blue bloaters" were described as patients with little weight loss, enlarged cardiac silhouettes, a history of heart failure, and polycythemia. These patients often were hypoxic and hypercapnic at rest. It has often been thought that patients with the "blue and bloated" (hypoxic/hypercapnic) pattern of COPD have more severe pulmonary hypertension than the "pink and puffing" (normoxic/normocapnic) pattern *(37,38)*. By virtue of changing the rheological properties of blood, polycythemia in the blue and bloated patients may contribute to greater pulmonary hypertension *(39)*. Further, early clinicophysiologic studies suggested that the pink-and-puffing pattern was associated with more emphysema and the blue-and-bloated pattern with more chronic bronchitis *(20,36,40)*. However, later studies relating pathologic estimation of tissue destruction with the clinical syndrome failed to confirm this notion *(41)*. In 1989, Biernacki et al. *(42)* examined the correlation between the radiologic (CT scan) extent of emphysema and the clinical spectrum of disease severity. There were no significant relationships between the CT estimated extent of emphysema and arterial blood gas tensions, mean PA pressure, cardiac output, or pulmonary vascular resistance at rest or during exercise. The authors concluded that "to equate 'pink puffers' with emphysema, and 'blue bloaters' as having little or no emphysema, is no longer valid" *(42)*. The study did find a good correlation between CO transfer coefficient and the CT density histogram, suggesting CO diffusion capacity is a good index of the extent of amputation of the pulmonary vascular bed in emphysema. This finding may be important in predicting the effects of LVRS on pulmonary hemodynamics as will be discussed later.

The question of differences between emphysema and the bronchitic syndrome in COPD patients remains open. Burrows et al. *(20)* reported that COPD patients with emphysema have lower cardiac outputs and higher pulmonary vascular resistance than COPD patients without emphysema. On the other hand, Boushy and North *(43)* reported no hemodynamic differences between emphysema and nonemphysema COPD patients. These authors found progressive decreases in cardiac output of 6–7% over 25 mo in both groups.

Other authors *(44,45)* emphasize the importance of exercise in bringing out abnormalities of pulmonary hemodynamics in mild to moderate COPD, even before the appearance of abnormal resting PA pressure. The more severe the disease pathologically, the more severe the exercise response *(44)*. In fact, because of parallel changes in PA and wedge pressures with exercise, Wright et al. *(44)* concluded that dynamic hyperinflation leads to increased alveolar and pleural pressure rather than obliteration of pulmonary vascular bed. The later work of Butler et al. *(15)* agrees with this explanation. Wright et al. *(44)* also found that exercise-induced increases in PA pressure were abolished with O_2 breathing. In this case, O_2 breathing might have shortened the time constants for ventilation in poorly ventilated lung units, which would in turn have led to less hyperinflation and less increase in wedge and PA pressures. Schulman et al. *(45)* found a correlation between CO diffusion capacity and the increase in PA pressures with exercise. This finding led them to conclude that pulmonary hypertension in mild to moderate emphysema was due to obliteration of pulmonary vascular bed.

Oswald-Mammosser et al. *(46)* investigated pulmonary hemodynamics in a large (151 patients) series of normoxic and normocapnic emphysema patients with moderate to severe emphysema (mean FEV_1 1.2 L). Thirty-one of 151 patients (20.5%) had resting pulmonary hypertension (mean PA pressure >20 mmHg) and 99/151 (65.5%) had pulmonary hypertension during exercise. Resting PA pressures were well correlated with CO diffusion capacity, and FEV_1, but only poorly correlated with resting PO_2 and PCO_2. These findings suggested that pulmonary hypertension was not a feature of most patients with moderate to severe emphysema, and that hypoxemia and hypercapnia were not important determinants of pulmonary hypertension. The correlation between measures of airflow obstruction (FEV_1) and PA pressure could have been related to hyperinflation and increased alveolar pressures. The correlation between PA pressure and CO diffusion capacity were similar to those of Biernacki et al. *(42)*, suggesting that CO diffusion capacity predicts the extent of capillary bed destruction in emphysema.

Left Ventricular Function in Emphysema

Decreased compliance of the LV has been demonstrated in patients with chronic cor pulmonale because of COPD *(47)*. This is likely a result of diastolic interdependence *(4,5)*. Additionaly, systolic interdepence has been described *(5)* by which increasing RV systolic pressure assists LV contraction. This works because the fibers of the LV and RV contract toward the same center of gravity and systolic forces are transmitted through the septum. However, as the septum hypertrophies, its stiffness increases and the transmission of systolic forces decreases *(5)*. There has been a good deal of debate in the literature concerning the effects of chronic cor pulmonale on LV function, and as to whether chronic RV overload leads to structural and functional changes in patients. Rao et al. *(48)* first reported depressed LV function in some patients with cor pulmonale and no other identifiable cause of LV failure. This was followed by other reports of decreased LV function measured by systolic time intervals or ejection fraction *(49–51)*. However, other studies have failed to find evidence of LV dysfunction in COPD patients with cor pulmonale in the absence of an identifiable cause of LV failure *(52–56)*. In a clinicopathologic study Kohama et al. *(57)* demonstrated myocardial fibrosis and cellular hypertrophy in the LV in COPD patients dying of heart failure with no other identifiable cause of heart failure. These changes might be related to hypoxemia, hypercarbia, acidosis, and chronic sympathetic overload. In this sense, the animal studies quoted before have direct relevance.

Patients with COPD generate large inspiratory negative swings in intrathoracic pressure *(46)*. As noted earlier, there are a number of factors that exaggerate inspiratory swings in intrathoracic pressure and that could influence ventricular function. These include increased venous return with flow-related RV overload *(58)* and increased LV afterload *(59,60)*. Regarding LV afterload, the effects of transient (inspiratory), as opposed to sustained, decreases in intrathoracic pressure are not well known in humans and are the subject of considerable debate in animal studies *(58)*. In normoxic chronic upper airway obstruction in rats (inspiratory intrathoracic pressure decrease to approx -30 mmHg), LV hypertrophy was not observed. These findings suggested that increasing negative intrathoracic swings *per se* are not sufficient to affect LV function *(61)*.

Smoking is by far the most common cause of emphysema and the overwhelming majority of patients presenting as candidates for LVRS have a long smoking history. Coronary artery disease is also known to be a major risk for surgery of any kind, and smoking is a major risk for coronary artery disease. Thus, it is to be expected that many patients with emphysema presenting for surgery will have a history of coronary artery disease. Surprisingly, there are few reports of concomitant coronary disease in previous studies of LVRS. This is because these patients are screened for coronary disease and excluded if this is found based on symptoms or history. Cardiac evaluation has generally been restricted to patients with apparent clinical indications. However, it is well known that the lack of cardiac symptoms does not exclude the presence of coronary disease in patients with obstructive lung disease. Thus, it might be expected that silent coronary disease could be a potential problem in patients presenting for LVRS. Thurnheer et al. *(62)* prospectively studied the prevalence of clinically silent coronary artery disease in LVRS candidates by angiography in 41 LVRS candidates. Six of these patients (15%) were found to have asymptomatic, but significant (defined as > 70% stenosis) coronary lesions. In five of these patients, the findings altered the clinical management of the patients. These patients were found to have higher cholesterol levels and greater smoking histories. The data do not allow one to say whether risk stratification is worthwhile for LVRS candidates or whether coronary revascularization prior to LVRS is indicated. Nevertheless, these intriguing findings do indicate that consideration of the possibility of silent coronary disease is indicated in evaluation of LVRS candidates.

There have been few studies of LV function in patients with the emphysema clinical syndrome, as opposed to chronic bronchitis. However, in severe emphysema, *Pw* has been reported in the minority of patients to be elevated although *Pw* generally increases with exercise *(21,38,42,46)*. Many authorities believe that increased *Pw* signals the

because LVEF in these patients was always normal. Thus, one of the other causes for increased Pw, downstream pulmonary shunts or hyperinflation, was likely the cause of increased Pw.

CONCLUSIONS

Generalizations about the effects of emphysema on hemodynamics must be made with caution. This is because of the variability of results found in different studies, which, in turn, often stems from variability in the definition, chronicity, and distribution of emphysematous changes within the lung. However, it appears that severe emphysema is capable of producing pulmonary hypertension in most patients, with limitation of peripheral O_2 delivery in some. This may be part of the reason for exercise limitation in emphysema patients. Further, pulmonary hypertension is likely to be a predictor of poor prognosis. In animal models and some human studies, it appears that pulmonary hypertension can be produced even if hypoxia is not a feature of the patient's illness. On the other hand, hypoxemia, if present, certainly will exacerbate the problem. Whereas pulmonary hypertension can be treated by lung transplantation, the effects of LVRS on pulmonary hemodynamics are not well known. The fact that different preliminary studies yield different results suggests the need for extensive evaluation of the effects of LVRS on pulmonary hemodynamics. Obviously, the opportunity to perform large-scale studies of the effects of emphysema and LVRS on pulmonary hemodynamic and cardiac function afforded by the NETT will add greatly to our understanding of this important problem.

REFERENCES

1. (1963) World Health Organization: Definition of chronic cor pulmonale: a report of the expert committee. *Circulation* 27: 594.
2. Laks M, Morady F, Adomian G, Swan J (1970) Presence of widened and multiple intercalated discs in the hypertophied canine heart. *Circ Res* 27: 391–402.
3. Laks M, Morady F, Swan J (1970) Canine right and left ventricular cell and sarcomere lengths after banding the pulmonary artery. *Circ Res* 24: 705–710.
4. Janicki JS, Weber KT (1980) The pericardium and ventricular interaction, distensibility and function. *Am J Physiol* 238: H494–H503.
5. Scharf SM (1994) Right ventricular load tolerance: role of left ventricular function. Perspectives en Réanimation, Les Interactions cardio-pulmonaires. Societé de Réanimation de langue francais, Arnette, Paris, pp. 17–28.
6. Whittenberger JL, McGregor M, Berglund E, Borst MC (1960) Influence of state of inflation of the lung on pulmonary vascular resistance. *J Appl Physiol* 15: 878–882.
7. Permutt S, Howell JBL, Proctor D, Riley RL (1961) Effects of lung inflation on static pressure-volume characteristics of pulmonary vessels. *J Appl Physiol* 16: 64–70.
8. Dhainaut JF, Aouate P, Brunet FP (1989) Circulatory effects of positive end-expiratory pressure in patients with acute lung injury. In: Scharf SM and Cassidy

SS, eds. *Heart-Lung Interactions in Health and Disease*. New York: Marcel Dekker, pp. 809–838.

9. Nakhjavan FK, Palmer WH, McGregor M (1966) Influence of respiration on venous return in pulmonary emphysema. *Circulation* 23: 8–16.

10. Fessler HE, Brower RG, Shapiro EP, Permutt S (1993) Effects of positive end-expiratory pressure and body position on pressure in the thoracic great veins. *Am Rev Resp Dis* 148: 1657–1664.

11. Robotham J, Scharf SM (1983) The effects of positive and negative pressure ventilation on cardiac performance. In: Matthay RA, Matthay MA, Dantzker D, eds. *Cardiovascular Pulmonary Interaction in Normal and Diseased Lung*. Philadelphia: W.B. Saunders, 161–187.

12. Fessler HE, Brower RG, Wise RA, Permutt S (1992) Effects of positive end-expiratory pressure on the canine venous return curve. *Am Rev Resp Dis* 146: 4–10.

13. Wallis TW, Robotham JL, Compear R, Kindred MK (1983) Mechanical heart-lung interactions with positive end-expiratory pressure. *J Appl Physiol* 54: 1039–1047.

14. Lloyd TC (1989) Mechanical heart–lung interactions. In: Scharf SM and Cassidy SS, eds. *Heart-Lung Interactions in Health and Disease*. New York: Marcel Dekker pp. 309–338.

15. Butler J, Schrijen F, Henriquez A, Polu JM, Albert RK (1988) Cause of the raised wedge pressure on exercise in chronic obstructive pulmonary disease. *Am Rev Resp Dis* 138: 350–354.

16. Albert RK, Muramoto A, Caldwell J, Koespell T, Butler J (1985) Increases in intrathoracic pressure do not explain the rise in left ventricular end-diastolic pressure that occurs during exercise in patients with chronic obstructive pulmonary disease. *Am Rev Resp Dis* 132: 623–627.

17. Snider GL, Kleinerman J, Thurlbeck Wmk et al. (1985) The definition of emphysema: Results of a National Heart, Lung and Blood Institute, Division of Lung Diseases, Workshop. *Am Rev Resp Dis* 132: 182–185.

18. Murphy ML, Bone RC (1984) *Cor Pulmonale in Chronic Bronchitis and Emphysema*. Mt Kisco, NY: Futura.

19. Traver GA, Cline MG, Burrows B (1979) Predictors of mortality in chronic obstructive pulmonary disease. *Am Rev Resp Dis* 119: 895–902.

20. Burrows B, Kettel LJ, Niden AH, Rabinowitz M, Diener CF (1972) Patterns of cardiovascular dysfunction in chronic obstructive lung disease. *N Engl J Med* 286: 912–918.

21. Mise J, Moriyama K, Itagaki S (1996) Clinical course and prognosis of chronic pulmonary emphysema with special reference to pulmonary circulatory disturbance. *Jpn Heart J* 7: 45–55.

22. Deschamps C, Farkas GA, Beck KC, Schroeder MA, Hyatt RE (1995) Experimental emphysema. *Chest Clin North Am* 5: 691–699.

23. Snider GL, Lucey EC, Stone PJ (1986) State of the Art: Animal Models of emphysema. *Am Rev Resp Dis* 133: 149–169.

24. Wright JL, Churg A (1991) Effect of long - term cigarette smoke exposure on pulmonary vascular structure and function in the guinea pig. *Lung Res* 17: 997–1009.

25. Sato S, Kato S, Arisaka Y, Takahashi H, Tomoike H (1994) Pulmonary haemodynamics in awake rats following treatment with endotracheal pancreatic elastase. *Eur Resp J* 7: 1294–1299.

26. Tseng SM, Qian S, Mitzner W (1992) Pulmonary vascular reactivity and hemodynamic changes in elastase-induced emphysema in hamsters. *J Appl Physiol* 73: 1474–1480.

27. Martorana PA, Wasten B, Van Evan P, Gîbel H, Schaper J (1982) A six-month study of the evolution of papain-induced emphysema in the dog. *Am Rev Resp Dis* 126: 898–903.

28. McFadden ER Jr, Braunwald E (1980) Cor pulmonale and pulmoanry thromboembolism. In: Braunwald E, ed. *Heart Disease, A Textbook of Cardiovascular Medicine*. Philadelphia: WB Saunders, 1643–1680.

29. Daly PA, Sole MJ (1990) Myocardial catecholanimes and the pathophysiology of heart failure. *Circulation* (suppl 1); 82: I34–I43.

30. Swedberg K, Enroth P, Kjekshus J, Wilhelmsen L (1990) Hormones regulating cardiovascular function in patients with severe CHF and their relation to mortality. *Circulation* 82: 1730–1736.

31. Mink SN, Gomez A, Whitley L, Coalson JJ (1986) hemodynamics in dogs with pulmonary hypertension due to emphysema. *Lung* 164: 41–54.

32. Gomez A, Unruh H, Mink S (1994) Left ventricular systolic performance is depressed in chronic pulmonary emphysema in dogs. *Am Heart J* 267 (Heart Circ Physiol 36): H232–H247.

33. Sagawa K, Suga H, Shoukas A, Bakalar K (1977) End-systolic pressure/volume ratio: new index of ventricular contractility. *Am J Cardiol* 40: 748–753.

34. Gomez A, Unruh H, Mink SN (1993) Altered left ventricular chamber stiffness and isovolumikc relaxation in dogs with chronic pulmonary hypertension caused by emphsema. *Circulation* 87: 247–260.

35. Scharf SM, Brown R, Warner KG, Khuri S (1989) Esophageal and pericardial pressures and left ventricular configuration with respiratory maneuvers. *J Appl Physiol* 66:481–491.

36. Filley GF, Beckwitt HJ, Reeves JT, Mitchell RS (1968) Chronic obstructive bronchopulmonary disease. Oxygen transport in two clinical tyupes. *Am J Med* 44: 26–37.

37. Bishop JM (1973) Cardiovascular complications of chronic bronchitis and emphysema. *Med Clinc North Am* 57: 771–780.

38. Matthay RA, Berger HJ (1981) Cardiovascular performance in chronic obstructive pulmonary disease. *Med Clin North Am* 65: 489–524.

39. Guidet B, Offenstadt G, Baffa G, et al. (1987) Polycythaemia in chronic obstructive pulmonary disease. *Chest* 92: 867–870.

40. Jones NL (1966) Pulmonary gas exchange during exercise in patients with chronic airways obstruction. *Clin Sci* 31: 39–50.

41. Mitchell AS, Stanford RE, Johnson JM, Silvers GW, Dart S, George MS (1976) The morphologic features of the bronchi, bronchioles and alveoli in chronic airway obstruction: a clinicopathologic study. *Am Rev Resp Dis* 114: 137–145.

42. Biernacki W, Gould GA, Whyte KF, Flenley DC (1989) Pulmonary hemodynamics, gas exchange, and the severity of emphysema as assessed by quantitative CT scan in chronic bronchitis and emphysema. *Am Rev Resp Dis* 139: 1509–1515.

43. Boushy SF, North LB (1977) Hemodynamic changes in chronic obstructive pulmonary disease. *Chest* 72: 565–570.

44. Wright JL, Lawson L, Parç PD, Hooper RO, Peretz DW, Nelems JM, Schulzer M, Hogg JC (1983) The structure and function of the pulmonary vasculature in mild chronic obstructive pulmonary disease. *Am Rev Resp Dis* 128: 702–707.

45. Schulman LL, Lennon PF, Wood JA, Enson Y (1994) Pulmonary vascular resistance in emphysema. *Chest* 105; 798–805.

46. Oswald-Mammosser M, Apprill M, Bachez P, Ehrhart M, Weitzenblum E (1993) Pulmonary hemodynamics in chronic obstructive pulmonary disease of the emphysematous type. *Respiration* 58: 304–310.

47. Krayenbuehl HP, Turino J, Hess O (1978) Left ventricular function in chronic pulmonary hypertension. *Am J Cardiol* 41: 1150–1158.

48. Rao BS, Cohn KE, Eldridge FL, Hancock HW (1968) Left ventricular failure secondary to chronic pulmonary disease. *Am J Med* 45: 229–241.
49. Hooper RG, Whitecomb ME (1974) Systolic time intervals in chronic obstructive pulmonary disease. *Circulation* 50: 1205–1209.
50. Chipps BE, Alderson PO, Roland JA, et al. (1979) Noninvasive evaluation of left ventricular function in chronic obstructive pulmonary disease. *J Pediatr* 95: 379–387.
51. Jardin F, Gueret P, Prost J-F (1984) Two dimensional echocardiographic assessment of left ventricular function in chronic obstructive pulmonary disease. *Am Rev Resp Dis* 129: 135–144.
52. Caldwell EN (1984) The left ventricle in chronic obstructive lung diseases. In: Rubin LJ, ed. *Pulmonary Heart Disease.* The Hague: Martinus Nijhoff, p. 247.
53. Fishman AP (1971) The left ventricle in chronic bronchitis and emphysema (editorial). *N Engl J Med* 285: 402.
54. Kachel RB (1978) Left ventricular function in chronic obstructive pulmonary disease. *Chest* 74: 286–290.
55. Weisse AB (1974) Contralateral effects of cardiac disease affecting either the left or right chambers of the heart. *Am Heart J* 87: 654–663.
56. Steele P, Ellis JH Jr, Van Dyke D, Sutton F, Creagh E, Davies H (1975) Left ventricular ejection fraction in severe chronic obstructive airways disease. *Am J Med* 59: 21–28.
57. Kohama A, Tanouchi J, Hori M, et al. (1990) Pathologic involvement of the left ventricle in chronic cor pulmonale. *Chest* 98: 794–800.
58. Scharf SM (1991) Cardiovascular effects of airway obstruction. *Lung* 169:1–23.
59. Scharf SM, Brown R, Tow DE, Parisi AF (1979) Cardiac effects of increased lung volume and decreased pleural pressure in man. *J Appl Physiol* 47:257–262.
60. Scharf SM, Bianco JA, Tow DE, Brown R (1981) The effects of large negative intrathoracic pressure on left ventricular function in patients with coronary artery disease. *Circulation* 63:871–875.
61. Salejee I, Tarasiuk A, Reder I, Scharf SM (1993) Chronic upper airways obstruction produces right but not left ventricular hypertrophy in rats. *Am Rev Resp Dis* 148: 1346–1350.
62. Thurnheer R, Muntwyler J, Stammberger U, Bloch K, Zollinger A, Weder W, Russi E (1997) Coronary artery disease in patients undergoing lung volume reduction surgery for emphysema. *Chest* 112: 122–128.
63. Mithoefer JC, Holford FD, Keighley JF (1974) The effect of oxygen administration on mixed venous oxygen in chronic obstructive pulmonary disease. *Chest* 66: 122–132.
64. Mithoefer JC, Ramirez C, Cook W (1978) The effect of mixed venous oxygenation on arterial blood in chronic obstructive pulmonary disease. *Am Rev Res Dis* 117: 259–264.
65. Stewart RI, Lewis CM (1986) Cardiac output during exercise in patients with COPD. *Chest* 89: 199–205.
66. Joint Statement of the American Society for Transplant Physicians (ASTP), American Thoracic Society (ATS), European Respiratory Society (ERS), International Society for Heart and Lung Transplantation (IHSLT) (1998) International guidelines for the selection of lung transplant candidates. *Am J Resp Crit Care Med* 158: 335–339.
67. Keller CA, Espiritu JD, Ohar J, Trello C, Osterloh J, Ruppel G (1996) Pulmonary function, gas exchange and hemodynamics in patients with smoking-

induced versus α-antitrypsin deficiency (α1-ATD) endstage emphysema. *Am J Resp Crit Care Med* 153 (4 Abstracts): A48.

68. Vigneswaran WT, McDougall JC, Olson LJ, et al. (1993) Right ventricular assessment in patients presenting for lung transplantation. *Transplantation* 55: 1051–1055.

69. Judson MA (1993) Clinical aspects of lung transplantation. *Clin Chest Med* 14: 335–362.

70. Keller CA, Ohar J, Ruppel G, et al. (1995) Rightr ventricular function in patients with severe COPD evaluated for lung transplantaion. *Chest* 107: 1510–1516.

71. Spinale FG, Smith AC, Carabello BA, et al. (1990) Right ventricular function computed by thermodilution and ventrulography. *J Thorac Cardiovasc Surg* 99: 141–152.

72. Spinale FG, Mukherjee R, Ryunhei T, et al. (1991) The effects of valvular regurgitation on thermodilution ejection fraction measurements. *Chest* 101: 723–731.

73. Morrison DL, Maurer JR, Grossman RF (1990) Preoperative assessment for lung transplantation. *Clin Chest Med* 11: 207–215.

74. Hoyos A, Demajo W, Snell G, et al. (1993) Preoperative prediction for the use of cardiopulmonary bypass in lung transplantation. *J Thorac Cardiovasc Surg* 106: 787–796.

75. Pasque MK, Trulock EP, Cooper JD, et al. (1995) Single lung transplantation for pulmonary hyptertension. *Circulation* 92: 2252–2258.

76. Keller CA, Naunheim KS, Osterloch J, et al. (1997) Hemodynamics and gas exchange after single lung transplantation and unilateral thoacoscopic lung reduction. *J Heart Lung Transplant* 16: 199–208.

77. Bjortuff O, Simonsen S, Geiran OR, et al. (1996) Pulmonary haemodynamics after single lung transplantation for end-stage pulmonary parenchymal disease. *Eur Resp J* 9: 2007–2011.

78. Rensing BJ, McDougall JC, Breen JF, et al. (1997) Right and left ventricular remodeling after orthotoic single lung transplantation for end-stage emphysema. *J Heart Lung Transplant* 16: 926–933.

79. Iqbal M, Keller C, Criner G, Fessler H, Berkoski P, Scharf S (2000) Pulmonary hemodynamics in patients with severe emphysema. *Am J Resp Crit Care Med* 2000; 161:A817.

80. Cooper JD, Trulock EP, Triantafillou AN, Patterson GA, Pohl MS, Deloney PA, Sundaresan RS, Roper CL (1995) Bilateral pneumonectomy (volume reduction) for chronic obstructive pulmonary disease. *J Thorac Cardiovasc Surg* 109:106–119.

81. Sciurba FC, Rogers RM, Keenan RI, Slivka WA, Gorcsan J, Ferson PF, Holbert JM, Brown ML, Landreneau RI (1996) Improvement in pulmonary flinction and elastic recoil after lung-reduction surgery for difflise emphysema. *N Engl J Med* 334 : 1095–1099.

82. Scharf SM, Rossoff L, Graver LM, McKeon K, Graham C, Steinberg H (1998) Changes in pulmonary mechanics following lung volume reduction surgery. *Lung* 176: 191–204.

83. Weg II., L Rossoff, McKeon K, Graver LM, Steinberg HN, Scharf SM (1999) Development of pulmonary hypertension following lung volume reduction surgery. *Am J Resp Resp Crit Care Med* 159: 552–556.

84. Oswald-Mammoser M, Kessler R, Massard G, Wihlm J-M, Weitzenblum E, Lonsdorfer J (1998) Effect of lung volume reduction surgery on gas exchange and pulmonary hemodynamics at rest and during exercise. *Am J Respir Crit Care Med* 158: 1020–1025.

85. Raper R, Sibbald W (1986) Misled by the wedge? The Swan-Ganz catheter and left ventricular preload. *Chest* 89: 427–434.
86. Jezek V, Herles F (1969) Uneven distribution of pulmonary arterial wedge pressure in chronic bronchitis and emphysema. *Cardiologia* 54: 164–169.
87. Hellens HR, Haynes FW, Dexter L (1949) Pulmonary "capillary" pressures in man. *J Appl Physiol* 2: 24–29.
88. Herles F (1966) The pulmonary artery wedge pressure: its origin and value in assessing pulmonary hemodynamics in emphysema. Editorial. *Cor Vasa* 8:161–166.

4 Radiologic Assessment of Emphysema in LVRS Candidates

John H. M. Austin, MD,
Gregory D. N. Pearson, MD,
Maria C. Shiau, MD,
and Yahya M. Berkmen, MD

CONTENTS

INTRODUCTION
CHEST RADIOGRAPHY
COMPUTERIZED TOMOGRAPHY (CT)
NUCLEAR IMAGING
ULTRASOUND
MAGNETIC RESONANCE (MR) IMAGING
REFERENCES

INTRODUCTION

Radiologic evaluation has long been pivotal in the evaluation of the patient with pulmonary emphysema. In the era of lung volume reduction surgery (LVRS), thoracic imaging provides valuable information about the extent of the disease, preoperative guidance for the surgeon, and prediction of clinical and functional outcomes *(1–7)*.

This chapter reviews pulmonary emphysema from the point of view of the major imaging modalities (chest radiography, CT scans, nuclear imaging, ultrasound, and MR imaging), each first in general terms, and then specifically in the context of LVRS.

From: *Lung Volume Reduction Surgery*
Edited by: M. Argenziano and M. E. Ginsburg © Humana Press Inc., Totowa, NJ

CHEST RADIOGRAPHY

End-inspiratory posteroanterior and lateral chest X-rays (CXR) have long been considered as insensitive, but specific, indicators of pulmonary emphysema *(8–14)*. The major CXR finding of pulmonary emphysema relates to destruction of pulmonary parenchyma, as manifested by changes in pulmonary parenchymal blood vessels. When the destruction of the lung is moderate to severe, peripheral pulmonary vessels become sufficiently attenuated that a decrease in their number and caliber is evident on CXR (*see* Fig. 1) *(8–14)*. In regions of the lung where pulmonary parenchymal destruction is absent or minimal, redistribution of pulmonary blood flow is found, which may enhance the CXR observation of parenchymal vascular heterogeneity *(4,8,12)*. However, regions of mild emphysematous destruction of the lung usually appear normal on CXR because the predominant patterns of parenchymal destruction in pulmonary emphysema are multifocal and permeative. Bullae, which are evident radiographically as thin-walled, air-containing, and nearly spherical regions of the lung, are seen on CXR in only a minority of patients with pulmonary emphysema *(8)*.

After Gough and Wentworth reported in 1949 the development of paper-mounted thin sections of whole lung for examination by the naked eye *(15)*, correlations of radiologic and morbid anatomic findings in chronic bronchitis and emphysema were stimulated *(16–18)*. However, false-positive and false-negative interpretations, as well as inter- and intraobserver variation among radiologists have been features of a number of CXR studies *(9,13,16)*. Moreover, correlations of functional and CXR findings of pulmonary emphysema show a considerable range of variation *(4,11,14)*.

Increased lung volume, including a low, flat diaphragm and increased anteroposterior diameter of the chest, is a common finding in severe pulmonary emphysema, but these findings are usually only marginally evident in patients with emphysema of mild-to-moderate severity *(8,11)*. In 1978, the eminent Canadian chest pathologist, W. M. Thurlbeck, and the eminent British chest radiologist, George Simon, reported that in severe pulmonary emphysema, CXR showed the right hemidiaphragm in the midclavicular line at or below the sixth rib anteriorly in 95% of subjects and at or below the seventh rib anteriorly in 55% of subjects *(13)*. On the other hand, "The level of the diaphragm, although low, is not as important as its flattening" *(12)*. For the diaphragm to be considered flat, the convention is to draw an imaginary line on the lateral CXR between the anterior and posterior ends of the diaphragm; if the maximum distance of a line perpendicular to this imaginary line to the actual diaphragm is less than 1.5 cm, then the diaphragm may be regarded as flat *(10)*.

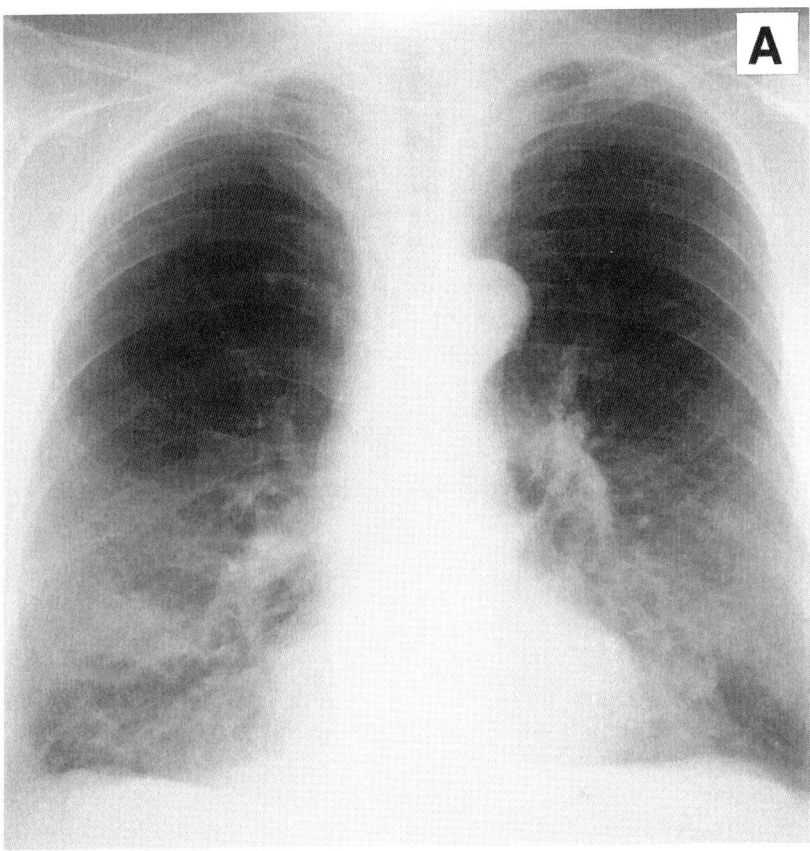

Fig. 1. *(this page and next 2 pages)* Pulmonary emphysema in a 68-yr-old man. (A) Posteroanterior chest radiograph shows severe pulmonary emphysema in the upper-lung zones, as manifested by marked attenuation of upper-lung zone vessels, combined with crowding ("compression") of lower-lung zone vessels. These signs correlate with favorable response to LVRS *(4)*. Note that the transverse diameter of the trachea is slightly decreased ("saber-sheath trachea") *(24)*. CT scans at upper (B), middle (C), and lower (D) thoracic levels (slice thickness, 5 mm) demonstrate attenuation of pulmonary vessels and ill-defined lucent foci, severe in the upper zones (B), severe in the right mid-lung zone (C), moderately severe in the left mid-lung zone (C), and mild in the lower-lung zones (D). Also note"saber-sheath" configuration of the trachea (B). Immediately after LVRS, frontal chest radiograph (E) shows elevation of the diaphragm compared to preoperative hyperinflation (A).

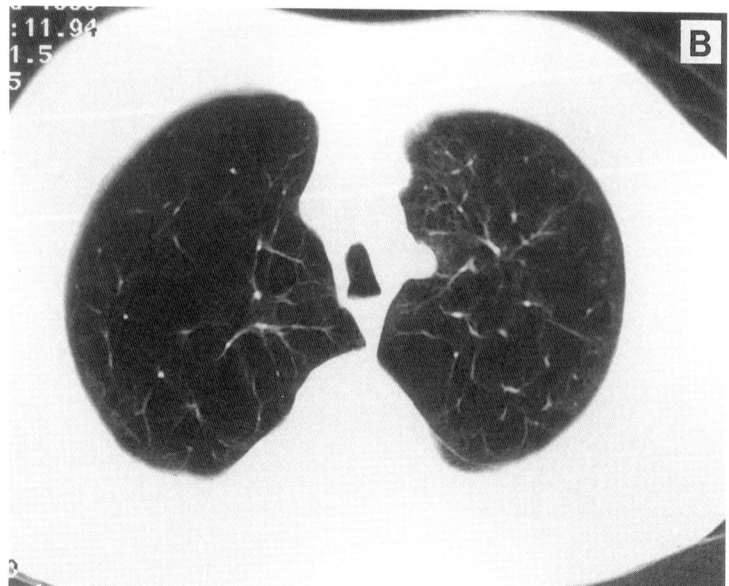

Fig. 1. (B)

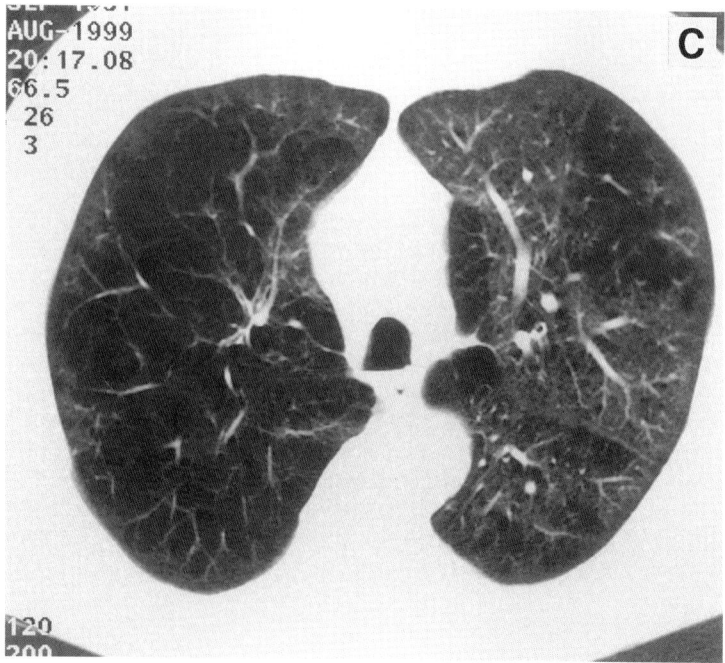

Fig. 1. (C)

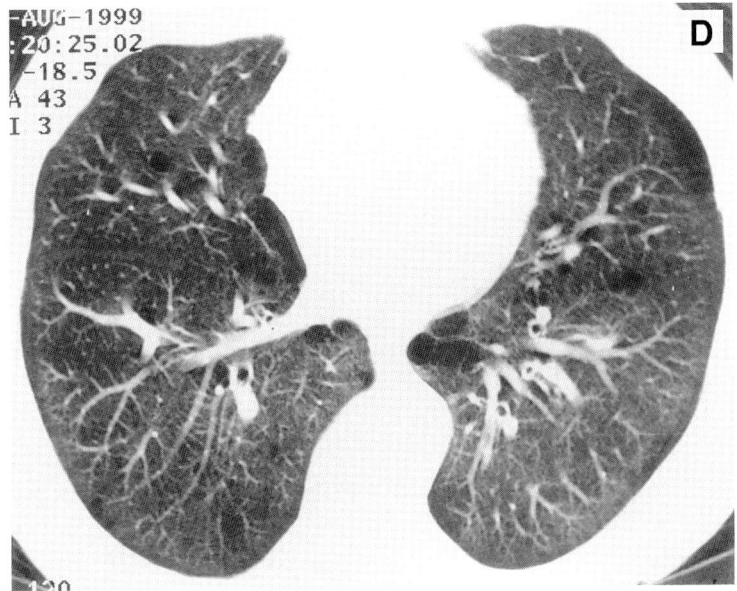

Fig. 1. (D)

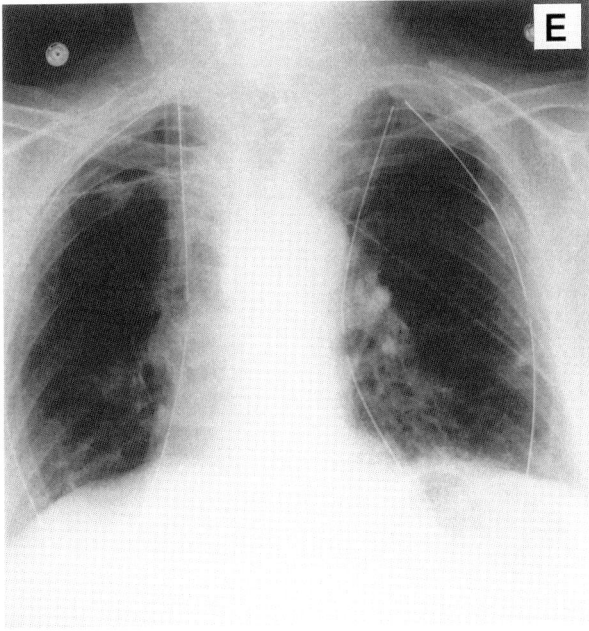

Fig. 1. (E)

The retrosternal space is defined (on lateral CXR) as the minimum anteroposterior distance from the inner aspect of the body of the sternum to the ascending aorta. Although this measurement may vary depending on body habitus, a distance of 2.5 cm is the accepted upper limit of normal in men *(12–14)*. In order for this to be considered reliable, however, the anterior margin of the ascending aorta must be clearly identifiable *(14)*. Simon noted that in emphysema, the retrosternal space "often measures 3 to 5 cm," but may be as small as "2.5 cm or less," and that the "retrosternal translucent zone also tends to extend down lower in emphysema than in a normal person, often reaching within 1 to 2 cm of the diaphragm in emphysema, whereas it is rarely lower than 3 cm in a normal person" *(8)*.

After reviewing these criteria involving chest wall and diaphragm, Thurlbeck and Simon concluded in 1978 that the subjective finding of "diminished or absent vascularity" remains the most important CXR sign of pulmonary emphysema *(13)*. Habitus affects the other CXR criteria substantially, and this conclusion has remained generally accepted over the last two decades.

Expiratory radiographs may also be obtained to assess motion of the diaphragm and chest wall between inspiration and expiration. Normal diaphragmatic excursion, however, ranges widely, from 2.5 to 8 cm *(19,20)*. Although vital capacity does not correlate closely with diaphragmatic motion, the amplitude of diaphragmatic contractions is inversely correlated with the severity of pulmonary emphysema *(12)*. As emphysema becomes severe, craniocaudal diaphragmatic motion is often in the range of 0–3 cm *(12)*.

Planimetric measurements of posteroanterior and lateral CXRs readily allow computerized calculation of lung volume *(21,22)*. Correlations among spirometric, plethysmographic, and CXR measures of lung volume are excellent (in the $r=0.9$ range), including CXR timed 1 s after initiation of forced expiration from total lung capacity (FEV$_1$ CXR) *(23)*. Narrowing of the trachea in the coronal plane ("saber-sheath trachea") (see Fig. 1A) is another radiographic finding often associated with chronic obstructive pulmonary disease, almost always in men over 50 yr of age *(24)*. Mechanisms of its development are unknown.

The distribution of pulmonary emphysema is almost always bilateral, although it is often asymmetric. The characteristic upper-lung zone predominance of centrilobular emphysema and lower-lung zone predominance of panacinar emphysema can often be appreciated on CXR, assuming that the disease is at least moderately severe *(13)*.

Smokers are well known to show more rapid decline in measures of pulmonary function than ex-smokers *(25)*, but CXR data have also shown that patients with predominant upper-zone emphysema deteriorate functionally and symptomatically more rapidly than patients with either generalized or predominant lower zone emphysema *(25)*.

Pulmonary hypertension secondary to pulmonary emphysema is commonly associated with severe hypoxemia *(26)*. Radiographic measurements of the caliber of the pulmonary artery and its major subdivisions do show statistically significant correlations with mean pulmonary artery pressure, but the data also show fairly wide scatter (r in the range of 0.5–0.7) *(26–28)*. The CXR prediction of the presence of pulmonary hypertension in a patient with pulmonary emphysema is, therefore, moderately accurate, but CXR analysis does not permit prediction of specific pulmonary arterial pressures as a function of specific central pulmonary arterial caliber.

Radiologists' patterns of visual search in pulmonary emphysema also include careful assessment of the spectrum of associated comorbid conditions, specifically including pulmonary infection, carcinoma of the lung, cardiomegaly, atherosclerotic calcification of the coronary arteries, and dilatation and atherosclerotic calcification of the thoracic aorta.

Chest Radiography in LVRS Patients

At the outset of the modern LVRS era, so-called heterogeneity of distribution of pulmonary emphysema was initially emphasized as a predictor of successful surgical outcome *(29)*. Four major CXR series have subsequently supported that view *(1,4,30,31)*. "Heterogeneity" refers to a pattern of emphysema in which severely involved pulmonary parenchymal destruction is present in some regions, usually in the upper zones, and minimal or no emphysema is present in other regions, usually in the lower zones. The rationale for lung removal is to reduce thoracic distention and allow the chest wall and diaphragm to return to a more normal configuration, improving lung recoil pressure and respiratory mechanics. Removal of the most emphysematous portion of the lung reduces air trapping and also may improve ventilation-perfusion matching" *(1)*.

Radiographic levels of heterogeneity correlate with postoperative functional (FEV_1, arterial oxygen saturation, 6-min walk distance) improvements, with Pearson correlation *(r)* coefficients in the range of 0.3–0.5 ($p < 0.01$) *(1)*. Moreover, radiographic upper vs lower zone radiographic emphysema scores correlate with post-LVRS improvement of FEV_1 (*r* values in the 0.5–0.7 range, $p < 0.001$) *(1,4)*.

The University of Pennsylvania group reported in 1999 that what they called "high disease heterogeneity" and "vascular crowding" (also called "lung compression") on CXR were each "100% predictive of a favorable outcome (FEV_1 increase, >30%)" after LVRS *(4)* (see Fig.

1A). On the other hand, they reported that a lack of heterogeneity on CXR was 94% predictive of an unfavorable outcome (postoperative FEV_1 increase <30%) and lack of lung compression was 92% predictive of an unfavorable outcome (postoperative increase of FEV_1 < 30%) after LVRS (4).

Because of its strong predictive value, "high disease heterogeneity" in that study (4) is worth considering in further detail. The frontal CXR was divided into three zones (upper, middle, lower) on each side, and then, in turn, each of the six zones was divided into medial and lateral subdivisions. The severity of emphysema in each of the 12 subdivisions was assessed subjectively on a brief scale of 0–3, in which 0 = normal lung, 1 = mild (estimated <25% emphysema), 2 = moderate (estimated 25%–75% emphysema), and 3 = severe (estimated >75% emphysema). The "heterogeneity score" was simply the difference between the greatest and least scores for all 12 subdivisions on the frontal CXR, i.e., 3 was the maximum score for heterogeneity. When the heterogeneity score was high (>2), all patients (n = 15) had a favorable outcome. When the score was low (<1), 94% (16 of 17) subjects did poorly (i.e., postoperative FEV_1 increase <30%).

An even simpler system of assessing heterogeneity by CXR was recently reported from Baylor (31). Each lung on the posteroanterior CXR was divided by a horizontal line halfway between the apex and the diaphragm, i.e., the two lungs become assessed as a total of four quadrants. The severity of emphysema was assessed in each quadrant on a 0–4 scale, in which a point was scored for each 25% of the quadrant that appeared emphysematous, i.e., a score of 3 meant 75% of the quadrant was emphysematous. The sum of the two lowest scores was then subtracted from the sum of the two highest scores, e.g., 8 was the index number for most heterogeneity possible. Patients with an index of 0 or 1 "tended to stay the same or get worse" after LVRS (31).

Hyperinflation, i.e., a low flat diaphragm as shown by CXR, appears not to be a strong predictor of a favorable response to LVRS (1,4,5,30) (e.g., r = 0.25 for hyperinflation as a predictor of favorable outcome in the Pennsylvania study). This result is entirely consistent with the result that heterogeneity distinguishes the subgroup of emphysema patients who will be responders to LVRS. Radiographic hyperinflation in severe pulmonary emphysema correlates merely with increased lung volume, but not with heterogeneous distribution.

Similarly, CXR in inspiration and expiration, which have only been assessed before and after LVRS in two series from one center (32,33), have not shown preoperative low diaphragmatic excursion as a predictor of postoperative favorable outcome, even when controlled for upper lobe vs lower lobe heterogeneity. However, entirely as would be expected, inspiratory CXR after LVRS does show decreases in antero-posterior dimensions of the chest *(34)* and of height of the lungs *(35)* (*see* Fig. 1E).

COMPUTERIZED TOMOGRAPHY (CT)

Computed tomography is a powerful tool for evaluation of pulmonary emphysema *(36–42)*. It provides an excellent anatomic display of normal and abnormal pulmonary structures and is highly sensitive to even minor pathologic changes. It is the best imaging modality for in vivo diagnosis of pulmonary emphysema.

CT assessment of emphysema on 10-mm-thick sections shows excellent correlation (r in the range of 0.8, $p < 0.001$) with airflow obstruction *(37)*. However, whether thick (10 mm) or thin (1–3 mm) sections are employed, the limit of CT detection is zones of emphysema >4 mm diameter *(43)*. CT, and especially thin-section CT, can readily distinguish among centrilobular, panacinar, bullous, and paraseptal emphysema when those patterns present in characteristic fashion, but when these types mix in patterns of severely permeative parenchymal destruction, then the characterization of subtypes becomes much less important than the overall quantitative extent of the destructive process *(40)*.

So-called high-resolution CT now refers to the combination of slice thickness of usually 1 mm (3 mm maximum), small field of view, and reconstruction using a bone algorithm. It is the optimal technique for the demonstration of centrilobular emphysema by CT *(40, 44)* (*see* Fig. 2).

Expiratory CT has occasionally been employed in assessing pulmonary emphysema *(3,45)*. Nishimura et al. have found that expiratory scans "appear to underemphasize the severity of emphysema," but also found that both inspiratory and expiratory CT appearances of emphysema correlated comparably well with diffusion capacity and total lung capacity *(45)*. They also found no significant difference between 5-mm- and 2-mm-thick scans in assessing emphysema *(45)*.

The diagnosis of emphysema on CT is based on detection of regions of distinctly lower attenuation than normal pulmonary parenchyma *(26,28–30,32,34)* (*see* Figs. 1–3). These regions are the CT equivalent of the CXR finding of regions of peripheral vascular deficiency. However, CT is far more sensitive than CXR in detecting emphysema, with a high degree of accuracy (CT-pathologic correlation coefficients in the 0.7–0.9 range, $p < 0.005$) *(43,46,47)*. Thus, when the diffusing capacity is low in a dyspneic patient who has an unremarkable CXR and normal FEV_1, CT not infrequently will show emphysema *(39)*.

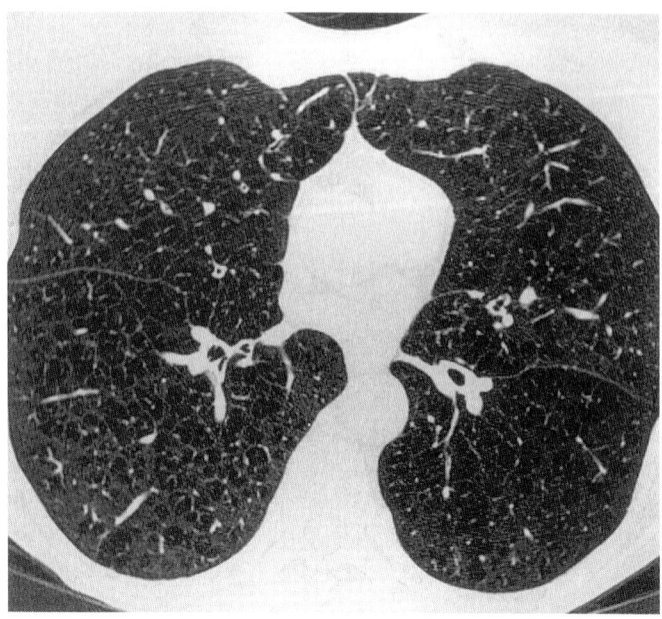

Fig. 2. Moderately severe centrilobular pulmonary emphysema in a 70-yr-old woman (CT scan, slice thickness 1 mm), as manifested by many intralobular rounded lucent regions.

Thin-section CT frequently demonstrates centrilobular emphysema as many small lucencies that are in centrilobular locations, usually patchy in distribution, and predominantly in the upper lobes and superior segments of lower lobes (*see* Fig. 2) *(13,40,47)*. When severe, the lucencies become confluent. Panlobular (panacinar) emphysema, which characterizes α-1-antitrypsin deficiency, equally destroys all parts of pulmonary lobules, and tends to involve preferentially the lower lobes *(13,40,48,49)*. Because panlobular emphysema involves lung in a "more or less diffuse" manner *(48)*, ". . . it is the most difficult form of emphysema to recognize on CT" *(49)*. Paraseptal emphysema, which is also readily shown by CT, is peripheral and seen as rounded lucencies that share very thin walls *(40)*. The abnormally low attenuation of pulmonary emphysema can be seen optimally at CT by use of low window levels, e.g., levels centered in the range of -600 to -800 Hounsfield Units (HU).

Bullous emphysema is most commonly a complication of centrilobular and paraseptal emphysema. By definition, a bulla is a sharply demarcated lucent zone, has a thin (<1 mm) wall, and is at least 1 cm in diameter *(50)*. The term "giant bullous emphysema" refers to bullae that occupy at least one-third of a hemithorax and are each on the order of 5–10 cm in diameter *(51)*. Giant bullous emphysema tends to be an asymmetric, progressive disease of the upper lobes in cigarette-smoking men in their middle years *(51)*.

CT also permits quantitative analysis of the severity of pulmonary emphysema, using a "density mask" technique, in which HUs of pixels lower than a given threshold limit are considered emphysematous *(38,41,52)*. Various threshold numbers in the range of -900 HU to -950 HU have been used by different authors, but the generally accepted value is -910 HU for end-inspiratory CT images *(38,41,51)*.

Lung volume is readily and accurately quantifiable by CT *(53)*. Indeed, CT may now be used as a research tool in patients with pulmonary emphysema to measure weight, tissue volume, and gas volume of the lungs *(54)*. Rib cage dimensions in hyperinflated subjects with severe pulmonary emphysema can readily be assessed by CT. Cassart et al. have shown that anteroposterior diameters of the chest in severe emphysema are increased by 2–3 cm, but that transverse dimensions remain normal, so that the cross-sectional shape of the thorax tends toward the circular in this population *(55)*. These investigators found the increased anteroposterior dimensions especially marked in the lower portions of the rib cage, suggesting that the diaphragm may be at a "greater mechanical disadvantage than expected" *(55)*.

CT also may be used to assess secondary pulmonary hypertension in patients with pulmonary emphysema, by measurement of the caliber of the main pulmonary artery. Diameter of the main pulmonary artery of at least 29 mm has been described as 87% sensitive and 89% specific for predicting pulmonary hypertension (mean pulmonary pressure of at least 20 mmHg) in patients with parenchymal lung disease *(56)*.

CT in LVRS Patients

The major role of chest CT in patients who are candidates for LVRS is to confirm the diagnosis of at least moderately severe pulmonary emphysema, as well as to evaluate any associated manifestations of chronic obstructive airway disease, e.g., bronchiectasis, chronic bronchitis, or respiratory bronchiolitis *(57)*. Carcinoma of the lung, which has a reported prevalence of 2–5% as Stage 1 disease in LVRS candidates *(32,58–61)*, also must be excluded.

CT assessment of the severity of pulmonary emphysema can be both subjective and objective. The subjective analysis in current use in the ongoing National Emphysema Treatment Trial (NETT) divides each lung into upper, middle, and lower zones and then assigns a score of 0–4 to each zone, so that the maximum possible severity score is 24 (*see* Fig. 3).

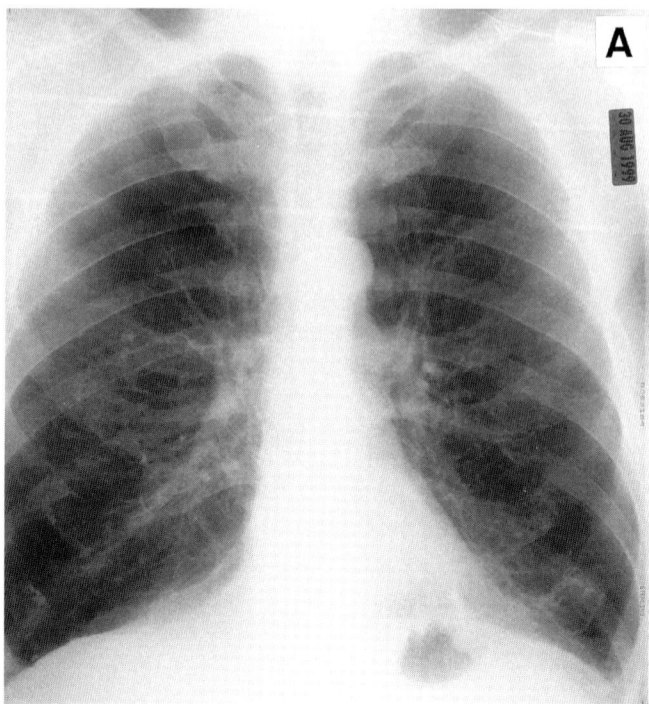

Fig. 3. (A) *(see this page and next page)*Diffuse severe pulmonary emphysema in a 66-yr-old man. (A) Posteroanterior radiograph shows generalized and severe attenuation of pulmonary vessels. The diaphragm is low and flat. CT scans at upper (B), and middle (C), and lower thoracic (D) levels (slice thickness, 1 mm) demonstrate widespread and severe replacement of normal lung architecture by ill-defined focal lucencies.

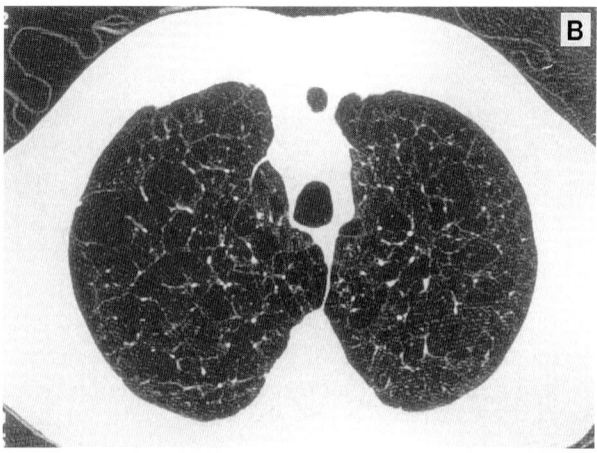

Fig. 3. (B)

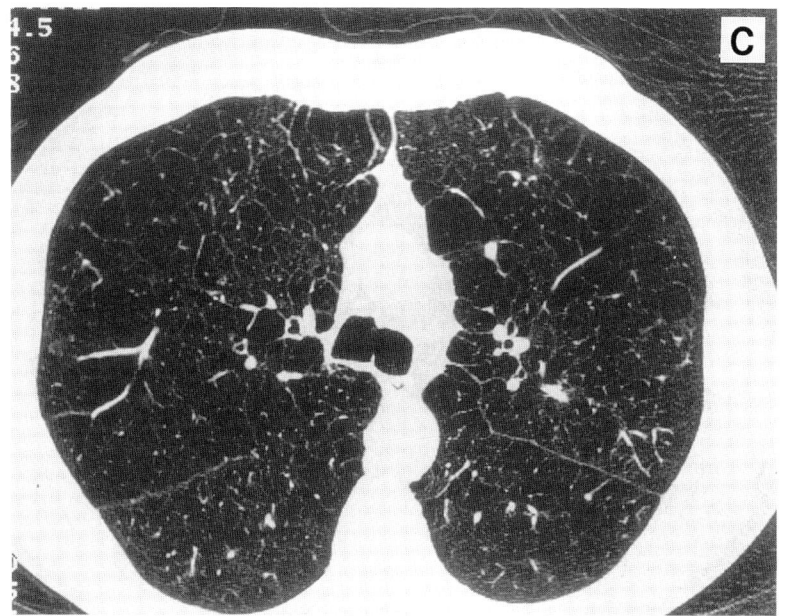

Fig. 3. (C)

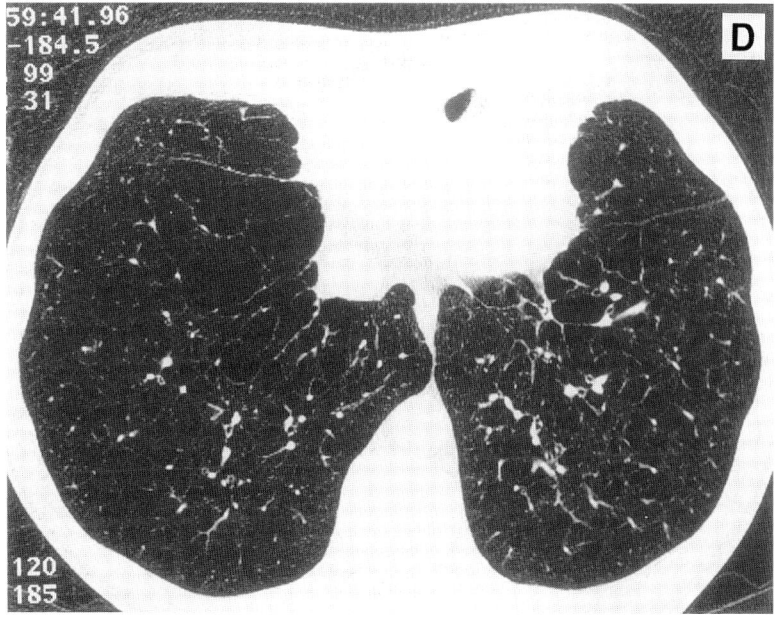

Fig. 3. (D)

Scoring is based on the system of Eda et al. *(62)* and is by subjective visual estimates, as follows: 0=no emphysema; 1=1%–25% emphysema; 2=26%–50% emphysema; 3=51%–75% emphysema; and 4=76%–100% emphysema. Objective analysis will consist of assessment of the percentage of lung in which pixels < –910 HU are considered as representing emphysema *(38,41,50)*. As of this writing, no results of the NETT are yet available.

CT quantitative analysis can employ inspiration and expiration images to compare functional and CT findings. For example, Eda et al. showed that the average CT numbers of each lung, when assessed as an expiratory to inspiratory ratio, correlated with both FEV_1 (% predicted) and also with the ratio of residual volume to total lung capacity, i.e., expiration : inspiration CT attenuation levels may be used as a surrogate for air trapping *(2)*. Subjective visual scoring, on the other hand, correlated best with diffusing capacity (% predicted), which may be used as a surrogate for the presence and severity of regional distribution of emphysema *(2)*.

Increased vital capacity after LVRS has been shown at inspiratory : expiratory CT by investigators at Washington University. They described the average CT lung volume after LVRS as decreasing from 7.5 L to 5.6 L (25% decrease) at inspiration and from 6.4 L to 3.8 L (41% decrease) at expiration, i.e., "increased air movement between respiratory cycles"*(2)*. Similarly, investigators at Columbia Presbyterian Medical Center have shown reduced air trapping after LVRS (10% decrease of residual volume/total lung capacity per operated lung), by analysis of inspiratory and expiratory CT scans *(3)*.

CT quantitative analysis has also been used to assess the effects of both unilateral and bilateral LVRS *(3)*. Because the mediastinum may shift after LVRS and the remaining lung may possibly expand after LVRS, the results of Becker et al. employing inspiration and expiration CT before and after LVRS, are of interest because they showed that "a lung's response to LVRS was independent from that of the contralateral lung" *(3)*.

Heterogeneous distribution of pulmonary emphysema, as assessed by CT, is associated with better post-LVRS results than is homogeneous disease *(3,7,63)* (*see* Figs. 1 and 3), confirming the similar results of CXR analysis of LVRS patients *(1,4,5,30)*. In this manner, the thoracic surgical group at University Hospital in Zürich, Switzerland, has reported interesting results: when 50 consecutive LVRS patients were divided by CT criteria into three groups (markedly, moderately, and minimally heterogeneous emphysema), FEV_1 increased at 3 mo post-LVRS by 81%, 44%, and 34%, respectively *(64)*. The authors concluded, contrary to the findings of the University of Pennsylvania investigators

(4), that "...even patients with homogeneous emphysema experienced a considerable subjective and functional benefit" *(64)*. However, the distribution of pulmonary emphysema more in the upper halves of the lungs than in the lower halves does appear to be a strong predictor of functional improvement (FEV_1, 6-min walk) after LVRS *(30)*.

Combining thin-section CT and physiologic data as a screening tool for LVRS has been suggested by Hunsaker et al. who reported an analysis of 16 subjects with moderate to severe emphysema by CT criteria. In this series, elevated inspiratory resistance (> 8.5 cm $H_2O/L/s$) predicted poor response to LVRS, whereas patients with inspiratory resistance < 8.5 cm $H_2O/L/s$ responded favorably *(65)*. These results suggest that some candidates for LVRS may have a component of fixed airway narrowing that will not respond to surgical intervention.

Is CT necessary to assess the distribution of emphysema in the lungs of LVRS candidates, compared to chest radiography? According to a review of 174 consecutive patients at the University of Michigan, the addition of CT to CXR analysis changed the ultimate assessment of distribution in 68 (39%) of the 174 patients *(66)*. Recent data from Pittsburgh and Vancouver show that when CT identifies regions of severe emphysema, excision of these specific regions correlates with postoperative reduction in total lung volume and postoperative improvement in cardiopulmonary exercise performance *(42)*. At the present juncture, however, the ideal imaging regimen—whether CT, CXR, or both—for assessing heterogeneity of emphysema, and for identifying optimal candidates for targeted lung resections, has not been established *(67)*.

NUCLEAR IMAGING

Perfusion scintigraphy is an excellent method for identifying regions of decreased or absent pulmonary perfusion in patients with pulmonary emphysema *(68)*. Perfusion scintigraphy is a widely accepted preoperative tool in the evaluation of patients with chronic obstructive pulmonary disease (COPD) who require a major lung resection for malignant disease *(69)*. Ventilation scintigraphy may also be useful *(68)*, but is generally regarded is less useful than perfusion scintigraphy as a predictor of postoperative status in emphysema patients who undergo pulmonary resection *(70)*.

Aerosol bolus dispersion is a test recently described to measure inhomogeneous distribution of ventilation *(71)*. Its role, if any, in diagnosis and management of pulmonary emphysema remains, however, to be defined.

Nuclear Imaging in LVRS Patients

According to Thurnheer et al., perfusion scintigraphy "may help to identify target areas for resection" *(6)*, but these same authors found better assessment of heterogeneity of emphysema by use of CT than scintigraphy *(6)*. Similarly, the Washington University group found that perfusion scintigraphy "can provide modest prognostic information" *(70)*. Quantitative analysis of perfusion scans has shown that the lower the ratio of perfusion in upper to lower halves of the lungs, the greater the improvement in dyspnea severity and FEV_1 after LVRS *(72)*. A recent multiinstitutional trial, however, has concluded that "perfusion scanning is superfluous in the preoperative evaluation of patients with emphysema for LVRS" *(73)*.

Ventilation scintigraphy, to our knowledge, has been studied in only one series of LVRS patients. Xenon-133 washout curves at Temple University showed a biphasic pattern in 29 LVRS patients with severe pulmonary emphysema *(74)*. The rapid first phase reflected emptying of large airways. The slow second phase was attributed to gas from small airways. After LVRS, the slow-phase washout increased and significantly correlated with increased FEV_1, implying enhanced function of small airways. This finding did not correlate anatomically with the sites of lung resection, suggesting that LVRS improves function in both operated and nonoperated regions of lung.

ULTRASOUND

Ultrasound can readily assess diaphragmatic contraction in vivo at the level of the zone of apposition between the periphery of the diaphragm and the thoracoabdominal wall *(75)*. Surface echocardiography in patients with severe pulmonary emphysema offers diagnostic advantages and limitations *(76)*. Echocardiography is a noninvasive means of assessing biventricular systolic function, including an estimation of pulmonary arterial pressure. It also allows evaluation of valvular heart disease, if present. Because anteriorly hyperexpanded lung may block transmission of sound waves, however, the quality of the images can be compromised. This limitation has been reported in 1–20% of subjects *(75–77)*.

Ultrasound Imaging in LVRS Patients

Standard surface echocardiography may be a useful test, but stress echocardiography utilizing dobutamine may be even more valuable. According to a recent study from the University of Michigan, dobutamine stress echocardiography provided "excellent negative predictive value" for both early and late adverse cardiac events *(78)*. Four (9%) of the 46 patients in that series showed ischemic changes during testing *(78)*. One of these four patients developed an episode of pulmonary edema after LVRS and two others had transient arrhythmias. No major cardiac complication developed after LVRS in the 41 patients with a negative test *(78)*.

MAGNETIC RESONANCE (MR) IMAGING

Magnetic resonance imaging (MRI) has several disadvantages that have made it unsuitable for the imaging of the pulmonary parenchyma in emphysema. First, MRI has lower spatial resolution than CT, and the direct dependence of signal amplitude on voxel size precludes the use of very thin sections. In addition, because the lung is comprised primarily of gas, the density of protons needed for conventional MRI is low. Because standard spin-echo imaging sequences require imaging times of several minutes, breath-hold imaging is not possible, and thus images are further degraded by respiratory motion. However, the development of fast-spin-echo and gradient-echo MRI techniques have overcome the problems of respiratory motion in all but the most dyspneic patients. MRI has thus proven most useful in imaging secondary effects of pulmonary emphysema: chest wall and diaphragmatic motion.

Resulting from its ability to scan in sagittal and coronal planes, MRI is ideally suited for evaluation of the diaphragm, which is difficult to image in the axial plane. Paiva et al. reported in 1992 studies on diaphragmatic shape using MRI in normal subjects *(79)*. Kenematsu et al. *(80)* and Giarada et al. *(81,82)* used fast gradient echo images to study diaphragmatic structure and motion, but both groups were unable to image all portions of the diaphragm in all subjects because of limitations in spatial resolution. Iwasawa et al. *(83)* used sequential fast MRI to demonstrate paradoxical chest wall motion in emphysema patients, as well as a "see-saw" motion of the diaphragm that they hypothesized was secondary to pendelluft ventilation, i.e., ventilation of varying time-constants in different regions of the lungs. Suga et al. *(84)* found that emphysema patients had reduced, irregular, or asynchronous chest wall and diaphragmatic motion, decreased amplitude of motions, and decreased length of apposition between the lung and diaphragm.

In the past decade, studies have also been initiated on the use of MRI in the evaluation of pulmonary perfusion. Kondo et al. *(85)* used velocity-encoded cine MRI images to analyze pulmonary flow and flow patterns in 10 patients with pulmonary hypertension, 5 of whom had emphysema. Peak flow correlated with the results of Doppler echocardiography, and patients with pulmonary hypertension had an inhomogeneous flow profile with greater retrograde flow after middle-to-late systole, correlating with elevated pulmonary vascular resistance. Silverman et al. *(86)* studied 13 patients with emphysema, using phase contrast cine MRI images, demonstrating high correlation between blood flow calculated from MRI and perfusion as determined by radionuclide perfusion scintigraphy. Berthezene et al. *(87)* used a dynamic gadolinium-enhanced inversion recovery turbo FLASH sequence with ultrashort TE to evaluate perfusion in patients with emphysema and with suspected pulmonary embolism, again showing good correlation between MRI and scintigraphy ($\kappa = 0.63$), although correlation was better in the upper lobes than in the lower lobes. These results suggest potential applicability of this modality in choosing suitable candidates for LVRS and for selecting regions of most severely diseased lung for resection.

Pulmonary ventilation has traditionally been evaluated via pulmonary function testing and scintigraphic ventilation scans using inhaled radionuclides. The use of MRI in the evaluation of pulmonary ventilation was first reported in the mid-1990s. In 1994, Albert et al. *(88)* used laser-polarized 129Xe as an MR contrast agent for pulmonary perfusion imaging, and Middleton et al. *(89)* reported the use of 3He as a contrast agent the next year. Edelman et al. *(90)* used inhaled molecular oxygen as a contrast agent and were able to demonstrate ventilation defects in a patient with bullous emphysema. Because scintigraphic ventilation scans are limited to planar projection images, MR ventilation techniques may offer improved spatial resolution and the ability to derive three-dimensional ventilation maps. Hyperpolarized 3He imaging also offers promise for the study of gas diffusion within the lung *(91–93)*.

MRI in LVRS Patients

Investigations into the use of MRI in preoperative and postoperative assessment of LVRS patients are only in an early stage. The potential use of MRI is intriguing, as no other technique alone can provide such a broad range of structural and functional data about the lungs, chest wall, diaphragm, heart, and pulmonary vasculature.

Several groups have used MRI to study respiratory mechanics in LVRS patients. Gierada et al. found that lung volumes calculated from fast-gradient echo breath-hold MRI were comparable to those derived from CT, but differed from those of plethysmography, and that the changes in thoracic dimensions after LVRS were consistent with improved respiratory mechanics *(94)*. Fujimoto et al. *(95)* found that thoracic movement was significantly increased after LVRS, as assessed on sagittal dynamic MRI at full inspiration and expiration, and that these changes correlated with decreased dyspnea and increased FEV_1. Suga et al. *(84)* showed significantly improved amplitude of diaphragmatic and chest wall motion and increased length of apposition of the diaphragm after LVRS.

The use of MRI perfusion imaging in the preoperative evaluation of emphysema patients is still undergoing preliminary investigation *(96,97)*. MR ventilation imaging before LVRS is also an area of active investigation, with hyperpolarized 3He the ventilation agent of choice due to its greater magnetic movement than 129Xe, slower depolarization, and lack of absorption *(93)*. DeLange et al. calculated MR ventilation/perfusion ratios as the ratio of signal on 3He to conventional proton MRI and found the results correlated with functional measurements, although only one patient was imaged both before and after LVRS *(97)*. However, until added value for MRI over more conventional and less expensive imaging techniques can be demonstrated, MRI is likely to remain experimental in the evaluation of LVRS patients.

REFERENCES

1. Slone RM, Pilgram TK, Gierada DS, Sagel SS, Glazer HS, Yusen RD, Cooper JD (1997) Lung volume reduction surgery: comparison of preoperative radiologic features and clinical outcome. *Radiology* 204: 685–693.
2. Bae KT, Slone RM, Gierada DS, Yusen RD, Cooper JD (1997) Patients with emphysema: quantitative CT analysis before and after lung volume reduction surgery. *Radiology* 203: 705–714.
3. Becker MD, Berkmen YM, Austin JHM, Mun IK, Romney BM, Rozenshtein A, et al. (1998) Lung volumes before and after lung volume reduction surgery: quantitative CT analysis. *Am J Respir Crit Care Med* 157: 1593–1599.
4. Maki DD, Miller WT Jr, Aronchick JM, Gefter WB, Miller WT Sr, Kotloff RM, et al. (1999) Advanced emphysema: preoperative chest radiographic findings as predictors of outcome following lung volume reduction surgery. *Radiology* 212: 49–55.
5. Austin JHM (1999) Pulmonary emphysema: imaging assessment of lung volume reduction surgery. *Radiology* 212: 1–3.
6. Thurnheer R, Engel H, Weder W, et al. (1999) Role of lung perfusion scintigraphy in relation to chest computed tomography and pulmonary function in the evaluation of candidates for lung volume reduction surgery. *Am J Respir Crit Care Med* 159: 301–310.
7. Hamacher J, Bloch GE, Stammberger U, et al. (1999) Two years' outcome of lung volume reduction surgery in different morphologic emphysema types. *Ann Thorac Surg* 68: 1792–1798.
8. Simon G (1964) Radiology and emphysema. *Clin Radiol* 15: 293–306.
9. Nicklaus TM, Stowell DW, Christiansen WR, Renzetti AD Jr (1966) The accuracy of the roentgenologic diagnosis of chronic pulmonary emphysema. *Am Rev Respir Dis* 93: 889–899.
10. Simon G (1971) *Principles of Chest X-Ray Diagnosis*, 3rd ed. New York: Appleton-Century-Crofts.
11. Simon G, Pride NB, Jones NL, Raimondi AC (1973) Relation between abnormalities in the chest radiograph and changes in pulmonary function in chronic bronchitis and emphysema. *Thorax* 28: 15–23.
12. Gamsu G, Nadel JA (1973) The roentgenologic manifestations of emphysema and chronic bronchitis. *Med Clin North Am* 57: 719–733.
13. Thurlbeck WM, Simon G (1978) Radiographic appearance of the chest in emphysema. *Am J Roentgenol* 130: 429–440.
14. Pratt PC (1987) Role of conventional chest radiography in diagnosis and exclusion of emphysema. *Am J Med* 82: 998–1006.
15. Gough J, Wentworth JE (1949) The use of thin sections of entire organs in morbid anatomical studies. *J Royal Microsc Soc* 69: 231–235.

16. Simon G, Galbraith NJ (1953) Radiology of chronic bronchitis. *Lancet* 2: 850–852.
17. Laws JW, Heard BE (1962) Emphysema and the chest film: a retrospective radiological and pathological study. *Brit J Radiol* 35: 760–761.
18. Reid L, Millard NJ (1964) Correlation between radiological diagnosis and structural lung changes in emphysema. *Clin Radiol* 15: 307–311.
19. Young DA, Simon G (1972) Certain movements measured on inspiration-expiration chest radiographs correlated with pulmonary function studies. *Clin Radiol* 23: 37–41.
20. Alexander C (1966) Diaphragm movements and the diagnosis of diaphragmatic paralysis. *Clin Radiol* 17: 79–83.
21. Glenn EW Jr, Greene R (1975) Rapid computer-aided radiographic calculation of total lung capacity (TLC). *Radiology* 117: 269–273.
22. Kilburn KH, Warshaw RH, Thornton JC, Thornton K, Miller A (1992) Predictive equations for total lung capacity and residual volume calculated from radiographs in a random sample of the Michigan population. *Thorax* 47: 519–523.
23. Gamsu G, Shames DM, McMahon J, Greenspan RH (1975) Radiographically determined lung volumes at full inspiration and during dynamic forced expiration in normal subjects. *Invest Radiol* 10: 100–108.
24. Greene R (1978) "Saber-sheath" trachea: relation to chronic obstructive pulmonary disease. *Am J Roentgenol* 130: 441–445.
25. Hughes JA, Hutchison DCS, Bellamy D, et al. (1982) Annual decline of lung function in pulmonary emphysema: influence of radiologic distribution. *Thorax* 37: 32–37.
26. Keller CA, Shepard JW Jr, Chun DS, et al. (1986) Pulmonary hypertension in chronic obstructive pulmonary disease: multivariate analysis. *Chest* 90: 185–192.
27. Matthay RA, Schwarz MI, Ellis JH Jr, et al. (1981) Pulmonary artery hypertension in chronic obstructive pulmonary disease: determination by chest radiography. *Invest Radiol* 18: 95–100.
28. Chetty KG, Brown SE, Light RW (1982) Identification of hypertension in chronic obstructive pulmonary disease from routine chest radiographs. *Am Rev Respir Dis* 126: 338–341.
29. Cooper JD, Trulock EP, Triantafillou AN, et al. (1995) Bilateral pneumectomy (volume reduction) for chronic obstructive pulmonary disease. *J Thorac Cardiovasc Surg* 109: 106–119.
30. Kazerooni EA, Curtis JL, Paine R III, et al. (1998) Long-term outcome after bilateral apical lung volume reduction surgery (LVRS) via median sternotomy. *Radiology* 209(P), Suppl. (Nov.): 257 (abstract).
31. Baldwin JC, Miller CC III, Prince RA, Espada R (2000) Chest radiograph heterogeneity predicts functional improvement with volume reduction surgery. *Ann Thorac Surg* 70: 1208–1211.
32. McKenna RJ Jr, Fischel RJ, Brenner M, et al. (1996) Combined operations for lung volume reduction surgery and lung cancer. *Chest* 110: 885–888.
33. McKenna RJ Jr, Brenner M, Fischel RJ, et al. (1997) Patient selection criteria for lung volume reduction surgery. *J Thorac Cardiovasc Surg* 114: 957–967.
34. Lando Y, Boiselle P, Shade D, et al. (1999) Effect of lung volume reduction surgery on bony thorax configuration in severe COPD. *Chest* 116: 30–39.
35. Takasugi JE, Wood DE, Godwin JD, et al. (1998) Lung-volume reduction surgery for diffuse emphysema: radiologic assessment of changes in thoracic dimensions. *J Thorac. Imaging* 13: 36–41.

36. Foster WL, Pratt PC, Roggli VL, Godwin JD, Halvorsen RA Jr, Putman CE (1986) Centrilobular emphysema: CT-pathologic correlation. *Radiology* 159: 27–32.

37. Sakai F, Gamsu G, Im J-G, Ray CS (1987) Pulmonary function abnormalities in patients with CT-determined emphysema. *J Comput Assist Tomogr* 11: 963–968.

38. Müller NL, Staples CA, Miller RR, Abboud RT (1988) Density mask: an objective method to quantitate emphysema using computed tomography. *Chest* 94: 782–787.

39. Klein JS, Gamsu G, Webb WR, Golden JA, Müller NL (1992) High-resolution CT diagnosis of emphysema in symptomatic patients with normal chest radiographs and isolated low diffusing capacity. *Radiology* 182: 817–821.

40. Webb WR, Müller NL, Naidich DP (2001) *High resolution CT of the Lung* (3rd ed.), Philadelphia, PA: Lippincott Williams & Wilkins 436–462.

41. Gevenois PA, Maertelaer Y de, De Voyst P (1995) Comparison of computed density and macroscopic morphometry in pulmonary emphysema. *Am J Respir Crit Care Med* 152: 653–657.

42. Rogers RM, Coxson HO, Sciurba FC, Keenan RJ, Whittall KP, Hogg JC (2000) Preoperative severity of emphysema predictive of improvement after lung volume reduction surgery: use of CT morphometry. *Chest* 118: 1240–1247.

43. Miller RR, Müller NL, Vedal S, Morrison NJ, Staples CA (1989) Limitations of computed tomography in the assessment of emphysema. *Am Rev Respir Dis* 139: 980–983.

44. Murata K, Khan A, Herman PG (1989) Pulmonary parenchymal disease: evaluation with high-resolution CT. *Radiology* 170: 629–635.

45. Nishimura K, Murata K, Yamagishi M, et al. (1998) Comparison of different computed tomography scanning methods for quantifying emphysema. *J Thorac Imaging* 13: 193–198.

46. Hruban RH, Meziane MM, Zerhouni EA, et al. (1987) High resolution computed tomography of inflation-fixed lungs: pathologic-radiologic correlation of centrilobular emphysema. *Am Rev Respir Dis* 136: 935–940.

47. Kuwano K, Matsuba K, Ikeda T, et al. (1990) The diagnosis of mild emphysema: correlation of computed tomography and pathology scores. *Am Rev Respir Dis* 141: 169–178.

48. Anderson AE Jr, Foraker AG (1973) Centrilobular emphysema and panlobular emphysema: two different diseases. *Thorax* 28: 547–550.

49. Spouge D, Mayo JR, Cardoso W, Müller NL (1993) Panacinar emphysema: CT and pathologic findings. *J Comput Assist Tomogr* 17: 710–713.

50. Austin JHM, Müller NL, Friedman PJ, et al. (1996) Glossary of terms for CT of the lungs: recommendations of the nomenclature committee of the Fleischner Society. *Radiology* 200: 327–331.

51. Stern EJ, Webb WR, Weinacker A, Müller NL (1994) Idiopathic giant bullous emphysema (vanishing lung syndrome): imaging findings in nine patients. *AJR* 162: 279–282.

52. Kinsella M, Müller NL, Abboud RT, Morrison NJ, DyBuncio A (1990) Quantitation of emphysema by computed tomography using a "density mask" program and correlation with pulmonary function tests. *Chest* 97: 315–321.

53. Brown MS, McNitt-Gray MF, Goldin JG, et al. (1999) Automated measurement of single and total lung volume from CT. *J Comput Assist Tomogr* 23: 632–640.

54. Coxson HO, Rogers RM, Whittall KP, et al. (1999) A quantification of the lung surface area in emphysema using computed tomography. *Am J Respir Crit Care Med* 159: 851–856.

55. Cassart M, Gevenois PA, Estenne M (1996) Rib cage dimensions in hyperinflated patients with severe chronic obstructive pulmonary disease. *Am J Respir Crit Care Med* 154: 800–805.

56. Tan RT, Kuzo R, Goodman LR, et al. (1998) Utility of CT scan evaluation for predicting pulmonary hypertension in patients with parenchymal lung disease. *Chest* 113: 1250–1256.

57. Gückel C, Hansell DM (1998) Imaging the "dirty lung"—has high resolution computed tomography cleared the smoke? *Clin Radiol* 53: 717–722.

58. Pigula FA, Keenan RJ, Ferson PF, Landrenau RJ (1996) Unsuspected lung cancer found in work-up for lung reduction operation. *Ann Thorac Surg* 61: 174–176.

59. Hazelrigg SR, Boley TM, Weber D, Magee MJ, Naunheim KS (1997) Incidence of lung nodules found in patients undergoing lung volume reduction. *Ann Thorac Surg* 64: 303–306.

60. Duarte IG, Gal AA, Mansour KA, Lee RB, Miller JI (1998) Pathologic findings in lung volume reduction surgery. *Chest* 113: 660–664.

61. Rozenshtein A, White CS, Austin JHM, Romney BM, Protopapas Z, Krasna MJ (1998) Incidental lung carcinoma detected at CT in patients selected for lung volume reduction surgery to treat severe pulmonary emphysema. *Radiology* 207: 487–490.

62. Eda S, Kubo K, Fujimoto K, Matsuzawa Y, Sekiguchi M, Sakai F (1997). The relations between expiratory chest CT using helical CT and pulmonary function tests in emphysema. *Am J Respir Crit Care Med* 155: 1290–1294.

63. Geddes D, Davies M, Koyama H, et al. (2000) Effect of lung-volume-reduction surgery in patients with severe emphysema. *N Engl J Med* 343: 239–245.

64. Weder W, Thurnheer R, Stammberger V, Burge M, Russi EW, Bloch KE (1997) Radiologic emphysema morphology is associated with outcome after surgical lung volume reduction. *Ann Thorac Surg* 64: 313–320.

65. Hunsaker A, Ingenito E, Topal U, Pugatch R, Reilly J (1998) Preoperative screening for lung volume reduction surgery: usefulness of combining thin-section CT with physiologic assessment. *AJR* 170: 309–314.

66. Adusumilli S, Kazerooni EA, Martinez FJ (1998) Distribution of pulmonary emphysema: comparison of chest radiography to CT. *Radiology* 209(P): Suppl. (Nov.): 256–257 (abstract).

67. Salzman SH (2000) Can CT measurement of emphysema severity aid patient selection for lung volume reduction surgery? *Chest* 118: 1231–1232.

68. Markos J, Mullan BP, Hillman DR, et al. (1989) Preoperative assessment as a predictor of mortality and morbidity after lung resection. *Am Rev Respir Dis* 139: 902–910.

69. Olsen GN, Block AJ, Tobias JA (1974) Prediction of postpneumonectomy pulmonary function using quantitative macroaggregate lung scanning. *Chest* 66: 13–16.

70. Wang SC, Fisher KC, Slone RM, et al. (1997) Perfusion scintigraphy in the evaluation for lung volume reduction surgery: correlation with clinical outcome. *Radiology* 205: 243–248.

71. Kohlhäufl M, Brand P, Rock C, et al. (1999) Noninvasive diagnosis of emphysema: aerosol mophometry and aerosol bolus dispersion in comparison to HRCT. *Am J Respir Crit Care Med* 160: 913–918.

72. Jamadar DA, Kazerooni EA, Martinez FJ, et al. (1998) Prediction of clinical outcome after LVRS; comparison of quantitative computer-generated ratio of upper/lower lung perfusion with semiqualitative scoring of perfusion defects in the upper and lower lungs on 99m-MAA technetium. *Radiology* 209 (P): Suppl. (Nov.): 213 (abstract).

73. Cleverley JR, Desai SR, Wells AU, et al. (1999) Evaluation of patients undergoing lung volume reduction surgery: ancillary information available from computed tomography. *Radiology* 213(P): Suppl. (Nov.): 343 (abstract).

74. Travaline JM, Maurer AH, Charkes ND, Urbain JL, Furukawa S, Criner GJ (2000) Quantitation of regional ventilation during the washout phase of lung scintigraphy: measurement in patients with severe COPD before and after bilateral lung volume reduction surgery. *Chest* 118: 721–727.

75. Ueki J, De Bruin PF, Pride NB (1995) In vivo assessment of diaphragm contraction by ultrasound in normal subjects. *Thorax* 50: 1157–1161.

76. Bach DS, Curtis JL, Christensen PJ, Iannettoni MD, Whyte RJ, Kazerooni EA, et al. (1998) Preoperative echocardiographic evaluation of patients referred for lung volume reduction surgery. *Chest* 114: 972–980.

77. Danchin N, Cornette A, Henriquez A, et al. (1987) Two-dimensional echocardiographic assessment of the right ventricle in patients with chronic obstructive lung diseases. *Chest* 92: 229–233.

78. Bossone E, Martinez FJ, Whyte RI, et al. (1999) Dobutamine stress echocardiography for the preoperative evaluation of patients undergoing lung volume reduction surgery. *J Thorac Cardiovasc Surg* 118: 542–546.

79. Paiva M, Verbanck S, Estenne M, Poncelet B, Segebarth C, Macklem PT (1992) Mechanical implications of in vivo diaphragm shape. *J Appl Physiol* 72: 1407–1412.

80. Kenematsu M, Imaeda T, Mochizuki R, et al. (1995) Dynamic MRI of the diaphragm. *J Comput Assist Tomogr* 19: 67–72.

81. Gierada DS, Curtin JJ, Erickson SJ, et al. (1995) Diaphragmatic motion: fast gradient-recalled-echo MR imaging in healthy subjects. *Radiology* 194: 879–884.

82. Gierada DS, Curtin JJ, Erickson SJ, et al. (1997) Fast gradient echo magnetic resonance imaging of the normal diaphragm. *J Thorac. Imag* 12: 70–74.

83. Iwasawa T, Kagei S, Gotcoh T, et al. (1999) Asynchronous respiratory motion of the chest wall and hemidiaphragm in patients with emphysema: detection with sequential MR imaging and quantitative analysis. *Radiology* 213 (P) Suppl. (Nov.): 553.

84. Suga K, Tsukuda T, Awaya H, et al. (1999) Impaired respiratory mechanics in pulmonary emphysema: evaluation with dynamic breathing MRI. *J Magn Reson Imag* 10: 510–520.

85. Kondo C, Caputo GR, Masui T, et al. (1992) Pulmonary hypertension: pulmonary flow quantification and flow profile analysis with velocity- encoded cine MR imaging. *Radiology* 183: 751–758.

86. Silverman JM, Julien PJ, Herfkens RJ, Pelc NJ (1993) Quantitative differential pulmonary perfusion: MR imaging versus radionuclide lung scanning. *Radiology* 189: 699–701.

87. Berthezene Y, Croisille P, Wiart M, et al. (1999) Prospective comparison of MR lung perfusion and lung scintigraphy. *J Magn Reson Imag* 9: 61–68.

88. Albert MD, Cates GD, Driehuys B, et al. (1994) Biological magnetic resonance imaging using laser-polarised 129Xe. *Nature* 370: 199–201.

89. Middleton H, Black RD, Saam B, et al. (1995) MR imaging with hyperpolarized He-3 gas. *Magn Reson Med* 33: 271–275.

90. Edelman RR, Hatabu H, Tadamura E, et al. (1996) Noninvasive assessment of regional ventilation in the human lung using oxygen-enhanced magnetic resonance imaging. *Nat Med* 2: 1236–1239.

91. Ebert M, Grossman T, Heil W, et al. (1996) Nuclear magnetic resonance imaging with hyperpolarised helium-3. *Lancet* 347(9011): 1297–1299.

92. Yablonskiy DA, Saam BT, Gierada DS, et al. (1999) Diffusion imaging of hyperpolarized 3He in patients with emphysema: changes in the structure of alveoli. *Radiology* 213(P) Suppl (Nov.): 344 (abstract).

93. DeLange EE, Mugler JP, Brookman JR, et al. (1999) Lung air spaces: MR imaging evaluation with hyperpolarized 3He gas. *Radiology* 210: 851–857.
94. Gierada DS, Hakimian S, Sloan RM, Yusen RD (1998) MR analysis of lung volume and thoracic dimensions in patients with emphysema before and after lung volume reduction surgery. *AJR* 170: 707–714.
95. Fujimoto K, Kubo K, Haniuda M, et al. (1999) Improvements in thoracic movement following lung emphysema: evaluation with dynamic breathing MRI. *J Magn Reson Imag* 10: 510–520.
96. Johkoh T, Müller NL, Mayo JR, et al. (1999) Scintigraphic and MRI perfusion imaging in the preoperative evaluation for lung volume reduction surgery: preliminary results. *Radiology* 213(P) Suppl (Nov.): 553 (abstract).
97. De Lange EE, Truwit JD, Christopher BS, et al. (1999) MR imaging with hyperpolarized Helium-3 gas: correlation with pulmonary function testing in healthy subjects and patients with chronic obstructive pulmonary disease. *Radiology* 213(P) Suppl (Nov.): 343–344 (abstract).

5 Medical Management of Emphysema and Chronic Obstructive Pulmonary Disease

Chun K. Yip, MD

CONTENTS

INTRODUCTION

Chronic obstructive pulmonary disease (COPD) is a disease process characterized by the presence of airflow obstruction secondary to emphysema or chronic bronchitis. It is this airflow obstruction that is the main culprit for the various symptoms manisfested by COPD patients. Consequently, one of the main objectives of medical treatment in COPD is to reduce airflow obstruction, which may be accompanied by airway hyperreactivity and, therefore, be partially reversible. Thus, bronchodilators are employed in the treatment of COPD. Furthermore, smoking cessation is the only currently available intervention that may slow progression of this disease. Besides pharmacotherapy, other medical treatments, such as oxygen therapy and pulmonary rehabilitation, have been proven to be beneficial to patients with COPD. Prevention and treatment of infection also plays an important role in reducing the frequency of acute exacerbations in these patients. Emphysema and chronic bronchitis usually coexist to different degrees in COPD patients *(1)*. Pharmacologic treat-

From: *Lung Volume Reduction Surgery*
Edited by: M. Argenziano and M. E. Ginsburg © Humana Press Inc., Totowa, NJ

ment of airflow obstruction is less effective in emphysema. This is because airflow limitation as a result of loss of elastic recoil in emphysema is irreversible. Because of the lack of effective medical therapy in severe emphysema, surgical interventions, such as lung volume reduction surgery (LVRS) and lung transplantation, are being explored as alternative treatment options in selected cases. Still, much can be done for most COPD patients by employing appropriate medical management techniques.

DIAGNOSIS OF COPD

In addition to a careful history and physical examination, spirometry and arterial blood gas measurements play an important role in the management of COPD. They not only help establish the diagnosis and assess the severity of the disease, but are also useful for monitoring the course of the disease. In addition, these objective measurements help suggest prognosis and guide medical therapy for these patients. In complex cases, more comprehensive pulmonary function testing, such as measurement of lung volumes and diffusing capacity (DLCO), as well as cardiopulmonary exercise testing, may be necessary. A chest radiograph should be done in all patients with symptoms of COPD to rule out other disease processes that can cause similar symptoms. Although most patients will not require a CT scan of the chest to establish the diagnosis of COPD, it provides a quantitative assessment of the degree of emphysema.

MEDICAL THERAPY OF COPD

The major goals in the management of patients with COPD are as follows:

1. To lessen or stop the rate of progression of the disease.
2. To decrease airflow limitation.
3. To prevent and shorten exacerbations of the disease.
4. To improve respiratory symptoms, exercise capacity, and quality of life.
5. To prolong survival.

There are a number of medical therapies available once a patient is diagnosed with COPD. These are discussed individually in the sections that follow.

Patient Education and Smoking Cessation

Patient education is an important part in the management of COPD. The patient should be educated about the disease and encouraged to take an active role in its management (2). Cigarette smoking is the most significant cofactor in the etiology of COPD. Consequently, cessation of smoking is the single most important therapeutic intervention in the management of COPD patients. This can reduce the progressive reduction in FEV_1 in smokers with established COPD *(3)*. Moreover, it is the only therapeutic intervention that can lessen or stop the rate of progression of COPD. Smoking cessation can be achieved by patients with the advice and support of their physician. If this is unsuccessful, other methods should be attempted, including nicotine replacement (in the forms of gum, transdermal patch, spray, or inhaler), bupropion, and/or professional counseling. Smoking cessation is crucial in the management of all stages of COPD, and patients should be encouraged to quit as soon as possible. It has been documented that mild pulmonary function abnormalities are completely reversible in smokers who have been smoking for a relatively short duration *(4)*.

Pharmacotherapy

Pharmacologic management of patients with COPD is mainly aimed at symptom relief, and thus at improving quality of life. Pharmacotherapy is directed against the reversible components of airway obstruction, namely, airway secretion, mucosal edema and congestion, cellular infiltration and inflammation, and bronchial smooth muscle spasm. By doing so, it decreases airflow limitation. In the management of these patients, it is important to remember that there is no pharmacologic treatment for the component of airway obstruction resulting from a loss of elastic recoil in emphysema. There are various potentially useful pharmacologic agents available in different preparations (*see* Table 1).

BRONCHODILATORS

Available bronchodilator agents include sympathomimetic drugs (β-agonists), anticholinergic agents, and theophylline. There is ample evidence supporting the usefulness of these agents in relieving the symptoms associated with COPD. Failure to respond to a single dose of bronchodilator on initial spirometric testing does not signify fixed airway obstruction *(5)*. It is also important to recognize that long-term bronchodilator therapy does not alter the natural history of COPD *(3)*.

SYMPATHOMIMETIC DRUGS

Sympathomimetic agents have been the mainstays of treatment for COPD. β-2 agonists, with fewer cardiac side effects, are the drugs of choice. Because of their rapid onset of action, they are preferred in treating acute bronchospasm. β-agonists have physiologic effects other than bronchodilation that may help patients with COPD. It has been shown that they enhance mucus clearance *(6)* and may improve endurance of fatigued respiratory muscles. β-agonists are available in the

Table 1
Pharmacotherapy in COPD

Bronchodilators

Sympathomimetic: β-agonist
(Aerosol or dry powder MDI, neubulized solution, oral
preparation,injectable)
Anticholinergic: Ipratroprium bromide
(MDI, nebulized solution)
Theophylline

Corticosteroids

Systemic aerosol or dry powder MDI
Oral-inhaled nebulized solution

following preparations: aerosol or dry powder via metered-dose inhaler (MDI), solution delivered by nebulizer, oral, and injectable preparations. The inhaled route of administration is preferred in order to maximize beneficial effects and minimize systemic adverse effects. Oral preparations should be avoided because of the high incidence of side effects, unless other modes of administration are impossible. Obtaining the maximal benefit from an aerosol MDI requires the proper use of the device. It is imperative that proper techniques be demonstrated to the patient. If necessary, a spacer can be employed. The dry powder inhaler is breath-activated, and therefore, no hand-breath coordination is required for its use.

ANTICHOLINERGIC AGENTS

Anticholinergic agents are effective bronchodilators in the treatment of COPD. Ipratropium bromide is a synthetic derivative of atropine given by inhalation. However, unlike atropine, it is free of anticholinergic side effects, because it is not absorbed from the airway. Its bronchodilation effect is thought to be a result of inhibition of cholinergically mediated bronchomotor tone. It has a slower onset and longer duration of action when compared to β-agonists. Ipratropium bromide does not significantly affect mucus production or its clearance from the airway. Ipratropium is available in MDI and nebulized solution. The recommended dose is 2 puffs 4-times/d (each puff contains 18 mcg). However, the drug is well tolerated in much higher doses, and therefore even up to 6 puffs 4 times/d can be given. Tachyphylaxis to ipratropium has not been demonstrated—its efficacy is not blunted with chronic use *(7)*. A long-acting anticholinergic agent, tiotropium bromide, may be available in the near future.

It is controversial whether a β-agonist or ipratropium is the drug of choice for the initial treatment of COPD. However, because of its many advantages (fewer cardiac side effects, greater effectiveness, longer acting, less sputum production without altering its viscosity), ipratropium is considered by many as the first-line therapy in COPD *(5)*. Because of their different mechanisms, sites, and duration of action, combination therapy with β-agonists and ipratropium may be beneficial. Studies have demonstrated that there is better response with combination therapy than either drug alone, without the risk of increased side effects.

THEOPHYLLINE

Although the use of theophylline in the treatment of COPD is controversial, mainly because of its narrow therapeutic index, several studies have shown that theophylline provides clear benefits to patients with COPD *(8)*. When used appropriately, theophylline remains a useful drug in the management of COPD. In addition to its bronchodilating effects, theophylline also enhances mucociliary clearance *(9)*, reduces pulmonary vascular resistance *(10)*, and stimulates central respiratory drive *(11)*. The ability of theophylline to increase diaphragmatic strength and endurance in COPD is debatable. Combination therapy, with theophylline plus a β-agonist or anticholinergic drug, produces more bronchodilation than either drug alone. Recognizing its potential toxicity, patients should be treated with lower dosage of theophylline, aiming for serum levels of 8–12 µg/mL. A number of slow-release long-acting anhydrous theophylline preparations are currently available.

CORTICOSTEROIDS

Both systemic and oral inhaled corticosteroids have been proven to be effective and beneficial in the treatment of bronchial asthma. However, despite years of study and use, their efficacy in COPD is still controversial, especially because of the potentially serious side effects of systemic corticosteroids. One of the rationales for the use of corticosteroids is the possible role of inflammation in the pathophysiology of COPD. Studies have shown objective and significant improvement in airway obstruction as determined by pulmonary function testing in some patients receiving corticosteroids *(12,13)*. It has also been suggested that improvement in FEV_1 after β-agonist therapy may predict response to corticosteroids *(12)*; but specificity is low. Even though the presence of emphysema does not preclude a response to corticosteroids, its injudicious use is discouraged, particularly in patients with predominantly emphysematous disease. Special attention must be paid when using systemic corticosteroids in this situation. It also appears that the degree of responsiveness to corticosteroids is dose dependent, and not an all-or-none phenomenon.

In COPD patients who are doing poorly despite adherence to an optimal bronchodilator regimen, a trial of corticosteroids is warranted. A dose of 40 mg of prednisone (0.5 to 1.0 mg/kg) per day can be given after baseline pulmonary function tests are obtained. If there is no improvement in the FEV_1 after 2–3 wk while on corticosteroids, the medication should be discontinued. If it is helpful, the drug should be tapered to the lowest dose that will sustain the improvement. The aim is to use the smallest effective dose of corticosteroids to minimize any potential adverse effects. An alternate day regimen should be considered in steroid-dependent patients.

The use of oral-inhaled corticosteroids is an attractive option for treatment of COPD because of a superior safety profile and high topical potency. These agents are frequently used in an attempt to reduce the dose of systemic corticosteroids. However, most published studies have shown that oral-inhaled corticosteroids are less effective than systemic corticosteroids in relieving airflow limitation and symptoms (14). Whereas some studies have shown little or no improvement with short-term treatment, there are reports showing definitive improvement in airflow obstruction, airway inflammation, and symptoms with oral-inhaled corticosteroids in COPD (15,16). The recent Lung Health Study reported that oral-inhaled corticosteroids do reduce the use of health care service for respiratory problems, and improve airway reactivity and respiratory symptoms in patients with COPD. But they do not slow the rate of decline in FEV_1 in these patients (17).

A therapeutic trial of oral-inhaled corticosteroids is reasonable in COPD patients who are symptomatic on optimal bronchodilator therapy. Assessment of improvement with treatment should be performed. Long-term chronic use of oral-inhaled corticosteroids should be prescribed only if there is evidence of clinical benefit in the individual patient. It is important to remind patients to rinse their mouths after inhaler use to decrease the risk of oral candidiasis and hoarseness. As with any MDI, proper techniques, including the employment of a spacer, is paramount to get the full benefit of the medication.

Control of Airway Secretions

Increased airway mucus production significantly contributes to the symptomatology of COPD patients. Controlling and clearing of excessive airway secretions decreases airflow limitation and thus improves symptoms. It is an important part of the overall medical management of COPD, but it is frequently overlooked. The most effective means of diminishing airway secretion is the avoidance of inhaled irritants, the most important of which is cigarette smoking. Use of air conditioners and air cleaners may also help reduce the effects of environmental air pollution. Various forms of chest physiotherapy are also effective in the mobilization and clearance of airway secretions. These techniques include proper controlled coughing, postural drainage, chest wall percussion, and vibration. Mucus clearance devices, such as the Flutter device and vibration vest, may be helpful *(18)*. There are also several mucoactive or mucolytic agents available to help diminish or clear airway secretions in patients with COPD.

EXPECTORANTS AND IODIDE PREPARATIONS

Oral expectorants, such as guaifenesin and glyceryl guaiacolate, have been shown to provide little or no benefit to COPD patients *(19)*. Iodide preparation, such as SSKI (saturated solution of potassium iodide), may be effective. This agent acts by decreasing the viscosity of mucus, facilitating the breakdown of proteins, and enhancing the rate of ciliary beating. The usual dose is 0.3–0.6 cc in a glassful of juice or water 4 times/d. Long-term use should be avoided because of its potential side effects.

β-AGONISTS

In addition to their bronchodilator properties, β-agonists have been shown to increase tracheobronchial mucociliary clearance, presumably by increasing ciliary beat frequency.

THEOPHYLLINE

As aforementioned, theophylline has also been shown to increase tracheobronchial mucociliary clearance.

ACETYLCYSTEINE

N-acetyl-L-cysteine breaks the disulfide bonds of mucoproteins. It liquefies and lowers the viscosity of mucus, and is given in 10–20% solution by nebulizer. It can cause bronchospasm, so it is usually given in combination with a β-agonist. Acetylcysteine can decrease the volume and viscosity of sputum.

PROSTAGLANDIN INHIBITORS

Bronchorrhea may be controlled by blocking the cyclooxygenase pathway using inhaled indomethacin *(20)*. This is because airway secretion may partially depend on endogenous prostaglandins.

ANTIBIOTICS

When increased airway secretion production is a result of an active bacterial infection, antibiotics should be used to combat the acute exacerbation.

There is some evidence that erythromycin and macrolide antibiotics may reduce mucus secretion independent of their antimicrobial activity *(21)*.

MISCELLANEOUS AGENTS

Various other medications, such as surfactant and recombinant human DNase have been suggested as mucolytic agents for COPD, but they are either not definitively beneficial or not readily available. In general, cough suppressants should be used cautiously to avoid impairing the clearance of secretions.

Prevention and Treatment of Infection

Prevention and early treatment of respiratory infections may help decrease the frequency, duration, and severity of acute exacerbations of COPD. Influenza vaccination should be performed annually in all patients, for it has been shown that it reduces morbidity and mortality during influenza seasons. Amantadine or rimantadine can be used for prophylaxis for those patients who are not immunized but are at high risk of contracting influenza, or for treatment of influenza A. A new class of antiviral agents, called neuraminidase inhibitors, has recently become available for the treatment of acute influenza A and B. These agents are available either as a pill (oseltamivir) or by inhalation (zanamivir). Clinical trials have shown that the neuraminidase inhibitors reduce the duration of both influenza A and B infection without significant side effects.

The efficacy of pneumococcal vaccine in preventing or reducing serious pneumococcal infections in patients with COPD remains controversial. Nonetheless, it is recommended for all COPD patients. Revaccination every 6–7 yr is recommended for asplenic patients or those at risk for a rapid decline in antibody levels *(22)*.

Most acute exacerbations of COPD are probably because of nonbacterial infections. Yet, empiric treatment with antibiotics has been shown to speed recovery and to shorten the duration of exacerbations caused by respiratory infection. Sputum gram staining, but not culture, may be helpful in the management of these presumed infections with antibiotics. Chronic prophylactic antibiotic use is usually not beneficial or indicated in COPD patients. However, this option can be considered in those patients who have demonstrated unusually frequent acute exacerbations secondary to recurrent infection.

α-1 Protease Inhibitor Replacement

α-1-antitrypsin deficiency leads to early development of pulmonary emphysema, together with liver disease. Replacement therapy or augmentation therapy is available, aiming at preventing the progression of pulmonary emphysema. The only form of augmentation therapy currently available is intravenous infusion of pooled human α-1 antiprotease. The goal is to raise the plasma level above the protective threshold of 11 μmol/L. The treatment appears to be safe and effective, but expensive. Recombinant DNA-produced α-1 antiprotease, aerosolized delivery of the enzymes, and gene therapy are all under active investigation.

Long-Term Supplemental Oxygen Therapy

Studies have confirmed the benefits of long-term oxygen therapy in the management of patients with severe COPD (23,24). It is the only therapy that increases the survival in hypoxemic patients with COPD, in addition to improving their symptoms and quality of life. The benefits of oxygen supplementation are proportional to the extent of use. That is, for patients who are oxygen-dependent, using the oxygen 24 h/d confers greater benefit than using it for 12 h/d.

Long-term oxygen therapy should be prescribed to patients, who, while breathing room air, have an arterial PO_2 (PaO_2) of 55 mm Hg or less, or an arterial oxygen saturation (SaO_2) of 88% or less (see Table 2). This could be at resting state, during exercise or during sleep. Oxygen supplementation is also indicated when the resting PaO_2 is between 56 and 59 mmHg or SaO_2 is 89%, with evidence of erythrocytosis (hematocrit greater than 56%), cor pulmonale, or right-sided heart failure. In addition, oxygen supplementation should be used during sleep when there is a drop of more than 10 mmHg in PaO_2 or 5% in SaO_2, in the presence of symptoms and signs of hypoxemia, such as impaired cognitive function, restlessness, or insomnia. Continuous oxygen therapy is not justified if hypoxemia is not present during awake hours or at rest, even though there is hypoxemia during sleep or exercise, which can be corrected by oxygen use during sleep or exercise only.

Many advances have been made recently in the various modes and systems of oxygen delivery. The most frequently used route to deliver oxygen is by nasal cannula at a flow rate to maintain a PaO_2 of 60 to 75 mmHg (SaO_2 of 90% or higher). It is a common practice to increase the resting oxygen flow rate by 1 L/min during sleep and exercise because of worsening of hypoxemia during these periods. But, titration of the oxygen dose required to maintain an adequate oxygen saturation during these periods should be performed.

STATIONARY SYSTEMS

Oxygen concentrators are the most commonly used stationary oxygen delivery systems, replacing the large compressed gas cylinders that are

Table 2
Indications for Long-Term Oxygen Therapy
in COPD

At Rest (room air)
PaO_2 = or < 55 mmHg; or SaO_2 = or < 88% PaO_2 = 56–59 mmHg; or SaO_2 = 89%; with: 　hematocrit > 56%, or 　cor pulmonale, or 　right heart failure
During Exercise (room air)
PaO_2 = or < 55 mmHg; or SaO_2 = or < 88%
During Sleep (room air)
PaO_2 = or < 55 mmHg; or SaO_2 = or < 88% PaO_2 drop > 10 mmHg; or SaO_2 drop > 5%; with 　symptoms and signs of hypoxemia

being used only as back-up units. They are electrically powered and provide an oxygen supply up to a flow rate of 4–6 L/min via a molecular sieve that separates nitrogen from oxygen in the air. Therefore, in the absence of power failure, these units provide an endless supply of oxygen.

Liquid oxygen (in canister form) is another stationary oxygen delivery system. However, these canisters need to be refilled frequently. One advantage is that smaller ambulatory units can be filled safely by the patient from the stationary unit.

PORTABLE SYSTEMS

These are usually steel tanks that weigh more than 10 lb. They are designed to be transportable on wheels and allow some degree of mobility. However, they are heavy and not easily carried or maneuvered by patients. There are portable oxygen concentrators that can be operated on rechargeable or car batteries and are thus useful for car travel away from home.

AMBULATORY SYSTEMS

These are systems that weigh less than 10 lb. They are designed to be easily carried by patients. These systems allow patients to be more mobile and active, and greatly improve their quality of life. In conjunction with an oxygen-conserving device, such as a demand oxygen delivery system or a reservoir pendant, each unit in these systems can last much longer (approx 8 h at 2 L/min). These systems include the ambulatory liquid system and the newest technological systems that make use of the lightweight aluminum or fiber-wrapped aluminum high-pressure cylinders.

TRANSTRACHEAL OXYGEN THERAPY

Transtracheal oxygen therapy appears to provide more advantages than oxygen therapy by nasal cannula *(25)*. One of the advantages is improved compliance. It provides obligatory 24-h oxygen therapy everyday, thus resulting in better improvement clinically and physiologically. It may also correct severe hypoxemia in COPD patients who remain hypoxemic despite high-flow oxygen therapy by nasal cannula. It is also aesthetically more pleasing. The disadvantages are that it is more invasive and may have complications relating to the insertion of the catheter or its maintenance.

AIR TRAVEL WITH OXYGEN

COPD patients on continuous oxygen therapy require higher oxygen supplementation during air travel to prevent arterial oxygen desaturation. As a general rule, the oxygen flow rate via nasal cannula while traveling in an airplane can be increased to 1.5 times that at sea level.

Pulmonary Rehabilitation

Pulmonary rehabilitation is covered in more detail in Chapter 6. It should be pointed out that pulmonary rehabilitation is an important and essential component of the comprehensive care of patients with severe COPD *(26)*. It attempts to get patients back to their best possible functional capacity. Many studies have confirmed the overall usefulness of a comprehensive pulmonary rehabilitation program. The benefits include improvement in dyspnea, exercise endurance, and quality of life *(27)*. It may also decrease the rate of repeated hospitalization and total hospital days. Notwithstanding these important benefits, pulmonary rehabilitation does not usually improve lung function.

There are certain components of pulmonary rehabilitation that specifically benefit COPD patients. Exercise conditioning, utilizing both general exercises and exercises of the lower and upper extremities, is the single-most important component in this respect. Controlled breathing techniques, such as pursed-lip breathing, are of value in reducing dyspnea and anxiety. Patient education and psychological support are additional components of pulmonary rehabilitation regimens that contribute to the overall beneficial effects of this therapy. Despite the salutary effects of pulmonary rehabilitation, gains in conditioning quickly dissipate if the exercise program is discontinued. Therefore, it is important for patients to continue their exercise program at home after they finish the formal pulmonary rehabilitation program.

Nutritional Support

A significant number of patients with severe COPD suffer from malnutrition. Studies have shown that these patients are at an increased mortality risk. Malnutrition and reduced body weight are associated with respiratory muscle wasting and weakness, impaired respiratory muscle function, and reduction of maximal exercise capacity. Increase in body weight in these patients appears to improve their muscle strength. Even though there is no convincing evidence that nutritional supplementation is directly beneficial in these patients, nutritional supplementation to increase calorie intake is recommended in malnourished patients with advanced COPD. The preferred method of nutritional support is via the oral or enteral route. Dietary counseling may be of help.

Miscellaneous Forms of Therapy

There are a few miscellaneous forms of medical treatment that are available for selected patients with COPD.

RESPIRATORY STIMULANTS

The use of analeptic agents, such as acetazolamide and medroxy-progesterone, to increase ventilation in COPD patients with hypercapnia are of doubtful value. They are not currently recommended.

PSYCHOACTIVE AGENTS

Patients with severe COPD frequently have psychosocial and emotional problems related to their disease. They frequently suffer from anxiety and depression, as well as other manifestations of psychiatric dysfunction. In addition to psychosocial support, careful use of psychoactive medications, such as anxiolytics and antidepressants, may be helpful in the overall care of these patients.

DRUG TREATMENT FOR DYSPNEA

For patients who have severe intolerable dyspnea, and are unresponsive to other treatment, opiates, such as hydrocodone and morphine, may improve their symptoms *(28)*. These agents must be used with great care because of their potential side effects.

ANTIOXIDANT THERAPY

Lung damage from oxidants has been proposed as a mechanism for the development of COPD. There are reports suggesting the use of antioxidants, such as vitamin C, vitamin E, and β-carotene, for lung protection and treatment of this disease *(29)*. Further studies and additional evidence are required before these are routinely recommended.

NONINVASIVE VENTILATORY SUPPORT

There are two types of noninvasive ventilatory support available for the treatment of acute and chronic respiratory failure in selected patients. The negative ventilation type includes the iron lung, cuirass, and poncho wrap. Iron lungs are largely unavailable. The other type is intermittent positive-pressure ventilation by nasal mask (BiPAP). Results of different studies of both types of noninvasive ventilation in chronic COPD are mixed. More studies are needed to evaluate their role in the treatment of chronic stable COPD.

MANAGEMENT OF ACUTE EXACERBATIONS

During an acute exacerbation, COPD patients suffer from acute worsening of their symptoms and pulmonary function. Acute exacerbations of COPD are usually precipitated by a respiratory infection or acute bronchospasm. Depending on the severity of the exacerbation the patient can be treated as an outpatient or inpatient. Indications for hospitalization include acute respiratory acidosis, worsening of hypoxemia, or coexisting comorbid conditions *(30)*. The objectives in the management of acute exacerbation in these patients are:

- Identifying and treating the precipitating event of the acute exacerbation.
- Optimizing pulmonary function.
- Providing adequate oxygenation.

Respiratory infection, either bacterial or viral, is the most common cause of acute exacerbation. If there is evidence of an infection, such as purulent sputum or increased sputum volume, antibiotics should be used. Antibiotics in such situations improve lung function and shorten the duration of exacerbations. Bronchodilators, either by MDI or nebulizer should be administered. Nebulizers may be more effective in patients whose pulmonary function is so severely compromised that they may not be able to use MDI. A short course of oral or parenteral corticosteroids may also be used in the treatment of an acute exacerbation. In patients with increased secretions, mucolytic agents and chest physiotherapy may be helpful, but this is controversial *(30)*. Oxygen supplementation is important in hypoxemic patients to achieve a PaO_2 of at least 60 mmHg, with careful monitoring of the pH and $PaCO_2$ level. For patients with severe acute respiratory failure during an acute exacerbation, mechanical ventilatory support may be needed. Recent studies have shown that the early use of noninvasive positive pressure ventilation may be effective in avoiding intubation *(31)*. In carefully selected patients, this mode of ventilatory support may be attempted prior to intubation.

SUMMARY OF GENERAL APPROACH TO MEDICAL MANAGEMENT OF COPD

After the diagnosis of COPD is established, education about the disease should be undertaken, so that the patient has a better understanding of the illness and can take an active role in its management. Smoking cessation should be emphasized and demanded. Pharmacotherapy is recommended in patients who are symptomatic. It should be instituted in a stepwise fashion according to the severity of symptoms and airway obstruction. In mild disease with only intermittent symptoms, inhaled β-agonists can be used on an as-needed basis. If the symptoms are more persistent, inhaled ipratropium bromide should be added on a regular basis. In more advanced disease stages with increasing symptoms, progressive addition of inhaled β-agonists (used on a regular basis or as long-acting preparations) and theophylline may be helpful. Dosage of these medications should be adjusted to minimize side effects. With severe disease and continued symptoms, a trial of inhaled or systemic corticosteroids is indicated.

During acute exacerbations, a short course of high-dose corticosteroids should be considered. Long-term systemic corticosteroids should only be used in the sickest patients who fail to respond to all other therapy and have shown objective improvement with this therapy. Antibiotics should be used early when a respiratory infection develops, and influenza and pneumo-coccal vaccines should be given routinely to all COPD patients.

If excessive secretions are present, measures to mobilize them, such as chest physiotherapy, can be instituted. Long-term oxygen therapy is indicated in COPD patients with hypoxemia. A pulmonary rehabilitation program is indicated in those patients who remain symptomatic and are restricted in their daily activities despite maximal pharmacotherapy and other treatment for their disease. Close attention to psychosocial problems and their appropriate treatment is also important in the overall medical management of patients with COPD.

REFERENCES

1. Burrows B, Bloom JW, Traver GA, et al. (1987) The course and prognosis of different forms of chronic airways obstruction in a sample from the general population. *N Engl J Med* 317: 1309–1314.
2. Make B (1994) Collaborative self-management strategies for patients with respiratory disease. *Respir Care* 39: 566–579.
3. Anthonisen NR, Connett JE, Kiley JP, et al. (1994) Effects of smoking intervention and the use of an inhaled anticholinergic bronchodilator on the rate of decline of FEV1: The Lung Health Study. *JAMA* 272: 1497–1505.
4. McCarthy DS, Craig DB, Cherniack RM (1976) Effect of modification of the smoking habit on lung function. *Am Rev Respir Dis* 114: 103–113.
5. Ferguson GT, Cherniack RM (1993) Management of chronic obstructive pulmonary disease. *N Engl J Med* 328: 1017–1022.
6. Santa Cruz R, Landa J, Hirsch J, et al. (1974) Tracheal mucous velocity in normal man and patients with obstructive lung disease: effects of terbutaline. *Am Rev Respir Dis* 109: 458–463.
7. Gross NJ (1988) Ipratropium bromide. *N Engl J Med* 319: 486–494.
8. Kirsten DK, Wegner RE, Jorres RA, Magnussen H (1993) Effects of theophylline withdrawal in severe COPD. *Chest* 104: 1101–1107.

9. Wanner A (1985) Effects of methylxanthines on airway mucociliary function. (1985) *Am J Med* 79: 16–21.

10. Matthay RA, Berger HJ, Davies R, et al. (1982) Improvement in cardiac performance by oral long-acting theophylline in chronic obstructive pulmonary disease. *Am Heart J* 104: 1022–1026.

11. Dowell AR, Heyman A, Sieker HU, et al. (1965) Effect of aminophylline on respiratory center sensitivity in Cheyne-Stokes respiration and in pulmonary emphysema. *N Engl J Med* 273: 1447–1453.

12. Mendella LA, Manfreda J, Warren CPW, et al. (1982) Steroid response in stable chronic obstructive pulmonary disease. *Ann Intern Med* 96: 17–21.

13. Callahan CM, Dittus RS, Katz BP (1991) Oral corticosteroid therapy for patients with stable chronic obstructive pulmonary disease. *Ann Intern Med* 114: 216–223.

14. Weir DC, Gove RI, Robertson AS, et al (1990) Corticosteroid trials in non-asthmatic chronic airflow obstruction: a comparison of oral prednisolone and inhaled beclomethasone dipropionate. *Thorax* 45: 112–117.

15. Thompson AB, Mueller MB, Heires AJ, et al. (1992) Aerosol beclomethasone in chronic bronchitis; Improved pulmonary function and diminished airway inflammation. *Am Rev Respir Dis* 146: 389–395.

16. Paggiaro PL, Dahle R, Bakran I, et al. (1998) Multicentre randomised placebo-controlled trial of inhaled fluticasone propionate in patients with chronic obstructive pulmonary disease. International COPD Study Group. *Lancet* 351: 773–780.

17. Wise RA, Connett JE, Weinmann G, et al. (2000) Effect of inhaled trinamcinolone on the decline in pulmonary function in Chronic Obstructive Pulmonary Disease. The Lung Health Study Research Group. *N Engl J Med.* 343:1902–1909.

18. Konstan MW, Stern RC, Doershuk CF (1994) Efficacy of the FLUTTER device for airway mucus clearance in patients with cystic fibrosis. *J Pediatr* 124: 689–693.

19. Clarke SW, Thomson ML, Pavia D (1980) Effect of mucolytic and expectorant drugs on tracheobronchial clearance in chronic bronchitis. *Eur J Respir Dis* 110(Suppl): 179–191.

20. Tamaoki J, Chiyotani A, Kobayashi K, et al. (1992) Effect of indomethacin on bronchorrhea in patients with chronic bronchitis, diffuse panbronchiolitis or bronchiectasis. *Am Rev Respir Dis* 145: 548–552.

21. Marom ZM, Goswami SK (1991) Respiratory mucus hypersecretion (bronchor-rhea): A case discussion – possible mechanism(s) and treatment. *J Allergy Clin Immunol* 87: 1050–1055.

22. Recommendation of the Immunization Practices Advisory Committee (1989) Pneumococcal polysaccharide vaccine. MMWR 38: 64–76.

23. Medical Research Council Working Party (1981) Long-term domiciliary oxygen therapy in chronic hypoxic cor pulmonale complicating chronic bronchitis and emphysema. *Lancet* 1: 681–686.

24. Nocturnal Oxygen Therapy Trial Group (1980) Continuous or nocturnal oxygen therapy in hypoxemic chronic obstructive lung disease. *Ann Intern Med* 93: 391–398.

25. O'Donohue WJ Jr (1992) Transtracheal oxygen: A step beyond the nasal cannula for long-term oxygen therapy. *Nebr Med J* 77: 291–295.

26. Hodgkin JE (1990) Pulmonary rehabilitation. *Clin Chest Med* 11: 447–460.

27. Niederman MS, Clemente PH, Fein AM, et al. (1991) Benefits of a multidisciplinary pulmonary rehabilitation program: Improvements are independent of lung function. *Chest* 99: 798–804.

28. Light RW, Muro JR, Sato RI, et al. (1989) Effects of oral morphine on breathlessness and exercise tolerance in patients with chronic obstructive pulmonary disease. *Am Rev Respir Dis* 139: 126–133.

29. Britton JR, Pavord ID, Richards KA, et al. (1995) Dietary antioxidant vitamin intake and lung function in the general population. *Am J Respir Crit Care Med* 151: 1383–1387.

30. Celli BR, Snider GL, Heffner J, et al. (1995) Standards for the diagnosis and care of patients with chronic obstructive pulmonary disease. *Am J Respir Crit Care Med* 152(suppl): S77–S121.

31. Keenan SP, Kernerman PD, Cook DJ, et al. (1997) Effect of noninvasive positive pressure ventilation on mortality in patients admitted with acute respiratory failure: a meta-analysis. *Crit Care Med* 25: 1685–1692.

6 Pulmonary Rehabilitation in Severe Emphysema

Matthew N. Bartels, MD, MPH

CONTENTS

INTRODUCTION

Chronic obstructive pulmonary disease (COPD) is the fourth most frequent cause of death in the United States, with an estimated national prevalence of 14 to 20 million persons *(1)*. Chronic disability caused by COPD ranks second only to cardiac disease in payments from Social Security for chronic disability. Most COPD is a result of chronic exposure to cigarette smoke, and 15% of all smokers will progress to COPD *(2)*. Most smokers who develop COPD have a history of smoking for 20 or more pack years. Because of the major role of smoking, counseling and smoking cessation should be considered an integral part of any pulmonary rehabilitation program.

Pulmonary rehabilitation in patients with COPD is a comprehensive modality that employs a multifaceted approach to treatment. The focus of the rehabilitation program is to alleviate the physiological effects of the disease process, as well as to help decrease the psychosocial effects

From: *Lung Volume Reduction Surgery*
Edited by: M. Argenziano and M. E. Ginsburg © Humana Press Inc., Totowa, NJ

of the illness on the individual. As an approach that addresses the disabling aspects of the disease process, the impact of the illness on social, vocational, and well being are also addressed. The history of pulmonary rehabilitation goes back approx 35 yr, with early mobilization programs running counter to the standard wisdom of the day, which advised restricted activity for individuals with respiratory limitations. The subjective beneficial effects of programs of increased activity were readily apparent, but the scientific evidence to support the ongoing use of pulmonary rehabilitation is still being developed, and only recently has there been an attempt to develop well-controlled clinical trials.

In 1994, in recognition of the need to form a consensus on pulmonary rehabilitation, the National Institutes of Health held a workshop on pulmonary rehabilitation research, which established the following definition of pulmonary rehabilitation:

> *Pulmonary rehabilitation is a multidisciplinary continuum of services directed to persons with pulmonary disease and their families, usually by an interdisciplinary team of specialists, with the goal of achieving and maintaining the individual's maximum level of independence and functioning in the community (3).*

The key aspects of the definition include the focus on the multidisciplinary approach, with a full range of services provided to the patient and their family. In the design and the maintenance of a pulmonary rehabilitation program, the emphasis on the team approach and the important interaction of all the team members is crucial for the successful delivery of services.

Because of the lack of irrefutable scientific evidence of the benefits of pulmonary rehabilitation, the ability to make sweeping and definitive statements regarding the effects of pulmonary rehabilitation in COPD is limited. The failings of research in pulmonary rehabilitation fall into two areas: 1) the lack of clearly consistent data, and 2) the lack of well-controlled longitudinal studies. However, the clear clinical consensus is that pulmonary rehabilitation is a useful part of the comprehensive treatment of the patient with severe COPD. In 1997, the American College of Chest Physicians (ACCP) and the American Association of Cardiovascular and Pulmonary Rehabilitation (AACVPR) released a joint ACCP/AACVPR statement of evidence-based guidelines regarding pulmonary rehabilitation *(4)*. The benefits seem to come in several areas, each of which will be discussed separately later. As each component of the comprehensive rehabilitation program is discussed, the pertinent existing scientific evidence and the areas for further investigation will be outlined.

BENEFITS OF PARTICIPATION IN PULMONARY REHABILITATION

Exercise Capacity

Because exercise capacity can be measured in several ways, it is often difficult to compare studies that have used different outcome measures. The most commonly used techniques are the 6- or 12-min walk and the symptom-limited maximum exercise test with the determination of maximum oxygen consumption (VO_2max). Although on first glance, these techniques may appear to resemble each other, they are, in fact, quite different. The 6- or 12-min walk is a submaximal exercise test that measures the greatest sustained comfortable effort that the individual can perform (obviously not the absolute maximum because the individual could not sustain that level of activity for longer than 1 min or so). The walk test must be performed meticulously in order to have validity. The conditions under which the test is taken should be reproduced, so that it is clear that there has been no alteration of the physiological parameters under which the test is performed. Although the test can measure efficiency of exercise, the improvement in efficiency that occurs in an individual who undergoes training should be seen, and any improvement in submaximal capacity resulting from efficiency will be measured. The training benefit, which is the goal of pulmonary rehabilitation, is to increase the efficiency of exercise at any submaximal level. The conditioning exercises that are part of a pulmonary rehabilitation program are designed to improve this efficiency, therefore the walk test is particularly well suited to assess the outcomes of a rehabilitation program.

The maximal exercise test evaluates the maximum capacity of the individual, and also can be used as a measure of efficiency in performing exercise. However, there are a number of issues to be considered in maximal testing. There is a safety risk to be considered, as a small number of maximal exercise tests can lead to complications or death. Another issue is the difficulty of performing the test on supplemental oxygen (special equipment) and the difficulty of interpreting the results of the exercise test afterward because the supplemental oxygen may alter the oxygen consumption numbers that are obtained. Additionally, there are problems in the interpretation of the numbers to identify anaerobic threshold and there may be issues with CO_2 retention causing VCO_2 values to be less reliable than in a normal population. The effort made by the patient during the test is also an issue, as a submaximal effort will yield less than adequate results.

Each of these techniques has its benefits and problems when applied to this population. There also have been somewhat unclear benefits of rehabilitation on VO_2 max capacities, whereas the outcomes of the walk tests have been more uniformly favorable after rehabilitation. These and other issues surrounding exercise testing are reviewed in detail in Chapter 2.

Dyspnea

One of the greatest benefits of pulmonary rehabilitation and exercise programs in COPD has been the improvement in dyspnea. Multiple studies, using reliable instruments to measure the levels of dyspnea in patients with COPD in rehabilitation have shown improvement in symptoms *(5–7)*. The improvement in symptoms of dyspnea are in both the performance of activities of daily living (ADL) and in the performance of exercise testing. With ongoing exercise in a maintenance program, this benefit of decreased dyspnea can then be sustained over time. The improvement in subjective symptoms of dyspnea are thought to be a result of several mechanisms. There may be an improvement in exercise performance, with improved efficiency and thus less effort required for all activities. There may also be a decrease in required ventilation with given activities, and this may contribute to a decrease in dyspnea, or there may be a process of desensitization with less subjective dyspnea for a given amount of ventilation *(8,9)*. Even though the measurement of dyspnea is a qualitative measure that is subjectively reported by the patient, the improvement in this symptom indicates that it is clearly an index that needs to be closely followed. Recently, the measurement of dyspnea has become one of the standard measures of success in pulmonary rehabilitation. The measures that can be used to assess dyspnea are either direct measures of dyspnea on a self-reported scale, or are indirect measures based on evaluation of selective activities. The commonly used scales for dyspnea and quality of life are outlined in Table 1.

Quality of Life

Medical science has come to appreciate that the goals of treatment need to assess the quality of life (QOL) that is provided by a treatment, as well as the improvement of clinical measures and length of life. Most of the studies of pulmonary rehabilitation that have assessed QOL have shown good subjective improvement in symptoms *(10–14)*. There have been issues regarding the quality of assessment instruments, which may call into question some reports of QOL improvement. With the validation of instruments for QOL assessment, the most recent studies have shown benefits, and yet other studies are currently underway. Table 1 lists these instruments and their areas of validity.

Table 1
Dyspnea and QOL Instruments

Measure	Direct/ Indirect	Validity	Specifics
Borg scale of percieved breathlessness	Direct	High for dyspnea, correlates with VE, VO$_2$, VAS	Modification of Borg scale of percieved exertion. 10-point scale.
Visual analogue scale (VAS)	Direct	High for dyspnea, correlates with VE, VO$_2$, VAS	Vertical analog scale of 100-m length. Subject indicat dyspnea by indicating a point on the line. Has good correlation with Borg scale.
Baseline and transitional dyspnea index (BDI)	Indirect	Has validity for dyspnea compared to CRQ, older studies, fair repeatability	Interview administered. Measures three components: functional impairment, magnitude of effort, magnitude of task. Focus is on activity that causes dyspnea.
Chronic respiratory disease questionnaire (CRQ)	Indirect	Has good clinical validity for dyspnea, has individualized dyspnea scale that makes comparisons difficult	20-item self-reported test, interview administered. Measures four dimensions—dyspnea, fatigue, emotional function, mastery of breathing. Evaluates five usual activities.
St. George's respiratory questionnaire (SGRQ)	Indirect	Fair for dyspnea, better for QOL. Good test retest reliability and good clinical correlation	Self-administered QOL questionnaire with 53 questions. Measures three areas —symptoms, activity, impact on ADL.
Pulmonary functional status and dyspnea questionnaire (PFSDQ)	Indirect	Fair for dyspnea, better for QOL. Good test retest reliability and good clinical correlation	Self-administered QOL questionnaire that evaluates 79 activities in six categories of activities: Self-care, mobility, eating, home management, social, and recreational.

Table 1 (cont.)
Dyspnea and QOL Instruments

Measure	Direct/ Indirect	Validity	Specifics
University of California, San Diego shortness-of-breath questionnaire (SOBQ)	Indirect	Newer instrument with reasonable repeatability	Patients indicate how they feel in 21 areas of ADL on a 6- point scale. Three questions are specifically aimed at shortness of breath, fear of harm from overexertion, and fear of shortness of breath.
Sickness impact profile	General	Multiple domains assessed, good validity. Not disease specific.	30-min self-administered. Covers many areas of function: social, ADL, mobility, vocational, communication, cognition, hygiene, emotional status.
Quality of well being (QWB)	General	Multiple domains assessed, good validity. Not disease specific.	15-min interviewer administered. Covers multiple areas: mobility, social, symptoms, physical activity.
Medical outcomes study—Short Form-36 (SF-36)	General	Multiple domains assessed, Good validity. Not disease specific.	10-min self-administered. Covers multiple areas of function: Role functioning, pain, health, vitality, social, mental health.

The general consensus is that pulmonary rehabilitation does result in significant clinical improvements, and that a comprehensive program will have the greatest impact on QOL. The following sections will deal with the specifics of the programs for pulmonary rehabilitation of the patient with COPD who is to undergo lung volume reduction surgery (LVRS). The benefits of the rehabilitation program are not only in the areas of function and QOL, but include the benefits of preparing the patient both physically and psychologically for the challenging and difficult recovery that awaits them after the completion of their surgery.

COMPONENTS OF A LVRS PULMONARY REHABILITATION PROGRAM

Smoking Cessation

The majority of COPD is caused by smoking. Cigarette smoking has been shown to be as addictive as alcohol or narcotic agents (15). This addictive power of tobacco explains the tendency of individuals to continue to smoke, even in the face of pulmonary disease. Because of this, it is crucial for interventions aimed at smoking cessation to be initiated and maintained. Quitting smoking is clearly in the patient's interest, and performing surgery or other therapeutic interventions in the face of continued smoking is self-defeating—the patient must actively participate in his or her care by not smoking. Direct confrontation and insistence on the cessation of smoking by the entire staff are critical components in the management of individuals with COPD in pulmonary rehabilitation. The involvement of the referring physician is important, as the physician's counseling and warning are important predictors of compliance with the program (16,17). The individuals who are to start a program of pulmonary rehabilitation should either have stopped smoking or commit to cessation during the rehabilitation program. The focus of the rehabilitation program then becomes one of support and education for the patient and the family. There are several roles that the rehabilitation program can play:

1. Support the initiation of smoking cessation.
2. Support the continuation of smoking cessation.
3. Integrate smoking cessation with the rehabilitation program.
4. Educate the patient and family in the maintainence of a smoke free environment (18).

Table 2 outlines the components of the smoking cessation program that should be associated with or incorporated into the rehabilitation program.

Table 2
Smoking Cessation Program

Steps	Involved Staff
Identify patients who are smoking	Physician, program coordinator, physical therapists
Confront patient	Treating physician and program coordinator
Establish quit date and form a "contract"	Treating physician
Arrange participation in a treatment program—either self-standing or part of a pulmonary rehabilitation program	Coordinator, physician, physical therapist
Continuous contact with individual after quit date, weekly for a month, then biweekly—provide supportive counseling as needed.	Coordinator, physical therapist, physician
Have medical Follow up within 2 mo of cessation. Assess compliance with testing as needed—carbon monoxide, cotinine levels. Reward compliance, provide strict guidelines, support for failure of abstinance.	Physician with assistance of the rehabilitation team
For failure of abstinance, consider nicotine replacements and/or pharmacological measures.	Physician
Use support group as available	Rehabilitation team, social worker, psychology
Ongoing follow-up after abstinence achieved with support and occasional screening testing, as required	Team and physician

Education

Education is one of the most important components of the pulmonary rehabilitation program in that it creates a more informed partner in the treatment plan who can more fully partake in the treatment plan. There are components to help the patient deal with the medications, oxygen equipment and mechanics of the disease, as well as components to help the individual live the best possible lifestyle they can within their physical capacities. Several studies have shown that there are benefits to education in patients with COPD, decreasing hospitalizations and ameliorating exacerbations (19,20). Education alone, however, has been shown in two separate studies to not provide the same benefits as education combined with a rehabilitation program (21,22). It is important to remember that education needs to be provided for both the patient and the family. Later, several of the key educational components of a pulmonary rehabilitation program are reviewed.

Energy Conservation

The concept of energy conservation is quite simple, and has often already been subconsciously incorporated into the everyday activities of a number of patients. The basic principle to impart on the participant is that they do not have a normal exercise tolerance and thus need to be aware of the ways in which they exert themselves and preserve energy in every possible way. A helpful analogy for individuals with COPD is to compare their energy state to a machine with limited battery storage. They do not have sufficient energy to achieve all tasks at full speed, and need to consider carefully how they will use the "charge" that is available to them. With appropriate rationing, they can achieve their goals and be able to achieve more than they thought possible—through being more "energy smart." Examples of energy conservation techniques are included in Table 3. This increase in efficiency is a very important part of the improvement of capacity that can be seen in patients with COPD, as the work efficiency of this group of patients has been shown to be a major component of the benefits seen after a program of rehabilitation *(23)*.

Medication Training

Medication training is an important part of allowing patients to take a greater part in their own management. Unfortunately, many patients do not fully understand the medication regimens they are on, and often do not use their inhaled medications properly *(24)*. The education should include discussions regarding the types of medications commonly used, discussed by class with in-depth review of mechanisms of action and side effects. Another important part of the education program is a review of drug interactions, especially with an eye to the issue of over-the-counter medications that often have significant effects that can harm the uninformed individual. A review of the proper use of inhaled medications is also appropriate as a part of the training program. Group education sessions can be used for the overall didactic portions of the program, whereas the inhaler education can often be best done in individual settings.

The overall goals of the medication education portion of the rehabilitation program is to help the patient take responsibility for their care and help them cope with their physical and functional status. By maximizing the involvement of the patient and their family in the management of medications, the patient is able to better manage their condition and

Table 3
Energy Conservation

Task	Energy Conservation Technique
Driving	Handicapped parking access
Grocery shopping	Use of a shopping cart to lean on
Performing daily errands	Planning all in a sequence rather than individual trips
Showering	Use a seat
Food preparation	Use a high stool to sit on or sit at table
Stair climbing	Plan ahead to minimize trips up/down stairs

make appropriate decisions. The informed patient is a better partner in the therapeutic relationship. Because each individual has different needs, there needs to be flexibility in the education process, and it is important to involve family members and caregivers in the process to assure adequate adherence to the prescribed regimen and to assess the efficacy of treatments *(25)*.

Oxygen Therapy

Oxygen therapy education is closely allied to medication education and has a number of essential components. Just like cigarette smoking cessation, oxygen therapy used correctly can have a direct effect on improving survival in end-stage lung disease *(26,27)*. The mechanisms of improved survival are through the prevention of pulmonary hypertension and polycythemia. The educational component regarding oxygen therapy should be performed in a combination of didactic and individual settings to assure that the patient has a good understanding of their oxygen equipment and also has a good understanding of safety and medical issues. Hands-on training under the observation of the therapist, as well as in one-on-one and group sessions are essential. Travel requirements, emergency procedures, and options available for the management of dyspnea are important topics for discussion. The actual titration of oxygen requirements with exercise and activity need to be determined on an individual basis. While performing exercise under the supervision of the physical therapist, the patient can learn how to appropriately titrate their oxygen to avoid hypoxemia, ergo not using more oxygen than required. The subjects should keep their oxygen saturation well above 85% or a pO_2 of 60 mmHg, as this is on the shoulder of the steep portion of the oxygen saturation curve. Although the medical needs of the maintenance of safety are crucial, it is to be remembered that a major goal of the education regarding oxygen use and equipment is to maximize the subject's independence.

Nutritional Counseling

Managing the nutritional requirements of individuals with COPD is an essential component of their treatment. The comprehensive pulmonary rehabilitation program is a good setting in which to introduce this part of the care of the patient. Either a nutritionist or another member of the team can be assigned to oversee this part of the program *(28,29)*. The intensity of the intervention can range from only education in a group setting for less severe cases, to an intensive one-on-one intervention for the patient with either severely increased or decreased weight.

The special nutritional requirements of an individual with COPD are based on specific metabolic issues. The COPD patient has an increased basal metabolic demand that may be related to both a higher energy cost of breathing at rest as well as with activity *(30)*. It has also been shown that with lower lean body mass, functional capacity *(31,32)*, and survival decrease *(33)*, independent of the FEV_1 or other indices. Attempts to treat the malnutrition and loss of lean body mass have focused on several interventions, including nutritional counseling. The use of anabolic steroids and growth hormone in combination with exercise have also been studied. The repletion of anabolic steroids has appeared to have a fair degree of safety so far, but there appears to be only an effect on the repletion of lean body mass and no effect on functional outcomes *(34)*. Because there are possible risks in increasing the metabolic demands of these patients, more research will need to be done before this can be considered a part of the regular treatment of individuals with COPD *(35)*. Likewise, growth hormone was initially thought to have a possible role in the treatment of COPD by helping to increase exercise tolerance and lean body mass. However, prospective studies failed to find a significant improvement in muscle strength or in exercise tolerance, even though the lean body mass increased *(36)*. In subsequent work, a large prospective study of growth hormone in Europe was terminated prematurely because of excess mortality, and this treatment has fallen out of favor. In the case of obesity, it is clear that the patient will require counseling to lose weight and approach ideal body weight. This should be done cautiously and in a balanced diet that will not cause a further loss of lean body mass.

Another aspect of nutritional counseling is to avoid the excess intake of carbohydrates and increase the reliance of the individual on fats and proteins to improve the respiratory quotient. Because the metabolism of fats and proteins yield a lower CO_2 load per unit of energy, these forms of nutrition place a lower respiratory burden on the individual. Appropriate intake of trace minerals, potassium, magnesium, phosphate, and calcium needs to be assured in order to avoid any negative impact on respiratory muscle function.

Disease-Specific Education

The role of education about the disease process and pathology of COPD are critical aspects of the pulmonary rehabilitation process. Nearly every review, study, or discussion of a comprehensive rehabilitation program emphasizes the importance of the disease-specific education component of the program. The latest recommendations for the development of a comprehensive rehabilitation program all include an educational component *(37,38)*. The form that this education takes can vary depending on the structure of the rehabilitation program, but usually includes both a didactic portion and a series of handouts or a textbook that the patient can refer to in order to reinforce the didactic materials from a lecture. Our own program has adapted materials from a number of programs into a loose-leaf binder to which sections are added during the course of the pulmonary rehabilitation program. In this fashion, as the lectures take place, the most up-to-date information can be passed on to the patient and can reinforce the lesson presented. In addition, we utilize a textbook to provide a further basis for the individual's education.

Stress Management

Stress management alone does not significantly alter the course or prognosis of COPD; however, as a component of the management program in a rehabilitation setting, it can improve a patient's function, possibly by allowing better coping with their disease *(39,40)*. In a meta-analysis of psychosocial interventions in COPD, the effect of relaxation training was confirmed to be most notable in the areas of subjective dyspnea and psychological well being *(41)*. There was also a trend toward less utilization of hospital services and toward a greater sense of independence in these studies. This is not necessarily surprising, as the patients who can remain calm and are able to relax are less likely to unnecessarily utilize emergency services. The effect of stress relaxation techniques on the utilization of sedative hypnotic medications in COPD has not been studied, but in our clinical experience, the need for these agents does seem to decline with the learning of appropriate relaxation maneuvers.

Because the comprehensive care of the patient with COPD in the pulmonary rehabilitation setting aims for achievement of the highest function possible, the psychosocial aspects of the program should not be neglected. The best form of relaxation technique is still a matter of controversy, and there is no clear recommendation to be made from a review of the literature. In reality, the availability of practitioners experienced in relaxation techniques will often limit the options at any one center, and each individual patient will respond differently to different treatment regimens. Techniques that are commonly used include hypnosis and autohypnosis, meditation, visualization, timed breathing, and relaxation audiotapes and videos. The goal is to allow the individual to find a tool that helps them to relax, and that can be used during exacerbations or periods of anxiety. Once the training has been achieved, the maintenance of the skill must be emphasized, as it is with all aspects of pulmonary rehabilitation.

Pulmonary Toilet

The severity and quantity of secretions in patients with COPD can range from non-existent to severe, especially in individuals with a bronchitic component to their disease. The pulmonary rehabilitation program can provide a great deal of benefit to help manage the secretions in the pre- and postoperative settings. The techniques of secretion management can often be taught to the individual and to caregivers, to be carried on after completion of the pulmonary rehabilitation program. The techniques of chest physical therapy are well described in other sources and will not be reviewed in detail here. They include percussion, postural drainage, and can also include suctioning and insufflation/exsufflation in selected patients *(42,43)*. Of course, any increase in sputum production or change in sputum quality should be treated aggressively to prevent a severe pulmonary infection. The role of respiratory muscle training has not been established to be definitively useful, although this modality may be indicated in individuals with clear muscular weakness *(44)*. The decision to use this type of treatment needs to be decided on a case-by-case basis.

PULMONARY REHABILITATION IN PATIENTS UNDERGOING LVRS

The rehabilitation of patients with COPD who are to undergo LVRS can be separated into four distinct phases: preoperative, perioperative, postoperative, and maintenance. Each of these phases is associated with special challenges, and often there is an overlap in services that allow for a reinforcement of previous training. Each phase will be discussed later.

Preoperative Rehabilitation

The ideal location for a pulmonary rehabilitation program for pre-LVRS care is in an outpatient hospital setting so that all the resources of the center are available, or in a satellite program with significant resources. The program for preoperative rehabilitation follows the basic outlines that any pulmonary rehabilitation program for COPD should follow. It is essential that it be a comprehensive program with a multidisciplinary approach. A proposed composition for a rehabilitation team is depicted in Table 4. This composition has to be altered to fit the demands of the program, as well as the resources of the institution. The demands of managed care and the limited resources usually available for pulmonary rehabilitation mean that most programs have members performing more than one task. In smaller settings, most of the tasks may be performed by one or two individuals. These pulmonary rehabilitation specialists are often physical therapists, respiratory therapists or nurses who take on certain aspects of the program outside of their area of normal expertise because specialists are not available. The combination of tasks is not necessarily detrimental as it can make a program more cohesive, but it does make a program vulnerable to staff attrition. The most important issue is to have a cohesive and enthusiastic team with a unified vision of providing excellent patient care. This then provides the patients and their families with a cohesive and organized program.

A comprehensive guidebook or compilation of instructional materials should be provided to each patient, along with a clear and uncluttered set of guidelines and a program schedule. A three-times-per-week program usually provides a sufficient degree of interaction and can be accommodated by most patients. Our program uses a loose-leaf binder that contains the complete materials of the program, and at the beginning, there is an outline of the program and introductory materials. As the educational components and the exercise program of the individual are developed, the patient can add those materials to the binder until, at the end of the program, the manual is complete. This technique allows each program manual to be tailored to the specific needs of the patient, and allows new material to be added as required without having to republish an entire manual.

Close contact with the primary physician is required as the continued compliance of the program will depend on the referring physician's support. There also is the need to coordinate the maximal medical management of the patient with the rehabilitation program, as oxygen requirements, inhaler dosing schedules, and need for parenteral steroids may change during the course of rehabilitation. It is best for the patient if these changes are enacted in coordination with the primary physician. Also, the patient may have a significant improvement and the treating physician needs to be kept abreast of the current status of the patient in order to recognize the early manifestations of an exacerbation.

Support groups need to be established and run in order to allow the patients to continue the lifelong program of pulmonary health manage-

Table 4
Rehabilitation Team Composition

Team Member	Training	Duties
Direct Team Members		
Physician Director	Pulmonary/chest medicine, rehabilitation medicine	Set priorities for program, evaluate and screen patients, Design rehabilitation programs, supervise rehabilitation program, continuing education for the rehabilitation staff
Rehabilitation Program Coordinator	Physical therapist, respiratory therapist, nurse, nurse practicioner	Arrange administrative issues of the program, scheduling of staff, coordination of activities within institution. Negotiate with providers/insurers. Provides day-to-day coordination.
Therapists	Physical therapist, respiratory therapist, nurse/nurse practicioner, occupational therapist	Provide one on one and group physical therapy. Education of patients and families, supervise home exercise program
Nutritionist	Certified nutritionist, dietitian	Provide group and individual nutritional counseling
Psychological Support	Psychologist/psychological social worker, psychiatrist	Provide group and individual psychological counseling. Run support groups. Help with smoking cessation program if such is part of the rehabilitation program.
Social Work	Certified social worker	Help patients and family deal with social issues, interface with equipment and insurance providers

Table 4 (cont.)
Rehabilitation Team Composition

Team Member	Training	Duties
Adjunct Members of Team		
Patient		Needs to be an active participant, has to agree to the course of rehabilitation and comply with the suggested program.
Primary Care Physician		Will need to be kept abreast of the patient progress and informed as to the treatment plan in order to allow for adequate adherence at end of rehabilitation program.
Patient Family		Will need to learn the patient's program and be able to support the treatment program of the patient. Essential role to allow for adherence to the prescribed program.

ment. The groups can be made general, especially in smaller programs, or can be tailored to specific groups. Smoking cessation groups and special support groups are particularly pertinent regarding pulmonary rehabilitation in preparation for LVRS. Outings and social events can also be planned in order to help the socialization of this very ill group of patients. The support groups can also be used as a center to continue the education of the participants, as members of the team can be asked to present special lectures on areas of interest to individuals with COPD.

The special additional areas of education for patients who are to undergo LVRS include a familiarization with the specifics of the surgery, and a program of preparation for the perioperative period. This includes education in secretion mobilization, familiarization with early postoperative mobilization, and introduction to the physical therapy staff who will participate in the early care after surgery. This introduction and education can make early mobilization easier as the staff that is asking the seemingly impossible of them is already familiar to the patient and has a therapeutic alliance already formed. The understanding of what is to come after the surgery also helps reduce patient anxiety. An outline of the goals and methods of the rehabilitation program are shown in Table 5. The rehabilitation program design includes the following features.

1. Patient Screening: This, essentially, is the selection of individuals for pulmonary rehabilitation. In the case of LVRS, any individual who is considered a candidate for surgery should undergo pulmonary rehabilitation. If an individual is in good conditioning at their evaluation, the duration of the program may be shorter, but the educational components of the program should be extended to help with the perioperative mobilization and postoperative recovery. The selection is often done on a team basis during regularly held conferences with the surgical and medical staff. These regular meetings also allow the rehabilitation staff to bring new issues, such as smoking or a decline in function, to the attention of the LVRS team.
2. Exercise Testing: This should be performed on all subjects prior to the initiation of training, as a symptom-limited VO_2 max determination will allow for an aggressive training program at 60% of the maximum exercise capacity. Six-minute-walk testing is also useful to help document progress.
3. Preoperative Exercise Prescription: A model for an exercise prescription template is included in Fig. 1. There is clear demographic data, as well as a clear indication of the contact numbers of the prescribing physician. As with all rehabilitation prescription it requires four elements:
    a. Diagnosis: This has to be accurate in order to help the team understand the patient's needs. This should also include the fact that an individual is to undergo LVRS.
    b. Specific Prescription: The prescription should describe in detail the rehabilitation program including the educational, psychosocial, and

Table 5
Goals and Methods of Pre-Operative Pulmonary Rehabilitation

Goals	Methods
Prevention	
Smoking cessation	Enroll in a cessation program, emotional support, monitor abstinence
Immunization compliance	Assure proper immunizations, communicate with primary physician
Prevent exacerbations	Self-assessment skills taught
	Self-intervention taught
	Instruct on accessing private physician
Appropriate medication use	Review medications and dosing schedules
	Review interactions and side effects
	Review appropriate use of inhalers and nebulizers
Pulmonary toilet	Review bronchial hygiene
	Teach proper cough techniques
	Use of chest physiotherapy as needed
	Teach chest physiotherapy techniques to family as appropriate
Appropriate use of oxygen therapy	Teach use with exertion
	Review self monitoring
	Review use of equipment
	Encourage acceptance of the need for O_2
	Review importance of use and consequences of failure to use oxygen
Nutritional Counseling	Counseling to achieve ideal body weight
	Counseling to avoid high carbohydrate diet
	Instruction in avoidance of high sodium diets
	Encourage balanced nutrition with avoidance of fad diets
Family Training	Teaching regarding: - COPD
	1) pulmonary toilet
	2) medication use
	3) oxygen use
	Family support group
	Counseling as needed
Dyspnea Relief - Exercise Training	
Exercise	Multifaceted program individualized to each patient's needs
- Strengthening	Emphasis on gradual increase in strength
	1) Focus on proximal muscle groups
	2) Avoid injury to weakened musculoteninous structures
	3) Focus more on high repetition, low intensity training

- Conditioning	Work to gradually increase exercise tolerance
	1) Cross training program
	2) Emphasis on the development of an independent training program
	3) Increase ambulation endurance with gait training
	4) Appropriate oxygen titration during exercise
- Respiratory muscle training	Inspiratory and expiratory muscle training
	1) Isocapnic hyperpnea
	2) Inspiratory resistance training
	3) Inspiratory threshold training
- Upper extremity training	1) Increase strength
	2) Increase capacity for sustained work
	3) Improve shoulder girdle strength
- ADL training	Energy Conservation techniques
	Adaptive techniques
	Relieve anxiety and stress
	Encourage pacing in activities
Breathing retraining	Pursed lip breathing
	Diaphragmatic breathing
Anxiety reduction	Stress relaxation techniques
	1) Paced breathing
	2) Autohypnosis
	3) Visualization
	Medications as needed
	1) Treat anxiety
	2) Treat depression
Improve confidence	Build compensatory techniques
	Build confidence in ability to exercise
Disease Management	
Disease acceptance	Education regarding disease process
	Reassurance about aggressive treatment
Coping Skills	Support group
	Psychology and social work intervention, as needed
	Treat depression, as needed
Quality of life improvement	Improve ADL tolerance
	Improve Coping skills
	Improve disease management
Advance directives review	Counseling regarding
	1) Health care proxy
	2) Resuscitation orders
	Help in preparing paperwork

Encouragement	Support group
	Social work support
	Psychological support
Continuing Compliance	Team encouragement
	Physician counseling
	Involve primary care physician in plan
	Family education

LVRS Specific Goals

Maximize exercise capacity	Perform high intensity exercise
	Increase diaphragmatic breathing strength
	Train in good pulmonary toilet
Education about surgery	Group or individual teaching
	Establish understanding of outcomes of surgery
Preparation for perioperative period	Education regarding early mobilization
	Introduction to therapy staff
Review postoperative rehabilitation program	May need to have inpatient rehabilitation initially
	Restoration of previous level of function
	Resumption of previous program
	Establishment of maintenance phase

nutritional needs of the patient. The exercise portion needs to specify both upper and lower extremity exercises and include both strengthening and conditioning exercises. The prescription should also state if exercise is to be done on oxygen, and at what level of supplementation. This is where a symptom limited VO_2 determination is helpful, as it allows the physician to specifically state a starting point and oxygen requirements for an aggressive rehabilitation program. The prescription should include the intensity, duration and goals of the program.

c. Frequency and Duration: The frequency of the patient attendance in the program needs to be specified, and is usually ordered in times per week. For most patients, four or five times per week is too strenuous and cannot be maintained. Three times per week is a usual program, although in some individuals lower frequencies may be required because of debility, travel distance, scheduling, or other factors. The planned duration of the program should also be specified. This is usually approx 6–8 wk, as that allows for 18 to 24 rehabilitation sessions. Maximal response to a conditioning program would take longer, but the realities of limited resources dictate that three to four month programs are essentially impractical.

d. Precautions: These need to be laid out in detail in the exercise prescription of individuals who are this fragile. The safe vital sign

Sample Pulmonary Rehabilitation Exercise Prescription

Human Performance Laboratory
Columbia Presbyterian Medical Center
The Atchley Pavilion – Room 316
Phone: 212-305-0483

Name:
ID:
Date:
Referring Physician:

Age:
Height (in):
Weight (lb):
Body Mass Index:

The patient is part of the Presbyterian Hospital Lung Volume Reduction Program.
Diagnosis: Chronic Obstructive Pulmonary Disease, Deconditioning, Osteoporosis, Steroid Myopathy
An aerobic exercise program is recommended.
Lower extremity exercise should be:
    Type: Continuous aerobic exercise with cross training on walking, bicycling, etc.
    Frequency: 3-4 times per week
    Duration: 20-30 minutes at the target intensity, with a 5 minute warm up and a 5 minute cool down.
    Intensity: Target heart rate of _____BPM (+/- 5BPM), Maximum work is _____METs, exercise should
    be performed at METs (+/- 0.5 METs). Exercise should begin at this intensity and be increased as
    tolerated.
Upper extremity endurance training:
    Type: Unsupported arm exercises, gradually increase weights by 0.5 pound increments.
    Frequency: 3 times per week
    Duration: 10-15 minutes per session
Strength Training:
    Type: Theraband, freeweight, or circuit training.
    Frequency: 3 times per week
    Duration: 10-15 minutes per session
Stretching Program:
    Type: Upper and Lower extremity stretching program.
    Frequency: 3 times per week
    Duration: 10 minutes per session
Education:
    Teaching regarding COPD, medications, oxygen therapy, nutrition, stress management, energy
    conservation and pulmonary toilet.
Precautions:
    Maximum Heart Rate: _____BPM
    Maximum Systolic Blood Pressure: _____mm Hg
    Maximum Diastolic Blood Pressure: _____mm Hg
    Minimum Oxygen Saturation: 90%
Supplemental Oxygen via nasal cannula from 1-6 liters per minute as needed during exercise to keep oxygen
saturation greater than 90%.
Nutritional Evaluation: Weight management program.
Psychosocial Support and Evaluation: Participation in support groups and educational activities
Overall ProgramFrequency: 3-5 times a week
Overall Program Duration: 6-8 weeks in a pulmonary rehabilitation program.

Matthew N. Bartels, MD, MPH

Fig. 1.

parameters need to be specified, as well as the lower limits of oxygen saturation. Once again, the symptom-limited exercise test allows for a greater degree of confidence in prescribing these limits.

The specific components of a rehabilitation program are well described in physical therapy textbooks and are beyond the scope of this chapter. The essential components of the exercise program are as follows.

1. Upper extremity exercises including strengthening and conditioning exercises. These are typically done with upper body ergometers (UBE) and with theraband and free weights.
2. Lower extremity exercises including strengthening and conditioning exercises. These are typically done with bicycle ergometers , treadmill exercise, and less frequently, with rowing machines of other equipment. The strength training is usually done and with theraband, free weights, and circuit training. The program should usually use the simplest equipment possible to allow the patient to develop an independent program that they can continue after completion of their training.
3. Educational components need to cover all the areas discussed before. It is important that the staff is well versed in LVRS so that they can allay patient anxieties and adequately prepare them for the surgery.
4. Psychological/social interventions also need to be specific to the individual patient needs. Depression and anxiety need active treatment and will often respond well to a combined supportive and pharmacological treatment.

Perioperative Rehabilitation Program

The perioperative program essentially consists of rapid mobilization after surgery, with "out of bed to chair" being the goal of the first day. The goal of subsequent days, up to the day of discharge, are to increase ambulation and to avoid complications. Ambulation should be started as soon as is possible from a point of medical stability. By the time of hospital discharge, an individual should be able to perform all of their basic ADL and also be able to ambulate independently. In individuals where complications or severe debility do not allow for rapid mobilization, the inability to progress rapidly may require consideration of an inpatient acute rehabilitation stay. Pulmonary toilet is a very important component in the prevention of postoperative pneumonia. Chest physical therapy should be aggressively provided by the nursing staff and by the physiotherapy staff to keep secretions well managed. The physiotherapy time devoted to pulmonary toilet should not detract from the time spent on patient mobilization.

The perioperative mobilization program should ideally consist of two sessions per day, and be undertaken 7 d/wk in order to maximize recovery. Therapist experience is essential, and designated therapists should provide these services. All patients need close monitoring of oxygen saturation, and in the case of cardiac arrhythmias or suspected ischemia, telemetric monitoring may also be necessary. The focus of this program is on ambulation and regaining ADL independence, so the main exercises include ambulation training, treadmill training, and bicycle ergometry. As soon as a patient has recovered sufficiently to transfer safely, a bedside bicycle ergometer is advised to allow for increased endurance training.

The educational components of the program at this time are limited. Social work and psychosocial interventions may need to be instituted for sudden family and patient crises. However, the need for intensive services at this time should be limited if a comprehensive preoperative rehabilitation program was followed and these issues identified at that earlier time.

Postoperative Rehabilitation Program

Usually, this is an outpatient program that is reinitiated at the site of preoperative program as soon as possible after the patient returns home. Because of complications or a prolonged recovery, selected patients will require inpatient rehabilitation prior to returning home. For individuals who require a prolonged wean from a ventilator, a rehabilitation center that provides physical and occupational therapy in addition to the basic weaning is necessary. For patients who are breathing independently, their rehabilitation should be done at a center with aggressive rehabilitation and experience in treating severe cardiac and pulmonary disease. Often a center performing a great deal of cardiothoracic surgery or with a large population of pulmonary patients will have established relationships with such centers. It is important to be sure that the rehabilitation is in an acute rehabilitation center, as a failure to be aggressive early on can lead to a prolonged rehabilitation with potentially increased complications.

The requirements of the outpatient program are essentially the same as those for the preoperative phase. The support groups should include other post-LVRS patients, or at least other postsurgical patients. The ongoing support will be best (and anxiety least) if the patient reestablishes contact with the same program. The exercise program here can often be done on a 1–2 times/wk basis, as the educational components have been covered, and supervised exercise is the main goal. By decreasing the intensity of the program somewhat, it may also allow the patient to have a somewhat longer duration of therapy, thereby allowing a better conditioning effect. Another goal of the postoperative program is to establish the patient in an independent and sustainable exercise program. The team needs to focus on the reassurance to the patient that gains will be realized through continued exercise and that failure to adhere to the exercise regimen will lead to a loss of function.

Maintenance

After postoperative rehabilitation is completed, the patient is discharged from rehabilitation and is expected to continue to maintain their previous level of functional gains. It is at this level that most rehabilitation failures occur, as many individuals do not continue their exercises. It is essential that the patient be given ongoing support from family, primary care physician, and other support groups in order to create an environment that will continue to encourage exercise compliance. Support groups that encourage continued attendance after the completion of the rehabilitation program are also useful, and the added benefit to the program is the ability to introduce current patients to graduates of the program. Many centers have started to use wellness centers, where a former patient can come for a nominal fee and exercise under a lowered level of supervision in the rehabilitation setting. This ongoing level of contact can help to increase compliance *(45)*. The establishment of an effective maintenance program for exercise conditioning is the greatest challenge faced in the rehabilitation of the patient with COPD. Successful solution of this dilemma will be one of the most important future developments in pulmonary rehabilitation.

CONCLUSIONS

The role of pulmonary rehabilitation in the treatment of COPD is important as a means to maximize the quality of life and the functional ability of the individual. In the case of the patient undergoing LVRS, rehabilitation has an important role in the preparation of a patient prior to LVRS, and then in the recovery and maximization of the benefits of surgery. The combination of pulmonary rehabilitation and LVRS has been shown to provide the greatest benefit for patients with severe emphysema, well above the effects of either intervention alone *(46)*. There is still a great need to further research the exact contributions that each can make to the well being of the patient. In the interest of providing the best care to all patients with severe COPD who will be undergoing LVRS, all patients should undergo intensive pulmonary rehabilitation. Maximal pulmonary rehabilitation before surgery will help prepare patients for the procedure, and maximize their conditioning in order to decrease complications. Aggressive perioperative rehabilitation will also help to prevent complications, and a consolidation rehabilitation program instituted postoperatively will allow a maximum benefit to be realized from the surgery.

REFERENCES

1. Celli BR, Snider GL, Heffner J, et al. (1995) Standards for the diagnoisis and care of patients with COPD. *Am J Respir Crit Care Med* 152 (suppl 5): S78–121.

2. Petty TL (1996) Thye worldwide epidemiology of chronic obstructive pulmonary disease. *Curr Opin Pulmon Med* 2: 84–89.
3. Fishman AP (1994) Pulmonary rehabilitaiton research NIH Workshop Summary. *Am J Respir Crit Care Med* 149(pt 1): 825–833.
4. Anonymous (1998) Guidelines for the management of chronic obstructive pulmonary disease. Working Group of the South African Pulmonology Society [see comments]. *S African Med J* 88: 999–1002, 1004: 1006–10.
5. Reardon J, Awad E, Normandin E, Vale F, Clark B, ZuWallack RL (1994) The effect of comprehensive outpatient pulmonary rehabilitation on dyspnea. *Chest* 105:1046–1052.
6. Wijkstra PJ, van der Mark TW, Kraan J, van Altena R, Koeter GH, Postma DS (1996) Long-term effects of home rehabilitation on physical performance in chronic obstructive pulmonary disease. *Am J Respir Crit Care Med* 153:1234–1241.
7. Ries AL, Kaplan RM, Limberg TM, Prewitt LM (1995) Effects of pulmonary rehabilitation on physiologic and psychosocial outcomes in patients with chronic obstructive pulmonary disease. *Ann Intern Med* 122:823–832.
8. Maltais F, LeBlanc P, Simard C, et al. (1996) Skeletal Muscle adaptation to endurance training in patients with chonic obstructive pulmonary disease. *Am J Respir Crit Care Med* 154; 442–447.
9. Carrieri-Kohlman V, Douglas MK, Gormley JM, et al. (1993) Desxensitization and guided mastery: treatment approaches for the management of dyspnea. *Heart Lung* 22: 226–234.
10. White B, Andrews JL, Jr., Mogan JJ, Downes-Vogel P (1979) Pulmonary rehabilitation in an ambulatory group practice setting. *Med Clin N Am* 63:379–390.
11. Strijbos JH, Postma DS, van Altena R, Gimeno F, Koeter GH (1996) A comparison between an outpatient hospital-based pulmonary rehabilitation program and a home-care pulmonary rehabilitation program in patients with COPD. A follow-up of 18 months. *Chest* 109:366–372.
12. Dekhuijzen PN, Folgering HT, van Herwaarden CL (1990) Target-flow inspiratory muscle training at home and during pulmonary rehabilitation in COPD patients with a ventilatory limitation during exercise. *Lung* 168:502–508.
13. Ojanen M, Lahdensuo A, Laitinen J, Karvonen J (1993) Psychosocial changes in patients participating in a chronic obstructive pulmonary disease rehabilitation program. *Respiration* 60:96–102.
14. Cox NJ, Hendricks JC, Binkhorst RA, van Herwaarden CL (1993) A pulmonary rehabilitation program for patients with asthma and mild chronic obstructive pulmonary diseases (COPD). *Lung* 171:235–244.
15. Herningfield JE, Nemeth-Coslet R (1988) Nicotine Dependence. Interference between tobacco and tobacco related disease. *Chest* 93:375–380.
16. Reis AL (1993) Preventing COPD: you can make a difference. *J Respir Dis* 14: 739–749.
17. Anonymous (1996) American Thoracic Society. Cigarette smoking and health: official statement of the American Thoracic Society. *Am J Respir Dis* 153:861–865.
18. Goldstein RS (1993) Candidate evaluation. In: Casaburi R, Petty TL, eds. *Principles and Practice of Pulmonary Rehabilitation*, Philadelphia: WB Saunders, pp. 317–321.
19. Atkins BJ, Kaplan RM, Timms RM, et al. (1984) Behavioral exercise programs in the management of chronic obstructive pulmonary disease. *J Consult Clin Psychol* 52: 591–602.
20. Make BJ (1994) Collaborative Self-management strategies for patients with respiratory disease. *Respir Care* 39: 566–569.

21. Ries AL, Kaplan RM, Linberg TM, et al. (1995) Effects of pulmonary rehabilitation on physiology and psychosocial outcomes in patients with chronic obstructive pulmonary disease. *Ann Intern Med* 122: 823–830.
22. Toshima M, Kaplan RM, Reis AL (1990) Experimental evaluation of rehabilitation in chronic obstructive pulmonary disease: short term effects on exercise endurance and health status. *Health Psychol* 9: 237–252.
23. Milani RV, Lavie CJ (1998) Disparate effects of out-patient cardiac and pulmonary rehabilitation programs on work efficiency and peak aerobic capacity in patients with coronary disease or severe obstructive pulmonary disease. *J Cardiopulmon Rehab* 18:17–22.
24. Gilmartin ME (1986) Pulmonary rehabilitation. Patient and family education. *Clin Chest Med* 7:619–627.
25. Resnikoff PM, Ries AL (1998) Maximizing functional capacity. Pulmonary rehabilitation and adjunctive measures. *Respir Care Clin N Am* 4:475–492.
26. Medical Research Council Working Party (1981) Long term domiciliary oxygen therapy in chronic hypoxic cor pulmonale complicating chronic bronchitis and emphysema. *Lancet* 1: 681–685.
27. Nocturnal oxygen therapy trial group (1980) continuous or nocturnal oxygen therapy in hypoxemic chronic obstructive airways disease: A clinical trial. *Ann Intern Med* 93: 391–398.
28. Owens MW, Markewitz BA, Payne DK (1999) Outpatient management of chronic obstructive pulmonary disease. *Am J Med Sci* 318:79–83.
29. San Pedro GS (1999) Pulmonary rehabilitation for the patient with severe chronic obstructive pulmonary disease. *Am J Med Sci* 318:99–102.
30. Creutzberg EC, Schols AM, Bothmer-Quaedvlieg FC, Wouters EF (1998) Prevalence of an elevated resting energy expenditure in patients with chronic obstructive pulmonary disease in relation to body composition and lung function. *Eur J Clin Nutr* 52:396–401.
31. Schols AM, Mostert R, Soeters PB, Wouters EF (1991) Body composition and exercise performance in patients with chronic obstructive pulmonary disease [see comments]. *Thorax* 46:695–699.
32. Schols AM, Soeters PB, Dingemans AM, Mostert R, Frantzen PJ, Wouters EF (1993) Prevalence and characteristics of nutritional depletion in patients with stable COPD eligible for pulmonary rehabilitation. *Am Rev Respir Dis* 147:1151–1156.
33. Schols AM, Slangen J, Volovics L, Wouters EF (1998) Weight loss is a reversible factor in the prognosis of chronic obstructive pulmonary disease. *Am J Respir Crit Care Med* 157:1791–1797.
34. Ferreira IM, Verreschi IT, Nery LE, et al. (1998) The influence of 6 months of oral anabolic steroids on body mass and respiratory muscles in undernourished COPD patients. *Chest* 114:19–28.
35. Casaburi R (1998) Rationale for anabolic therapy to facilitate rehabilitation in chronic obstructive pulmonary disease. *Baillieres Clin Endocrinol Metab* 12:407–418.
36. Burdet L, de Muralt B, Schutz Y, Pichard C, Fitting JW (1997) Administration of growth hormone to underweight patients with chronic obstructive pulmonary disease. A prospective, randomized, controlled study. *Am J Respir Crit Care Med* 156:1800–1806.
37. Celli BR (1996) Current thoughts regarding treatment of chronic obstructive pulmonary disease. *Med Clin North Am* 80:589–609.
38. Anonymous (1998) Guidelines for the management of chronic obstructive pulmonary disease. Working Group of the South African Pulmonology Society [see comments]. South Afr Med J 88:999–1002, 1004, 1006–1010.

39. Blake RL Jr, Vandiver TA, Braun S, Bertuso DD, Straub V (1990) A randomized controlled evaluation of a psychosocial intervention in adults with chronic lung disease. *Family Med* 22:365–370.
40. Sassi-Dambron DE, Eakin EG, Ries AL, Kaplan RM (1995) Treatment of dyspnea in COPD. A controlled clinical trial of dyspnea management strategies [see comments]. *Chest* 107:724–729.
41. Devine EC, Pearcy J (1996) Meta-analysis of the effects of psychoeducational care in adults with chronic obstructive pulmonary disease. *Patient Educat Counsel* 29:167–178.
42. Bach JR, Moldover JR (1996) Cardiovascular, pulmonary, and cancer rehabilitation. 2. Pulmonary rehabilitation. *Arch Phys Med Rehab* 77:S45–S51.
43. Bach JR (1992) Mechanical exsufflation, noninvasive ventilation, and new strategies for pulmonary rehabilitation and sleep disordered breathing. *Bull New York Acad Med* 68:321–340.
44. Anonymous (1997) Pulmonary rehabilitation: joint ACCP/AACVPR evidence-based guidelines. ACCP/AACVPR Pulmonary Rehabilitation Guidelines Panel. American College of Chest Physicians. American Association of Cardiovascular and Pulmonary Rehabilitation [see comments]. *Chest* 112:1363–1396.
45. Mahler DA (1998) Pulmonary rehabilitation. *Chest* 113:263S–268S.
46. Moy ML, Ingenito EP, Mentzer SJ, Evans RB, Reilly JJ Jr (1999) Health-related quality of life improves following pulmonary rehabilitation and lung volume reduction surgery. *Chest* 115:383–389.

II LUNG VOLUME REDUCTION SURGERY FOR EMPHYSEMA

7 The History of Surgery for Emphysema

Joseph J. DeRose, Jr., MD and Kenneth M. Steinglass, MD

INTRODUCTION

The first accounts of pulmonary emphysema can be found in Sir John Floyer's *A Treatise of the Asthma* (1698) *(1)*. In a description of an autopsy of a "broken winded" horse, Floyer vividly outlined the hyperinflation and airway obstruction that characterizes chronic obstructive pulmonary disease (COPD). Dr. Matthew Baillie is credited with the first anatomic description and illustration of pulmonary emphysema *(2,3)*. In *The Morbid Anatomy of the Human Body*, Baillie noted during a postmortem examination that "in opening into the chest it is not unusual to find that the lungs do not collapse but that they fill up the cavity completely on each side of the heart. When examined, their cells appear full of air so that there is seen upon the surface a prodigious number of small white vesicles." The autopsy description and accompanying illustration (*see* Fig. 1) are of the lungs of Dr. Samuel Johnson *(4)*.

From: *Lung Volume Reduction Surgery*
Edited by: M. Argenziano and M. E. Ginsburg © Humana Press Inc., Totowa, NJ

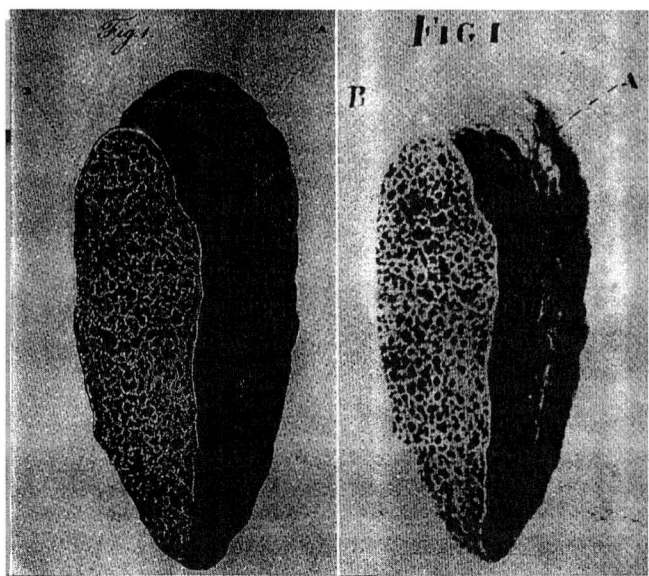

Fig. 1. Illustrations of the lung specimen from Samuel Johnson's autopsy. On the right is the original drawing by William Clift. The engraving on the right was made by William Skelton for Ballie's atlas.

The French physician and anatomist Rene Laennec is credited with the first systematic, clinical, and pathologic description of emphysema *(5,6)*. In his famous treatise on auscultation, Laennec noted that "in pulmonary emphysema the size of the vesicles is much increased and less uniform. The greater number equal or exceed the size of a millet seed while some attain the magnitude of a hemp seed, cherry stone, or even fresh beans." This work also introduced for the first time a method for percussion and auscultation of the chest using Laennec's own invention, the stethoscope. Concerning physical examination of the patient with emphysema, Laennec wrote "the whole chest yields a very distinct sound, and instead of its natural compressed shape it exhibits an almost round or globular outline, swelling out both before and behind. This conformation of the chest is sufficiently remarkable to have enabled me sometimes to announce the existence of emphysema from simple inspection."

These pathologic descriptions served as the basis for understanding the emphysematous disease process in the early part of the 20th century. It was not until the latter half of the century that the pathophysiology of COPD was fully elucidated. Nonetheless, a myriad of operations aimed at correcting the anatomic and structural consequences of emphysema were attempted beginning in the early 1900s. The failure of most of these procedures was rooted in an improper understanding of the pathophysiology of the disease. The initial vigor with which most experimental emphysema operations were extolled serves as a sobering lesson for critical, prospective, and randomized evaluation of all emerging new technology. However, it was the resurrection of a once-criticized and formerly abandoned operation described by Brantigan and Mueller that serves as the basis for modern lung volume reduction surgery (LVRS) *(7–9)*.

CHEST WALL SURGERY

Costochondrectomy

The misbelief that the thoracic cage was too small to accommodate full expansion of the emphysematous lung led to the development of several operations aimed at lessening the stiffness of the chest wall. In 1908, Freund and Seidel proposed a division of 4–6 costal cartilages in an attempt to increase the size of the rib cage *(10)*. The operation was performed under local anesthesia on one or both sides and in one or more sittings. It remained a popular approach for nearly two decades. Several surgeons even attempted to improve on the usual cause of relapse, which was thought to be bony reunion, by adding a transverse sternotomy. Costochondrectomy was reported to result in great relief of dyspnea and an immediate increase in vital capacity. These results were attributed to "freedom of movement of the soft parts beneath permitting the pleura to bulge in paradoxical fashion" *(11)*.

Thoracoplasty and Phrenicectomy

Recognition that enlargement of the thorax and descent of the diaphragm were the result, and not the cause, of emphysema led to the use of several procedures designed to reduce the volume of the thoracic cavity. In 1927, Voelcker suggested a posterior paravertebral thoracoplasty in an attempt to change the angle of the ribs to the more downward slanting position found in the normal chest *(10,12)*. Other similar procedures involved excising the third to seventh ribs and the corresponding intercostal nerves *(10,13)*. The rationale for phrenicectomy was that overinflated bullae might stimulate Hering-Breuer reflexes with consequent limitation of the depth of respiration. In 1947, Allison reported that he was able to increase ventilation and vital capacity by phrenic paralysis in a few selected patients *(14)*.

These operations were soon abandoned as surgeons began to realize that loss of integrity of the chest wall and diaphragm resulted in more profound interference with respiratory function and worsened dyspnea.

In a 1972 review of surgery for emphysema, LaForet wrote of thoraco-plasty and phrenicectomy, "The alleged benefits of those manoeuvres were frequently lost on patients whose worsened dyspnea left them little energy to debate with their surgeons" *(15)*.

PROCEDURES DIRECTED AT THE DIAPHRAGM

Abdominal Belts

The low, flat, immobile diaphragm seen in the emphysematous patient results in an altered intraabdominal–intrathoracic pressure relationship. Based on this concept, it was postulated that elevating the diaphragm might improve its level of contraction and function. Alexander and Kountz proposed the use of an abdominal belt in order to keep the diaphragm in an elevated position *(16)*. A screw bolt was fashioned to the belt and was used to keep a constant and comfortable pressure for the patient. Of 25 patients fitted with these belts over a 2–6 mo period, 73% reported subjective improvement with an average increase in vital capacity of 39%. These belts, however, proved impractical for daily use, and results remained difficult to reproduce.

Pneumoperitoneum

Reich was the first to describe the use of artificial pneumoperitoneum for the treatment of emphysema in 1924 *(17)*. The technique involved the instillation of 300–500 mL of air into the abdomen after which significant elevation of the diaphragm was noted to occur. Reich reported an increase in diaphragmatic excursion with a consequent increase in minute venti-lation, a reduction in dyspnea, and greater ease in raising secretions.

In 1950, Carter refined the technique of pneumoperitoneum and also subjected the procedure to objective evaluation *(18)*. His technique involved an initial fill of 700–1000 mL of a mixture of helium (80%) and room air (20%). Patients were then given refills every other week in order to maintain the pneumoperitoneum. Ten of 16 patients who under-went this protocol (63%) demonstrated subjective improvement with a reduction in dyspnea, increased exercise tolerance, and improved ability to clear secretions. These subjective improvements were supported by a 356-mL increase in vital capacity, an increase in maximal breathing capacity from 19 to 37 L/min and fluoroscopy, which demonstrated a significant increase in diaphragmatic motion. Unfortunately, future investigators were unable to reproduce these objective results, and criteria for patient selection remained absent *(19,20)*. Furthermore, the need for constant maintenance of the pneumoperitoneum, as well as the associated abdominal pain, hastened the abandonment of pneumoperi-toneum in the treatment of emphysema.

OPERATIONS ON THE PLEURA

In 1952, Crenshaw and Rowles proposed parietal pleurectomy and talc pleurodesis as a technique for increasing systemic-to-pulmonary collateral blood flow to emphysematous lung tissue *(21)*. The operation was based on the mistaken belief that emphysema was the end result of hypovascularity secondary to endarteritic changes within the bronchial arteries. In their initial report of 11 patients, surgery was tolerated well, and subjective improvement was noted in most patients. However, the realization that increased blood flow to poorly aerated lung tissue did not improve lung function soon resulted in the abandonment of this procedure.

OPERATIONS ON THE NERVOUS SYSTEM

Abbott et al. were the first investigators to propose denervation of the lung as a treatment for emphysema *(22)*. Such operations were undertaken in an attempt to decrease bronchospasm and secretions, as well as to improve pulmonary circulation. Abbot's technique included pulmonary plexectomy, pulmonary artery periarterial sympathectomy, upper dorsal sympathectomy and partial lung resection. Brantigan and Mueller likewise added a complex denervation procedure to their partial lung resection *(7–9)*. This procedure included complete removal of the posterior pulmonary plexuses by ligation of all branches of the vagus nerve to the heart, lung, and mediastinum, as well as an extensive perivenous and peribronchial stripping of symppathetic nerve fibers (see Fig. 2). The numerous different techniques and the lack of adequate control groups made it difficult to interpret the results of these operations and appropriate patient selection criteria were never identified.

Nonetheless, these lung denervation operations were soon followed by nearly 4000 cases in Japan of glomectomy for the treatment of asthma and emphysema *(23)*. A subsequent report by Overholt included more than 800 cases *(24)*. The rationale for carotid body resection was to abolish both the hypoxic respiratory drive and bronchospasm associated with asthma and some forms of COPD. Of interest, nearly two-thirds of patients in both series noted subjective improvement from this procedure even though there is no physiologic basis for its effect. It was not until several randomized, double-blind studies were performed in which patients were subjected to either glomectomy or a sham operation that this procedure was proved worthless.

OPERATIONS ON THE LUNG
Surgery for Giant Bullae

The compression of normal lung tissue by single or multiple giant bullae has led many surgeons to decompress or resect these lesions in an

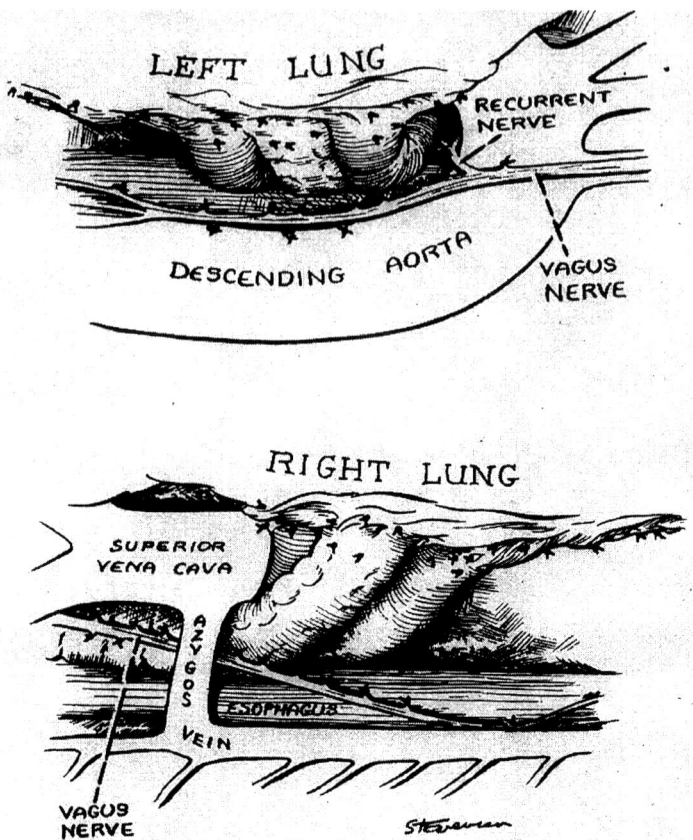

Fig. 2. Drawing from Brantigan's paper illustrating a method of denervation of the lung. The branches of the vagus nerve were excised from the thoracic inlet to the inferior pulmonary ligament. A stripping of the pulmonary artery, the bronchus, and the pulmonary veins was also performed.

attempt to improve pulmonary function. Monaldi initially described intracavitary suction and drainage as a procedure to relieve tension in tuberculous cavities *(27)*. Head and Avery later applied the technique to bullous lung disease with subjective improvement in many patients *(28)*. However, aspiration of giant bullae typically provided only temporary relief, and the sometimes disastrous results of tension pneumothorax led to the abandonment of this procedure.

As thoracic surgical techniques improved, operations aimed at resecting giant isolated bullae were developed. Plication, bullectomy, and anatomic resection were all applied with both subjective and objective improvement in pulmonary function *(11)*. Although selection criteria have remained elusive, resection of giant bullae remains an important option in patients with compromised pulmonary function. It was this early promising experience with giant bullae resection that fostered the birth of resectional surgery for emphysema.

LUNG VOLUME REDUCTION FOR EMPHYSEMA

The modern concepts and techniques of LVRS find their origin in Otto Brantigan's 1959 publication *A Surgical Approach to Emphysema* *(9)*. Brantigan's initial experience with giant bullae resection and a subsequent 8-yr period of trial and error resulted in the formulation of theories explaining the pathophysiologic processes characteristic of emphysema. Brantigan proposed that emphysema impaired the pulmonary elasticity and circumferential pull, which holds the bronchioles open. This elasticity is lost to the greatest extent during expiration resulting in functional expiratory obstruction. He likened the condition to "stuffing an inelastic lung of 6000 or 7000 cc into a pleural space of 5000 cc capacity." Brantigan also made the observation that the emphysematous disease process was frequently heterogeneous with the more severely damaged lung existing at the apex and the periphery. By resecting these areas of "functionless" lung tissue, "normal" lung would be allowed to expand, and radial traction on the terminal bronchioles would be re-established. In addition, Brantigan et al. postulated that volume reduction elevated the diaphragm and improved the contractility of the diaphragm and intercostal muscles.

The operation consisted of reducing the volume of the lung "to the capacity that fits the volume of the pleural space on full expiration." Resection was carried out with a clamp and suture method with reduction being accomplished as much by constriction of a running suture as by the volume of lung tissue removed (*see* Fig. 3). Anatomic resections were never performed for fear of removing "normal" lung tissue. An extensive lung denervation was also added to the lung volume reduction in order to relieve bronchospasm, decrease secretions, and increase pulmonary blood flow. Although Brantigan suggested that the operation be performed in a bilateral staged fashion, only half of the patients reported in his series had a bilateral operation.

Brantigan reported the results of 33 patients undergoing this operation with symptomatic improvement in all but one patient *(9)*. Although the paper mentions isolated instances of improved postoperative pulmonary function tests no effort was made to systematically evaluate the results. An 18% postoperative mortality rate prompted leading authorities of the day to dismiss volume reduction as an inappropriate surgical option in emphysema. However, Brantigan himself reported that there

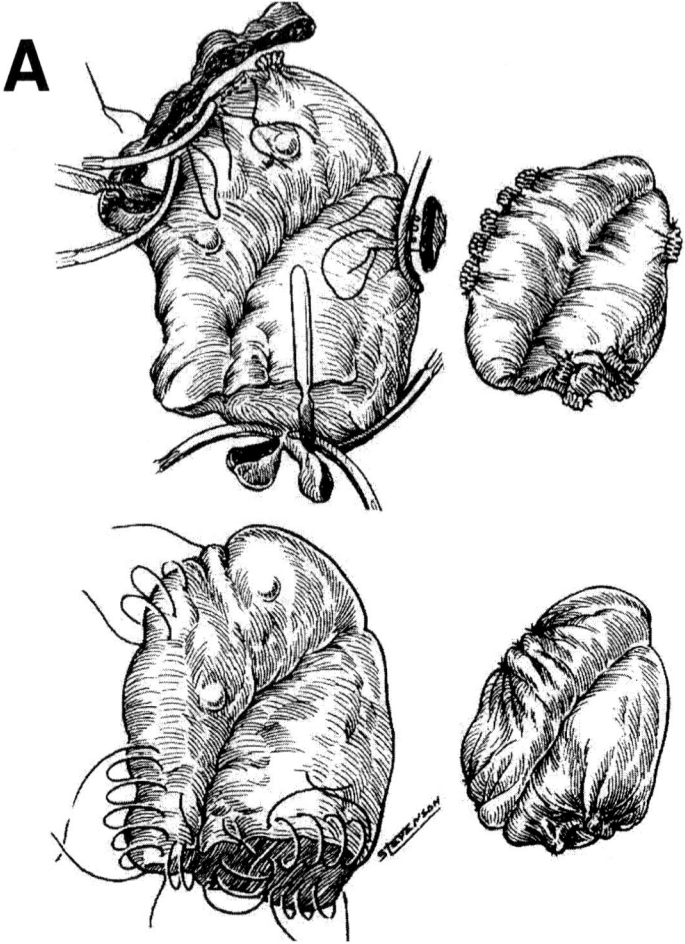

Fig. 3. (A) Illustration from Brantigan's paper demonstrating the "clamp and suture method" of lung resection.

was a steep learning curve in his 8-yr experience, with an understanding of the mechanism of improvement coming only in the last 18–24 mo.

Limited interest in Brantigan's operation persisted and, in 1980, Debesse theorized that removal of the worst areas of diffusely emphysematous lung might be equivalent to resection of isolated giant bullae *(29)*. Debesse et al. reported results on 10 patients and although there were only minimal improvements in postoperative spirometry, there were significant improvements in cardiac output and pulmonary artery pressure. In 1987, Dahan et al. reported significant increases in post-operative FEV$_1$ following surgery and coined the term "lung volume

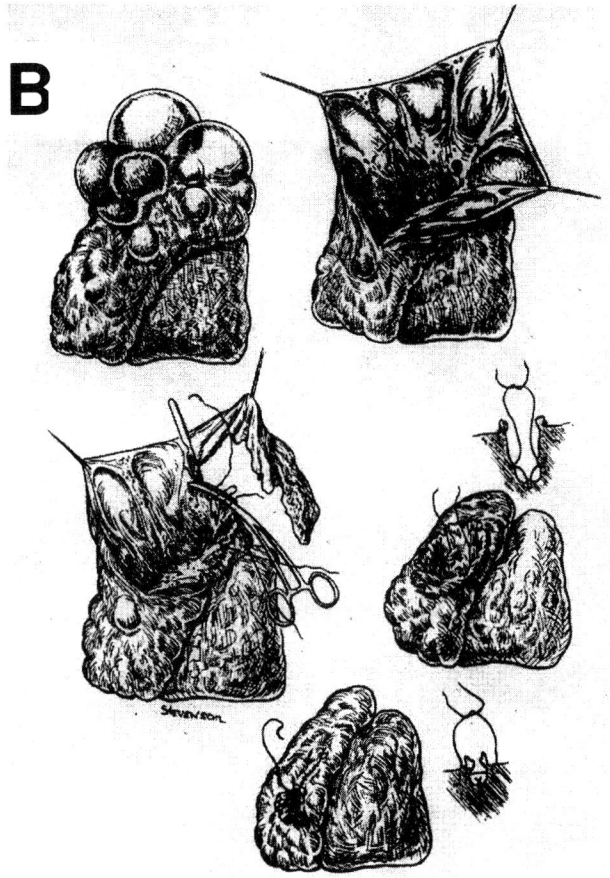

Fig. 3. (B) Brantigan's illustration of opening bullae and oversewing via plication during lung reduction surgery.

reduction"*(30)*. Wakabayashi et al. in 1992 reported on hundreds of patients undergoing thoracoscopic laser shrinkage of target areas with profound symptomatic improvement, but the report was marred by incomplete follow-up and poor objective assessment *(31)*.

The modern technique of LVRS is attributed to Cooper et al. From certain observations made in his lung transplant candidates, Cooper postulated that Brantigan's approach might be valuable as a "bridge" or alternative to lung transplantation. The operation was initially described through a median sternotomy with resections being performed with multiple firings of pericardial-lined stapling devices *(32)*. Cooper transformed the operation into a team-dependent, systematic approach based on sophisticated patient selection, preoperative preparation, modern postoperative care, and detailed follow-up. The first LVRS operations performed by Cooper's group were done in 1993 and the first published report appeared in 1995. In this first series of 20 patients, there were no early or late postoperative deaths and an impressive 82% improvement in FEV_1 was reported at 3 mo *(32)*.

CONCLUSIONS

The checkered history of surgery for emphysema serves as a sobering reminder of the value of objective and randomized studies for emerging clinical techniques. An understanding of the pathophysiology of the disease process has propelled the quest for surgical palliation of emphysema. Nonetheless, the role of surgery in postponing death from emphysema remains unclear. Undoubtedly, new techniques and concepts await their place in the unfolding history of emphysema surgery.

REFERENCES

1. Townsend GL (1969) Sir John Floyer (1649–1734) and the discovery of pulmonary emphysema. *Mayo Clin Proc* 44:484–488.
2. Baillie M The morbid anatomy of some of the most important parts of the human body. London: Printed for J. Johns and G. Nicol 793, p.314.
3. Cooper JD (1997) The history of surgical procedures for emphysema. *Ann Thorac Surg* 63:312–319.
4. McHenry LC Jr (1967) Dr. Samuel Johnson's emphysema. *Arch Int Med* 119:98–105.
5. Laennec RTH (1834) A treatise on the diseases of the chest and of mediate auscultation. Translated by John Forced, MD, FRS. 4th ed. London: Whittaker.
6. Rosenblatt MB (1972) Emphysema: historical perspective. *Bull N.Y. Acad Med* 48:823–841.
7. Brantigan OC (1954) Surgical treatment of pulmonary emphysema. *W Virginia Med J* 50:283–285.
8. Brantigan OC (1957) Surgical treatment of pulmonary emphysema. *Maryland Med J* 6:409.
9. Brantigan OC, Mueller E, Kress MB (1959) A surgical approach to pulmonary emphysema. *Ann Rev Respir Dis* 80:194–206.
10. Deslauriers J (1996) History of surgery for Emphysema. *Semin Thorac Cardiovasc Surg* 8:43–51.
11. Knudson RJ, Gaensler EA (1965) Surgery for emphysema. *Ann Thorac Surg* 1:332–362.
12. Voelcker H (1927) Behandlung des asthma bronchiale durch paravertebrale pfeilerresektion. *Arch Clin Chir* 148:522–527.
13. Phillips EW, Merle Scott WJ (1929) The surgical treatment of bronchial asthma. *Arch Surg* 19:1425–1456.
14. Allison PR (1947) Giant bullous cysts of the lung. *Thorax* 2:169.
15. LaForet EG (1972) Surgical management of chronic obstructive lung disease. *N Engl J Med* 287:175–177.

16. Alexander HL, Kountz WB (1934) Symptomatic relief of emphysema by an abdominal belt. *Am J Med Sci* 187:692–700.
17. Reich L (1924) Der einfluss des pneumoperitoneums auf das lungen-emphysema. *Wien Arch Finn Med* 8:245–260.
18. Carter MG, Gaensler EA, Kyllonen A (1950) Pneumoperitoneum in the treatment of pulmonary emphysema. *N Engl J Med* 243:549–558.
19. Becklake MR, Goldman HI, McGregor M (1954) The effects of pneumoperitoneum on lung function in pulmonary emphysema. *Thorax* 9:222–225.
20. Mann B, Murphy EA (1953) The treatment of hypertrophic emphysema by pneumoperitoneum. *Thorax* 9:87–90.
21. Crenshaw GL, Rowles DF (1952) Surgical management of pulmonary emphysema. *J Thorax Surg* 24:398–410.
22. Abbott OA, Hopkins WA, Guilfoil PH (1950) Therapeutic status of pulmonary autonomic nerve surgery. *J Thorac Cardiovasc Surg* 20:571–583.
23. Nakayma K (1961) Surgical removal of the carotid body for bronchial asthma. *Dis Chest* 40:595–604.
24. Overholt RH (1961) Glomectomy for asthma. *Dis Chest* 40:605–610.
25. Curran WS, Oser JF, Longfield AN, et al. (1966) Glomectomy for severe bronchial asthma. A double-blind study. *Am Rev Respir Dis* 93:84–89.
26. Curran WS, Graham WGB (1971) Long-term effects of a glomectomy. Follow-up of a double-blind study. *Am Rev Respir Dis* 103:566–568.
27. Monaldi V (1947) Endocavitaryaspiration. Its practical application. *Tubercle* 28:223–228.
28. Head JR, Avery E (1949) Intracavitary suction (Monaldi) in the treatment of emphysematous bullae and blebs. *J Thorac Cardiovasc Surg* 18:761–76.41.
29. Even P, Sors H, Safran D. Reynaud P, Venet A, Debesse B (1980) Hemodynamique de bulles d'emphyseme nouveau syndrome: la tampanode cardiaque emphysemateuse. *Rev Fr Mal Respir* 8:117–120.
30. Dahan M, Salerin F, Berjaud J, Renella Coll J, Galliard J (1989) Interet de l'exploration hemodynamique dans les indications chirurugicales des emphysemes. *Ann Chir* 43:669–672.
31. Wakabayshi A (1995) Thoracoscoplc laser pneumoplasty in the treatment of diffuse bullous emphysema. *Ann Thorac Surg* 60:936–942.
32. Cooper JD, Trulock EP, Triantafillou AN, et al. (1995) Bilateral pneumectomy (volume reduction) for chronic obstructive lung disease. *J Thorac Cardiovasc Surg* 109:106–119.

8 Lung Volume Reduction Surgery
Open Technique

Antonio L. Visbal, MD,
Claude Deschamps, MD, *and James P. Utz,* MD

INTRODUCTION

In the late 1950s, Brantigan *(1–4)* proposed that the removal of lung tissue would increase the circumferential pull on small airways and thereby relieve bronchial obstruction and dyspnea. He proceeded through a posterolateral thoracotomy. Although many of his patients reported symptomatic benefit, he made no attempt to document improvements in lung function. Because of this and a perioperative mortality rate of 18%, the Brantigan procedure was not widely accepted and the concept was viewed as ill-conceived by leading authorities of the time *(5)*. Limited interest in Brantigan's ideas persisted until the mid-1970s.

In 1977, Delarue *(6)* published a surgical series of 47 emphysema patients. He characterized emphysema as either focal or multifocal, with or without space occupation. He found it difficult preoperatively to distinguish bullae from more diffuse "cotton candy" changes and ended up resecting lung in patients without giant bullae. The approach was through a thoracotomy. The perioperative mortality was 21% and long-term improvement occurred in 45% of patients. Objective testing was not provided to support the claim of improved pulmonary function.

From: *Lung Volume Reduction Surgery*
Edited by: M. Argenziano and M. E. Ginsburg © Humana Press Inc., Totowa, NJ

In 1980, a French group headed by Debesse *(7)* theorized that the removal of the worst areas of diffusely emphysematous lung might result in a similar benefit as the removal of a single lesion in patients with the giant bullae syndrome. Based on their experience in 10 patients with giant bullae, Debesse et al. described a new syndrome of "emphysematous cardiac tamponade." These patients had experienced minimal improvements in spirometry, but significant increases in cardiac output and characteristic changes in the pulmonary artery pressure waveform. Between 1985 and 1987, Dahan et al. *(8)* tested Debesse's theory by operating on 10 patients with diffuse emphysema who exhibited the hemodynamic changes described in Debesse's paper. The operation, through a posterolateral thoracotomy, was coined "intervention chirurgicale de reduction du volume pulmonaire," which translates to "lung volume reduction surgery (LVRS)." Five patients were subjectively improved with increases in FEV_1 from 10% to 62%.

In 1992, Crosa-Dorado *(9)* published a description of a surgical suturing technique for excision of bullae or sectors of the lung destroyed by emphysema. The open surgery was performed in 76 patients over an 11-yr period and was described as "lung remodeling" in patients with diffuse disease, a concept similar to Brantigan's. No outcome data were presented.

The contemporary version of LVRS by open surgical resection has been championed by Cooper et al. Their experience grew from observations made in patients undergoing lung transplantation for chronic obstructive pulmonary disease (COPD). Initial LVRS operations were performed in 1993, information began to be disseminated at national meetings in 1994, and the first peer-reviewed manuscript was published in January 1995 *(10)*. According to this report on the first 20 patients, LVRS by median sternotomy produced an impressive 82% improvement in FEV_1 6 mo after surgery.

SURGICAL TECHNIQUE
Median Sternotomy (10–12)

Before the operation, while the patient is still awake, a thoracic epidural catheter is inserted for intraoperative and postoperative analgesia. Initially, a 6–8 cm^3 bolus of a mixture of bupivacaine (0.25%) and fentanyl (75–100 mcg) is injected in the epidural catheter followed by a continuous infusion of a solution of bupivacaine (0.075%) and fentanyl (5 mcg/cm^3) at a rate of 8–10 cm^3/h. A double-lumen tube is used for selective ventilation. The vertical skin incision is made shorter than the sternotomy itself to minimize the risk of postoperative sternal infection in the event that a tracheostomy is required during the postoperative period (see Fig. 1). A small sponge is placed on a ring forcep and inserted

double lumen tube

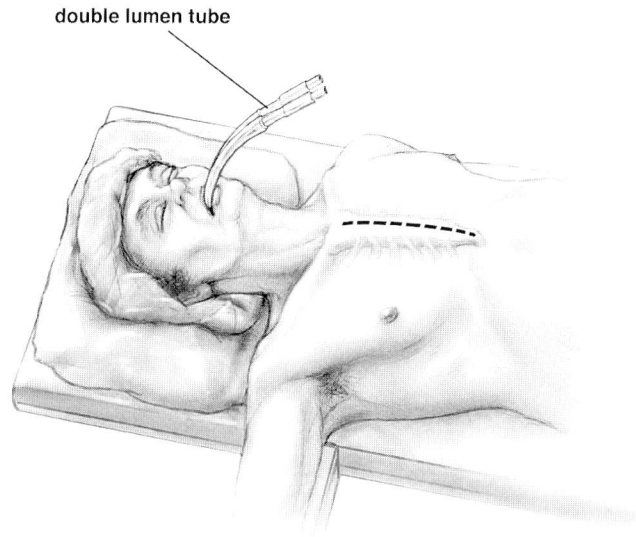

Fig. 1. Median sternotomy incision (broken line) starts 2 cm below the edge of the manubrium and ends at the level of the xiphoid process. Note patient is intubated with a double-lumen tube.

under the xiphoid process and is used to gently sweep the pleura laterally on each side. Ventilation is temporarily halted during the actual sternotomy. These maneuvers decrease the odds of penetration of the pleural space when the sternum is divided with the saw. The sternum is handled delicately and hemostasis is achieved with electrocautery. Pads are placed on the sternal edges to minimize potential damage by the retractor, which can be standard or internal mammary retractor (Delacroix Chevalier, France) (see Fig. 2).

The procedure is initiated on the more severely diseased lung, which is disconnected from the ventilator and allowed to deflate. Ventilation is continued on the contralateral lung. After 5–10 min, the areas of the lung with the most perfusion will be deflated, whereas the areas most affected by emphysema will remain inflated. The pleura is opened carefully to avoid damage to the lung parenchyma. At the beginning of our experience, we routinely attempted to mobilize a portion of the apical parietal pleura to create a pleural tent, hoping to decrease the postresection residual pleural space. More often than not, the fragility of the tissue resulted in a fenestrated pleural tent. As this defeats the purpose of the pleural tent, we have since abandoned this fruitless exercise. The pleural space is inspected and the lung is palpated

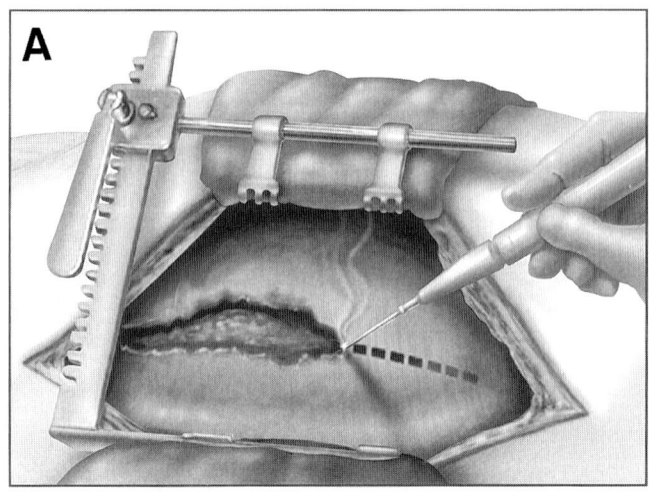

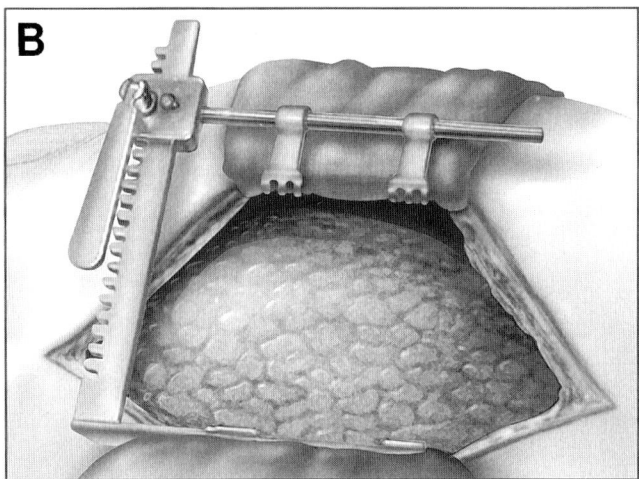

Fig. 2. (A) The broken line shows the intended incision of the mediastinal pleura. (B) An internal mammary retractor is used to elevate the sternum to favor exposure of the operative side.

delicately and thoroughly in search of unexpected pathology. When present, adhesions are meticulously divided with the electrocautery as far from the lung as possible to avoid tears in the pulmonary parenchyma. Manipulations and electrocautery are avoided in the neighborhood of the phrenic nerve. Next, the inferior pulmonary ligament is divided under direct vision with the electrocautery to favor optimal reexpansion following the procedure. Although this maneuver can cause hypotension, it is usually transient and well-tolerated. The pleural cavity is then half-filled with saline solution, elevating the lung into the wound. This minimizes manipulation of the fragile emphysematous lung and decrease the chances of prolonged air leak or pulmonary contusions.

The areas of intended resection are usually identified prior to operation, by review of computed tomography (CT) and perfusion scans. Frequently, the disease is most advanced in the apices. The lung to be resected is grasped with several Duvall clamps (*see* Fig. 3) and the resection is effected by three to five applications of a linear 90-mm GIA device with 4.8-mm staples, resulting in the removal of approx 50% of the upper lobe. Whereas the goal of LVRS is to remove 20%–30% of each lung *(10)*, it is unclear exactly how this number was adopted. Even if one accepts this number on faith, it is difficult if not impossible to measure the resected lung volume during surgery. The resected lung tissue is sometimes weighed, but at the time of surgery there is no way of knowing the specific density of the lung removed relative to that of the lung left behind. The resection follows an inverted "U" shape pattern, in order to avoid significant mismatch between the contour of the new lung apex and the chest wall (see Fig. 4). The staple line is buttressed with bovine pericardial strips (Peri-strips Dry™, Bio-Vascular, St. Paul, MN) to minimize postoperative air leaks. Staple lines may also be reinforced by other commercially available materials, such as polytetrafluoroethylene (PTFE). If pleural adhesions are too dense in the area of intended resection, extrapleural dissection is recommended and the parietal pleura adherent to the lung is included in the resected specimen. When the disease is most severe in the lower lobes, as in α-1 antitrypsin deficiency *(13)*, the resection follows the contour of the underlying diaphragm.

The volume-reduced lung is then gently reexpanded under saline solution to check for air leaks. Although minimal leaks are tolerated, every effort is made to address significant leaks with either reapplication of the stapling device, careful suturing of the parenchyma with nonabsorbable sutures or—ideally—application of one of the recently FDA-approved lung sealant products (e.g., FocalSeal™, Focal, Inc, Lexington, MA). The saline solution is suctioned, hemostasis is verified, and the pleural space is drained with a single 32-Fr. chest tube, inserted laterally with the tip positioned at the apex. No specific effort is made to close the pleura because it is rarely possible to achieve a hermetic seal. The contralateral lung is then deflated and the procedure is repeated in a similar fashion. The sternum is closed with at least seven stainless steel wires and the rectus abdominis aponeurosis is reapproximated with interrupted sutures. Each of the chest tubes is connected to its own collection system and is left on water seal postoperatively.

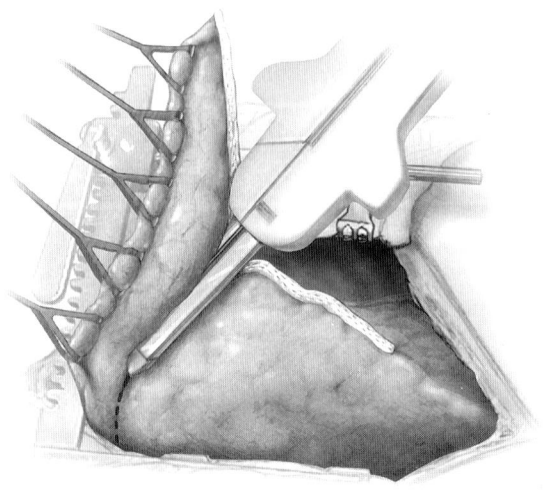

Fig. 3. Several Duvall clamps are gently applied along the area to be resected. The stapling device is oriented in such a manner to effect an inverted "U" shape excision of the parenchyma.

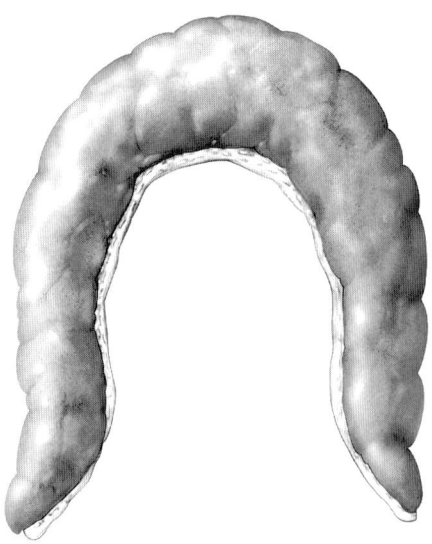

Fig. 4. Typical specimen from LVRS of the upper lobe.

Throughout the operation, optimal communication with the anesthesiologist is of the utmost importance. The timing of the lung reexpansion, the maximum airway pressure (< 25 cm H_2O), and the timing of extubation (usually in the operating room at the conclusion of skin closure) are key points where coordination between the surgical team and the anesthesiologist is vital.

Other Techniques

A variety of other techniques are available to perform LVRS. Laser ablation of pulmonary tissue is still promoted by some *(14)*, but most have abandoned this procedure *(1)*. In the only randomized study comparing laser ablation with surgical stapling, McKenna et al. compared unilateral stapled lung reduction with unilateral laser bullectomy for diffuse emphysema *(15)*. The authors of this study concluded that unilateral stapled lung reduction was superior to unilateral laser bullectomy.

Surgeons who use sternotomy for lung reduction surgery generally perform bilateral reductions. It appears that bilateral procedures tend to result in greater improvements in lung function, but there may be a role for unilateral stapling in selected patients *(16–18)*. When unilateral LVRS is indicated, posterolateral thoracotomy should be considered only if video-assisted thoracic surgery (VATS) is contraindicated *(18)*. Anterior bilateral thoracotomies through the clamshell approach may allow a better exposure of the lower lobes and the posterior lung field *(19)*. However, there is little justification to use this approach instead of the more simple midline sternotomy. There is no consensus on whether VATS stapling vs stapling via median sternotomy is superior. Some have suggested that this depends upon surgeon preference *(20)*. Several nonrandomized studies have suggested that equivalent results are achieved with VATS staple reduction and staple reduction via median sternotomy *(16,17,21)*. Selected studies that reported their results with the open approach are listed in Table 1.

POSTOPERATIVE CARE *(22)*

The patient is extubated in the operating room and observed carefully in the post-anesthesia recovery unit, and then transferred for overnight stay in the intensive care unit. Postoperative acidosis and hypercarbia are common in the first 12–24 h. This usually improves with time, as the effects of anesthesia gradually disappear and better pain control is achieved. Postoperative pain management consists of thoracic epidural analgesia. It can be supplemented by patient-controlled intravenous morphine analgesia and nonsteroidal antiinflammatory agents.

Table 1
Series of LVRS Through the Open Approach *(11)*

Authors	Patients (n)	Technique	Mortality(%)	Increased FEv$_1$(%)
Cooper et al. *(23)*	150	Bilateral	5.0	51
Miller et al. *(24)*	100	Bilateral	5.2	97
Daniel et al. *(25)*	26	Bilateral	3.8	40
Argenziano et al. *(26)*		Both*	7.1	61
Miller et al. *(27)*	53	Both*	5.2	97
Bousamra *(28)*	37	Both*	6.7	59
Date *(29)*	39	Bilateral	0	41
Demertzis *(30)*	25	Both*	0	50
Bagley *(31)*	55	Bilateral	0	27

* include bilateral and unilateral approach

A cephalosporine antibiotic is administered from the time of induction of general anesthesia until the last chest tube is removed. We have a low threshold for empiric treatment with large spectrum antibiotics when a new infiltrate is noted on the daily chest X-ray or when a change occurs in the appearance of the sputum. Oxygen saturation is monitored continuously and kept above 90% at all times. Chest tubes are kept on water seal and should not be removed before any air leaks have stopped and drainage is less than 300 mL over 24 h. In the presence of a prolonged air leak (greater than 7 d), a Heimlich valve can be used to allow for dismissal home, provided the lung remains expanded while on water seal. Early ambulation is encouraged and an exercise bicycle or treadmill is used 2–4 times/d, as tolerated, starting on the second postoperative day. In patients using inhaled bronchodilators preoperatively, that medication is resumed on the first postoperative day. Rarely, parenteral steroids will be required to manage an acute exacerbation of bronchospasm.

REFERENCES

1. Utz JP, Hubmayr RD, Deschamps C. (1998) Lung volume reduction surgery for emphysema: out on a limb without a NETT. *Mayo Clin Proc* 73:552–556.
2. Brantigan OC, Mueller E. (1957) Surgical treatment of pulmonary emphysema. *Am Surg* 23:789–801.
3. Brantigan OC, Mueller E, Kress MR. (1959) A surgical approach to pulmonary emphysema. *Am Rev Respir Dis* 80:194–206.
4. Brantigan OC, Kress MB, Mueller EA. (1961) The surgical approach to pulmonary emphysema. *Diseases Chest* 39:485–501.
5. Knudson RJ, Gaensler EA. (1965) Surgery for emphysema. *Ann Thorac Surg* 1:332–362.

6. Delarue NC, Woolf CR, Sanders DE, Pearson, FG, Henderson RD, Cooper JD, et al. (1977) Surgical treatment for pulmonary emphysema. *Can J Surg* 20:222–231.
7. Even P, Sors H, Safran D, Reynaud P, Venet A, Debesse B. (1980) Hemodynamique des bulles d'emphyseme - un nouveau syndrome: La tamponnade cardiaque emphysemateuse. *Revue Francaise des Maladies Respir* 8:117–120.
8. Dahan M, Salerin F, Berjaud J, Renella Coll J, Gaillard J. (1989) Interet de l'exploration hemodynamique dans les indications chirurgicales des emphysemes. *Ann Chirurgie* 43:669–672.
9. Crosa-Dorado VL, Pomi J, Pérez-Penco EJ, Carriquiry G. (1992) Treatment of dyspnea in emphysema: pulmonary remodeling: hemo- and pneumostatic suturing of the emphysematous lung. *Res Surg* 4:152–155.
10. Cooper JD, Trulock EP, Triantafillou AN, Patterson GA, Pohl MS, Deloney PA, et al. (1995) Bilateral pneumonectomy (volume reduction) for chronic obstructive pulmonary disease. *J Thorac Cardiovasc Surg* 109:106–116.
11. Shrager JB, Kaiser LR, Edelman JD. (2000) Lung volume reduction surgery. *Curr Probl Surg* 37:290–301.
12. Deschamps CD, Rocco G. (1999) La pneumoplastica riduttiva, trattamento dell'enfisema polmonare in stadio avanzato. *Leadership Medica (Italy)* 2:4–9.
13. Krowka MJ, Utz JP, Hyatt RE, Hubmayr RD, Deschamps C. (1997) Lung volume reduction surgery in alpha-1 antitrypsin deficiency. *Am J Respir Crit Care Med* 155:A795.
14. Wakabayashi A. (1995) Thoracoscopic laser pneumoplasty in the treatment of diffuse bullous emphysema. *Ann Thorac Surg* 60:936–942.
15. McKenna RJ Jr, Brenner M, Gelb AF, Mullin M, Singh N, Peters H, et al. (1996) A randomized, prospective trial of stapled lung reduction versus laser bullectomy for diffuse emphysema. *J Thorac Cardiovasc Surg* 111:317–322.
16. Kotloff RM, Tino G, Bavaria JE, Palevsky HI, Hansen-Flaschen J, Wahl PM, et al. (1996) Bilateral lung volume reduction surgery for advanced emphysema: A comparison of median sternotomy and thoracoscopic approaches. *Chest* 110:1399–1406.
17. Wisser W, Tschernko E, Senbaklavaci O, Kontrus M, Wanke T, Wolner E, et al. (1997) Functional improvement after volume reduction: Sternotomy versus videoendoscopic approach. *Ann Thorac Surg* 63:822–828.
18. Argenziano M, Thomashow B, Jellen PA, Rose EA, Steinglass KM, Ginsburg ME, et al. (1997) Functional comparison of unilateral versus bilateral lung volume reduction surgery. *Ann Thorac Surg* 64:321–327.
19. Bains MS, Ginsberg RJ, Jones WG, et al. (1994) The clamshell incision: An improved approach to bilateral pulmonary and mediastinal tumors. *Ann Thorac Surg* 58:30–33.
20. Naunheim KS, Ferguson MK. (1996) The current status of lung volume reduction operations for emphysema. *Ann Thorac Surg* 62:601–612.
21. Travaline JM, Furakawa S, Kuzma AM, O'Brien GM, Cordova FC, Criner GJ. (1997) Bilateral lung volume reduction surgery via median sternotomy versus video-assisted thoracoscopic surgery. *Am J Respir Crit Care Med* 155:A973.
22. Cooper JD, Patterson GA. (1995) Lung-volume reduction surgery for severe emphysema. *Chest Surg Clin North Am* 5:815–831.
23. Cooper JD, Patterson GA, Sundaresan RS, Trulock EP, Yusen RD, Pohl MS, et al. (1996) Results of 150 consecutive bilateral lung volume reduction procedures in patients with severe emphysema. *J Thorac Cardiovasc Surg* 112:1319-29.
24. Miller DL, Dowling RD, McConnell JW, Skolnick JL. (1996) Effects of lung volume reduction surgery on lung and chest wall mechanics. Presented at the 23rd Ann Mtg The Soc Thorac Surg; Jan 25–31, 1996; Orlando, FL.

25. Daniel TM, Chan BB, Bhaskar V, Parekh JS, Walters PE, Reeder J, et al. (1996) Lung volume reduction surgery: Case selection, operative technique, and clinical results. *Ann Surg* 223:526–531.

26. Argenziano M, Thomashow B, Jellen PA, Rose EA, Steinglass KM, Ginsburg ME, Gorenstein LA. (1997) A functional comparison of unilateral versus bilateral lung volume reduction surgery. Ann Thorac Surg 64:321–326, discussion 326–327.

27. Miller JI, Lee RB, Mansour KA. (1996) Lung volume reduction surgery: lessons learned. *Ann Thorac Surg* 61:1464–1469.

28. Bousamra M, Haasler GB, Lipchik RJ, et al. (1997) Functional and oximetric assessment of patients after lung reduction surgery. *J Thorac Cardiovasc Surg* 113:675–682.

29. Date H, Goto K, Souda R, et al. (1998) Bilateral lung volume reduction surgery via median sternotomy for severe pulmonary emphysema. *Ann Thorac Surg* 65:939–942.

30. Demertzis S, Wilkens H, Lindenmeir M, et al. (1998) Lung volume reduction surgery for severe emphysema. *J Cardiovasc Surg* 39:843–847.

31. Bagley PH, Davis SM, O'Shea M, et al. (1997) Lung volume reduction surgery at a community hospital: program development and outcomes. *Chest* 111:152–159.

9

Lung Volume Reduction Surgery
Video-Assisted Thoracoscopic Approaches

Joshua R. Sonett, MD *and Mark J. Krasna,* MD

LVRS: SURGICAL APPROACHES

Surgical approaches to lung volume reduction surgery (LVRS) continue to evolve and be debated along with the broader questions of the longevity, cost effectiveness, optimal selection criteria of this operation. Otto Brantigan's pioneering, and perhaps premature, work in LVRS described resection of 30% of the hyperinflated lung by thoracotomy *(1)*. However, at that time, advanced stapling devices, thoracic anesthesia, and intensive care practices were still in evolution and his patients succumbed to an unacceptably high mortality. Renewed acceptance of the procedure was heralded by the work of Cooper et al. *(2)*, who reported dramatic improvements in pulmonary function in patients undergoing bilateral simultaneous volume reduction surgery by median sternotomy, with resection of 30% of the each lung. Since then, surgeons have proven that the procedure can be performed safely and effectively either by sternotomy or by thoracoscopy.

Video-assisted LVRS was initially performed as a unilateral procedure, and with the use of the YAG laser *(3)*. Clinical experience with this approach quickly led to the use and adaptation of stapling devices and

From: *Lung Volume Reduction Surgery*
Edited by: M. Argenziano and M. E. Ginsburg © Humana Press Inc., Totowa, NJ

149

to simultaneous reduction of both lungs. Superiority of stapled lung reduction vs laser bullectomy was demonstrated by McKenna et al. *(4)*, in a prospective randomized trial. In this study, 72 patients were randomized to unilateral stapled reduction or neodymium: yttrium aluminum garnet (YAG) contact laser surgery. Although no significant difference was seen in operating time, hospital days, and air leakage, the mean postoperative improvement in FEV_1 was significantly greater for patients who received stapled reduction (32% vs 13%). The excellent results seen with the use of unilateral LVRS quickly led to the adaptation and wide-spread clinical implementation of simultaneous thoracoscopic volume reduction. Multiple clinical series have shown significantly greater gains in FEV_1, and 6-min walk parameters with bilateral volume reduction vs unilateral surgery, with no increase in morbidity or mortality, leading to the wide-spread implementation of the bilateral procedure *(5–7)*. Interestingly, the greater gains in postoperative function may not necessarily lead to superior long-term survival. In a large retrospective (multiinstitutional study involving 673 patients) no survival benefit could be found for bilateral thoracoscopic volume reduction vs unilateral thoracoscopic lung volume reduction *(8)*.

In more than 150 cases of LVRS at the University of Maryland, the surgical approach to LVRS has evolved from sternotomy and unilateral thoracoscopy, to bilateral thoracoscopic LVRS in the supine position. Our current technique described later involves bilateral LVRS in the supine position for the majority of patients. Patients with severely affected lower lobes and/or α-1 antitrypsin deficiency are approached in a sequential fashion, with unilateral procedures performed alternately in the right and left lateral decubitus position. Some authors advocate a bilateral anterior thoracosternotomy (clamshell incision) for these patients *(9)*. After intubation with a double-lumen tube, patients are positioned supine. The patient's arms are supported above the head utilizing an ether screen (see Fig. 1). The arms are carefully padded to protect ulnar nerves. Optimal positioning involves extending the humerus past the 90° position above the head to allow free access to and use of an axillary port. If this is not done, long thoracoscopic instruments cannot be fully maneuvered, as they will be impeded by the ether screen. The position of the three ports is depicted in Fig. 2. The ports are located in an elliptical arrangement around the inframammary crease. The camera port may be placed one interspace lower than depicted depending on the body habitus of the patient. The left-sided ports may be shifted laterally in patients with a large cardiac silhouette. The lung that is to be resected is grasped using the 5-mm axillary port and a conventional spongestick (without a sponge); great effort is made to

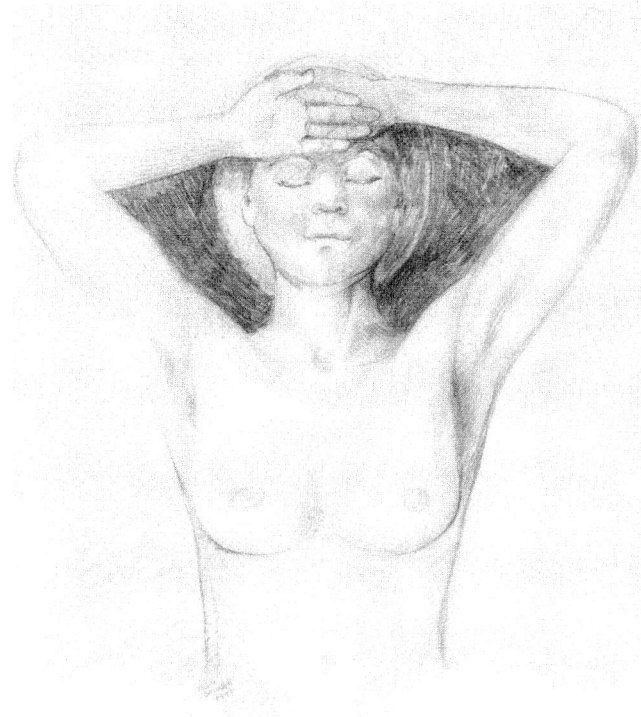

Fig. 1. Supine position for bilateral thoracoscopic approach to LVRS.

avoid grasping lung tissue that is not to be resected. Using the most medial inframammary port, an EZ-45 stapling device (Ethicon, Somerville, NJ) with buttressing material is then used to resect a large portion of the upper lobe. When using the EZ-45 stapler, a small 12-mm access incision is used rather than a complete thoracoscopic port, to allow passage of the oversized stapler head and buttress material. In general, we try to begin the stapling in a gradual fashion and progress to deeper parenchyma with each successive staple firing (see Fig. 3). The apex of the lung is resected by directing the stapler posteriorly at the level of the azygous vein. After the lung has been resected, it is always removed from the chest in a protected fashion using a sterile specimen bag (see Fig. 4). The final specimen can be seen in Fig. 5, and clearly resembles lung resected from an open sternotomy incision (see Fig. 6). After one side is completed, a single 28 Fr. chest tube is placed under direct vision through the lateral camera port trocar, the lung is reinflated, and the magnitude of air leak is assessed by connecting the chest tube to the pleural drainage system while the patient is still prepped and

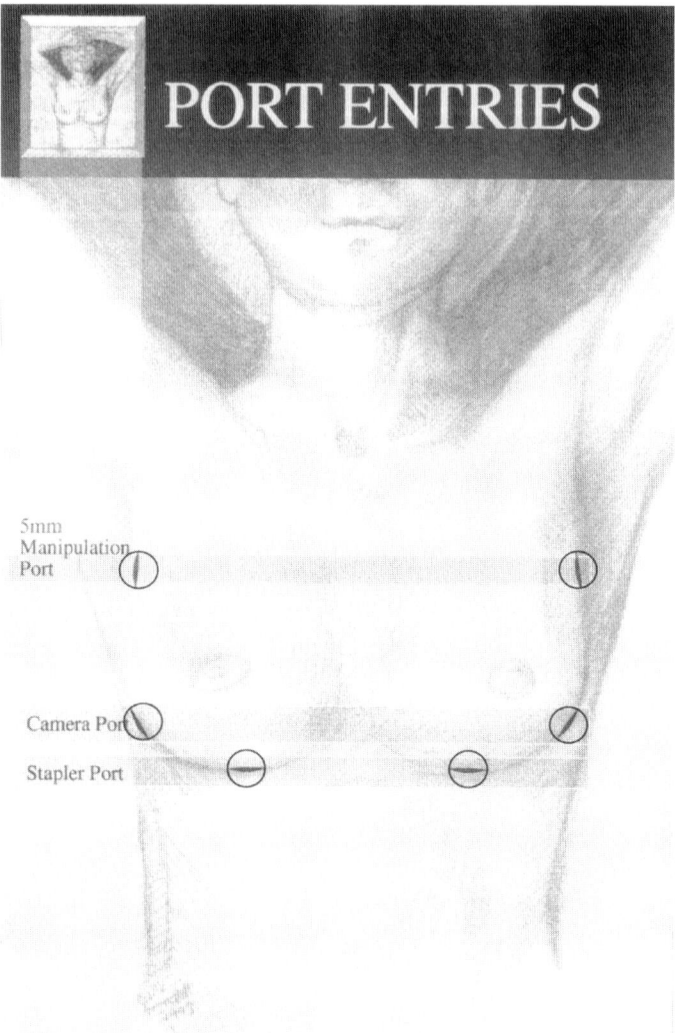

Fig. 2. Ports placement for supine bilateral LVRS.

sterile. If a large air leak is present, reassessment of the lung and staple line may be easily performed at that time. A similar procedure is then performed on the contralateral lung, and the patient is extubated in the operating room. Epidural pain control is used for all patients, and chest tubes are placed to water seal immediately. Patients immediately start chest physical therapy and are gotten out of bed at least once each shift.

The procedure can be performed in the full lateral decubitus position as well, using a standard three-port approach. Again, in this technique,

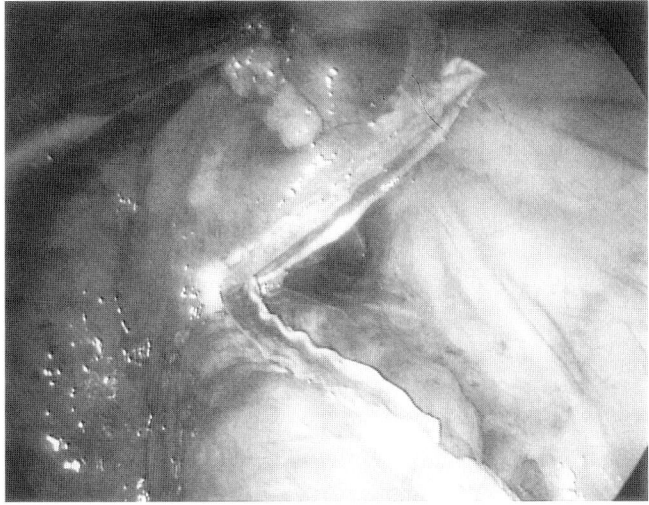

Fig. 3. Initial thoracoscopic staple line, phrenic nerve can be seen in mediastinum.

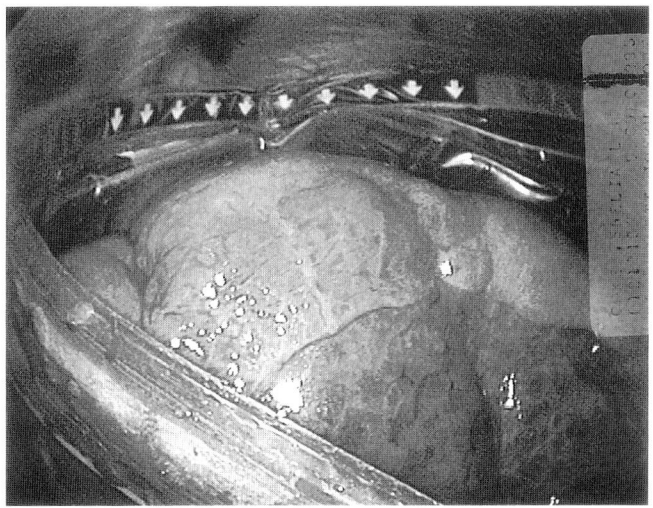

Fig. 4. Retrieval of lung specimen in protected bag.

a 5-mm port or access incision is placed superiorly for manipulation of lung tissue, a camera port is placed laterally, and the working stapling port is positioned in the inframammary crease in the anterior axillary line. This technique affords better access to the lower lobes, but requires repositioning and reprepping of the patient, adding a considerable amount of time to the procedure.

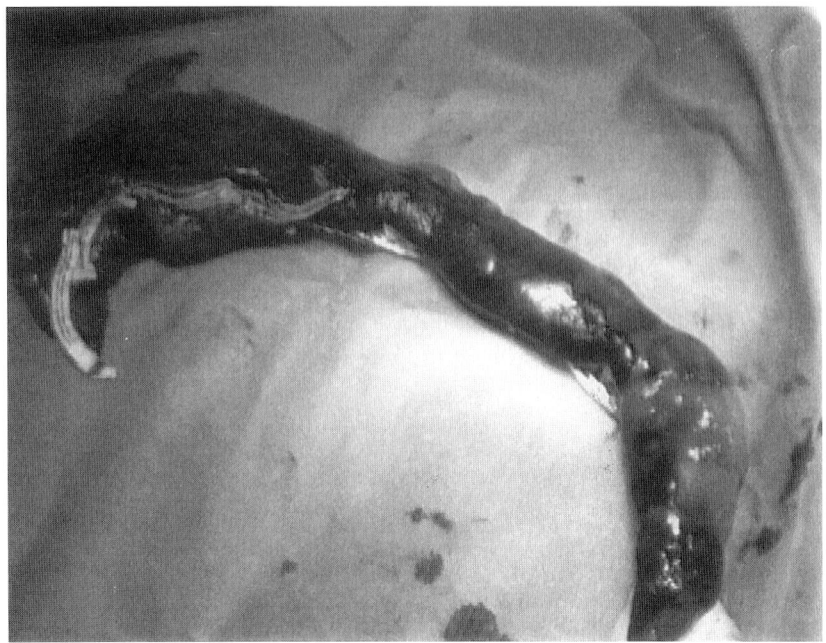

Fig. 5. Final specimen, showing complete extent of resection.

RESULTS

At the University of Maryland, the last 26 consecutive patients having LVRS for upper lobe predominant emphysema (all non-NETT and non-α antitrypsin deficiency patients) were operated on via the bilateral thoracoscopic approach in the supine position. The median length of hospital stay of the patients was 9 d, with a median ICU time of 2 d. Operating time averaged 119 min, and this included several patients with significant adhesions. FEV_1 increased from a mean of 25.3% of predicted to a mean of 38.3% of predicted, a relative increase of 58%. DLCO increased from an average of 31.2% of predicted to 42.0% of predicted, and the residual volume decreased from 250% of predicted to 175% of predicted. Fourteen of the 25 patients had an air leak lasting greater than 4 d, and one patient required thoracoscopic reexploration for hemothorax. There were two deaths in the series (7.6%): one from a cerebral hemorrhage on postoperative day 4, and one secondary to progressive postoperative pneumonia and respiratory failure.

DISCUSSION

Although the minimally invasive approach to LVRS is appealing and has now been performed by multiple institutions with excellent results, it has not clearly been shown to confer any advantage over median sternotomy. Proponents of median sternotomy note the technical ease of the incision and open procedure, and note that median sternotomy is an extremely well-tolerated incision in terms of pain and morbidity. In one retrospective study comparing a single institution's experience with sternotomy vs thoracoscopy, bilateral LVRS performed thoracoscopically offered equivalent functional outcome with potentially decreased morbidity and mortality (10). Presently, a prospective randomized trial at some centers in the NETT study is underway to more formally compare the two approaches. Critics of the thoracoscopic approach note the potential difficulty of VATS in the face of pleural adhesions. However, a recent review by Mineo et al. (11) demonstrated the feasibility of VATS LVRS in the presence of severe adhesions.

Other surgical issues that are independent of the surgical approach, but of significant import, include the volume of lung to be resected, and the need for pleural buttressing. Both in a rabbit model and in a clinical series, investigators at UC Irvine have attempted to address the amount of lung that should be resected during LVRS. In their clinical series they found a correlation between the amount of tissue resected (as measured in grams) and improvement in FEV_1 (12), with generally greater improvements in FEV_1 with greater volumes of lung resected. However, the better gains in FEV_1 were not translated into better long-term survival in this group, indicating factors other than the volume of resected lung play a part in the outcome after LVRS. A follow-up study by the same group using an animal model of emphysema may have offered some insight into their clinical observations, as larger resections of tissue in the animal model resulted in similar improvements in FEV_1, but decreases in DLCO (13). Thus, in some patients, the benefits derived from improved expiratory flow may, in fact, be limited by a concomitant worsening of diffusion capacity secondary to loss of pulmonary parenchyma. Another yet unanswered question regards the use of buttressed stapled lines to decrease air leaks, a practice which adds considerable expense to the procedure. A recent series by Stammberger et al. (14) presents 42 patients undergoing thoracoscopic LVRS in whom no such buttress was utilized. In this and another series in which no buttressing technique was used (15), the air leak rate and duration of chest tube duration was similar to that in series utilizing buttressed stapled lines. However, given the overall appeal and apparent logic of using buttressed stapled lines in these challenging patients, the abandonment of this technique will require further randomized studies supporting its exclusion during LVRS.

One of the most important advances in our management of patients undergoing thoracic surgical procedures has been the realization that air leaks can be managed conservatively. Accordingly, in current practice, patients are often discharged from the hospital even before complete resolution of air leaks, as long as the affected lung is expanded and the pleural space is adequately drained. Ambulatory pleural drainage has been facilitated by the use modalities such as the Heimlich valve. Numerous reports have now been published showing the efficacy of this approach, which is now widely utilized throughout the thoracic surgical community for non-LVRS patients.

REFERENCES

1. Brantigan OC, Mueller E (1957) Surgical treatment of pulmonary emphysema. *Am Surg* 23: 789–804.
2. Cooper JD, Trulock RP, Triantafillou AN, et al. (1995) Bilateral pneumectomy (volume reduction) for chronic obstructive pulmonary disease. *J Thorac Cardiovasc Surg* 109: 106–116.
3. Wakabayashi A, Brenner A, Kagaleh R, et al. (1991) Thoracoscopic carbon dioxide laser treatment of bullous emphysema. *Lancet* 337: 881–883.
4. McKenna RJ Jr., Brenner M, Fischel RJ, et al. (1996) Should lung volume reduction surgery be unilateral or bilateral? *J Thorac Cardiovasc Surg* 112: 1331–1339.
5. Serna DL, Brenner M, Osann KE, et. al. (1999) Survival after unilateral versus bilateral lung volume reduction surgery for emphysema. *J Thorac Cardiovasc Surg* 118: 1101–1109.
6. Hazelrigg SR, Boley TM, Grasch A, Shawgo T. (1999) Surgical strategy for lung volume reduction surgery. *Eur J Cardiothorac Surg* 16 Suppl 1:S57–S60.
7. Klepetok W. (1999) Surgical aspects and techniques of lung volume reduction surgery for severe emphysema. *Eur Respir J* 13(4): 919–925.
8. Naunheim KS, Kaiser LR, Bavaria JE, et al. (1999) Long-term survival after thoracoscopic lung volume reduction: a multiinstitutional review. *Ann Thorac Surg* 68(6): 2026–2031; discussion 2031–2032.
9. Argenziano M, Moazami N, Thomashaw B, Weinberg AD, Edsall J, Yip C, Prager KM, Gorenstein LA, Rose EA, Steinglass KM, Ginsburg ME (1996) Extended indications for lung volume reduction surgery in advanced emphysema. *Ann Thorac Surg* 62:1588–1597.
10. Roberts JR, Bavaria JE, Wahl P, et al. (1998) Comparison of open and thoracoscopic bilateral volume reduction surgery: complications analysis. *Ann Thorac Surg* 66(5): 1759–1765.
11. Mineo TC, Pompeo E, Rogliani P, et al. (1999) Thoracoscopic reduction pneumoplasty for severe emphysema: do pleural adhesions affect outcome? *Thorac Cardiovasc Surg* 47(5): 288–292.
12. Brenner M, McKenna RJ Jr, Chen JC, et al. (2000) Relationship between amount of lung resected and outcome after lung volume reduction surgery. *Ann Thorac Surg* 69(2): 388–393.
13. Chen J, Brenner M, Huh J, et al. (1998) Effect of lung volume reduction surgery on pulmonary diffusion capacity in a rabbit model of emphysema. *J Surg Res* 78: 155–160.

14. Stammberger UZ, Thurnheer R, Konrad E, et al, (1997) Thoracoscopic bilateral lung volume reduction for diffuse pulmonary emphysema. *Eur J Cardio Thorac Surg* 11: 1005–1010.
15. Naunheim KS, Keller CA, Singh A, et al. (1996) Unilateral video-assisted thoracic surgical lung reduction. *Ann Thorac Surg* 61: 1092–1098; Brantigan OC, Mueller E. (1957) Surgical treatment of pulmonary emphysema. *Am Surg* 23: 789–804.

10 Anesthetic Management of the Patient Undergoing Lung Volume Reduction Surgery

Ellise S. Delphin, MD, MPH

CONTENTS

INTRODUCTION
PREOPERATIVE EVALUATION
THE DAY OF SURGERY
POSTOPERATIVE PAIN MANAGEMENT
REFERENCES

INTRODUCTION

Advances in monitoring, equipment, pharmacologic agents, and perioperative pain management over the past 10 yr have provided the anesthesiologist with new clinical tools, allowing fine adjustment of care to critically ill patients undergoing surgery. The postoperative survival and well being of the patient undergoing lung volume reduction surgery (LVRS) continues to improve owing to perioperative clinical advances. Continuous monitoring of oxygen saturation and end-tidal carbon dioxide allow continual adjustment of intraoperative ventilation. Short-acting anesthetic agents have improved the possibility of early extubation. Intra- and postoperative pain control can be managed on an individual basis in order to optimize ventilation. These changes in clinical management have prevented complications and improved outcome in this critically ill population.

From: *Lung Volume Reduction Surgery*
Edited by: M. Argenziano and M. E. Ginsburg © Humana Press Inc., Totowa, NJ

PREOPERATIVE EVALUATION

From an anesthetic perspective, patients with end-stage pulmonary disease are unstable, even with optimal medical therapy for their disease. Unfortunately, our ability to correctly identify patients at high risk for deterioration during and after surgery remains limited. Preoperative evaluation of LVRS patients is optimally performed within 2 wk of the planned procedure, with reevaluation on the day of surgery. The preoperative visit is a time for patient evaluation, as well as instruction.

A careful history and physical examination are routine parts of any preoperative anesthetic evaluation. A history of previous general anesthetics, and, in particular, any difficulty with intubation or emergence from general anesthesia is noted. Airway anatomy is evaluated by the usual Mallampati criteria. Preoperative respiratory evaluation allows assessment of baseline breathing, laboratory values, and respiratory capacity. Attention to the degree of bullous disease, hyperinflation, bronchospasm, and resting oxygen requirements will allow preoperative plans to focus on problems that may occur during the period of anesthesia. This information is especially critical to the management of ventilation during the procedure and at the time of emergence and extubation. Preoperative blood gas analysis, in particular the degree of hypercarbia, may provide some guidelines for expectations at the time of extubation. All preoperative medications are noted at this time and the patient should be instructed to continue these up to the morning of surgery. Bronchodilators, steroids, and cardiac medications may need to be administered during the procedure and should be consistent with the patients prior therapeutic regimen. Landmarks for monitoring lines and the epidural catheter are noted during the physical examination *(1–4)*.

Evaluation of the cardiovascular system will often reveal primary disease or disease as a complication of respiratory failure. Coronary artery disease is common in this patient population because of advanced age and shared risk factors with emphysema. The nature and stability of ischemic disease must be evaluated with attention to left ventricular function. Pulmonary hypertension secondary to end-stage pulmonary disease, with or without associated right ventricular failure, is common and may require additional intra- and postoperative monitoring *(5,6)*.

Patient instruction begins with a discussion of the preinduction period. The patient is reminded to maintain all preoperative medication in their usual doses until the morning of surgery. An explanation of all required monitoring, including arterial, central venous, and Swan-Ganz catheters, as well as transesophageal echocardiography is given. If thoracic epidural analgesia is to be used, an explanation of awake catheter insertion and patient-controlled analgesia is given. Detailed instruction about the need for early postextubation, concentration on deep breathing, coughing, and incentive spirometry are included with emphasis on the need for early ambulation and postoperative pulmonary rehabilitation.

THE DAY OF SURGERY
Immediate Preinduction Management

Successful management of the patient undergoing LVRS requires the availability of specialized equipment. The anesthesia machine must be able to deliver long expiratory times and high gas flows, and include a mechanical ventilator that can provide pressure-controlled ventilation. An I:E ratio no greater than 1:3 (and often lower, with very long expiratory time) is necessary to prevent air trapping, pneumothorax and the development of auto-PEEP with its deleterious hemodynamic effects. Pressure-controlled ventilation will limit the possibility of air leaks and pneumothorax during the entire procedure. Fiberoptic bronchoscopy is a necessity in assuring proper placement of the double-lumen endotracheal tube. Breath sounds in the patient with emphysema and hyperinflation are often inaudible and serve as an inaccurate guide to tube placement.

Standard monitoring equipment, as recommended in the American Society of Anesthesiologists Standards for Intraoperative Monitoring, is required. Minimal mandatory additional monitoring includes an indwelling arterial catheter for continuous monitoring of arterial blood pressure and intermittent blood gas analysis. Central venous catheterization may be necessary for either vascular access or the administration of vasoactive medication that cannot be administered through a peripheral line. Patients with significant pulmonary hypertension, right or left ventricular dysfunction, or ischemic heart disease require a Swan-Ganz catheter and perhaps transesophageal echocardiography.

Immediately prior to the induction of anesthesia, there are several considerations to be made. Narcotics and sedatives producing respiratory depression should be withheld as they may prolong the time to extubation at the end of the procedure. Prophylactic antibiotics are given prior to incision. Perioperative steroid administration is utilized in the patient population receiving preoperative steroids. Deep vein thrombosis prophylaxis is initiated. A fluid bolus is considered in order to prevent the development of hypotension on induction. The hypotension may be worsened by a test dose of local anesthetic that has been administered after epidural placement. The decision as to whether to administer fluid or vasopressor is dependent upon the necessity of controlling fluid administration and is patient-specific *(7)*.

Induction of Anesthesia

The choice of an anesthetic induction agent is, as always, determined by the medical condition of the patient about to undergo surgery. LVRS patients are often cachectic, hypovolemic and many have cardiac disease. Although no specific agent has been scientifically proven to be superior in this patient population, low doses of agents that maintain hemodynamic stability have been successfully used. In particular, slow titration of propofol or etomidate seem to provide hemodynamic stability in this setting. Hypotension remains a significant problem during induction because of the side effects of pharmacologic agents and the initiation of positive pressure ventilation. α-agonist agents represent a rapid antidote to this complication. Muscle relaxants should be chosen with the same hemodynamic goals in mind, and in addition should be of intermediate duration of action and easily reversible.

Positive pressure ventilation, prior to intubation, begins in a controlled manner. In order to prevent an increase in air trapping (which may cause hypotension caused by decreasing venous return), the ratio of inspiration to expiration should be no higher than 1:3. In addition, limitation of the peak inspiratory pressure is necessary to prevent pneumothorax. In fact, the abrupt development of cardiovascular collapse during induction should raise the suspicion of tension pneumothorax, particularly if the hypotension is unresponsive to volume infusion and vasopressor administration. The diagnosis of this entity may be challenging because of the extreme difficulty associated with auscultation of the lungs in severe emphysema.

A left-sided double-lumen endotracheal tube is placed in order to allow selective lung ventilation. This will improve surgical exposure for either a median sternotomy or video assisted thoracoscopic (VATS) approach. It is also important to allow for selective ventilation if persistent air leaks develop intraoperatively. As aforementioned, confirmation of tube position is most accurately accomplished by fiberoptic bronchoscopy, as auscultion of breath sounds is unreliable (8).

Maintenance of Anesthesia

The anesthetic plan for maintenance is formulated with the goal of extubation of the patient in the operating room at the end of the procedure. Total intravenous anesthesia, as well as inhalational agents have been used successfully. Intermediate-acting muscle relaxants that are easily reversible are recommended. The intraoperative use of the thoracic epidural catheter in patients undergoing median sternotomy allows the anesthesiologist to moderate the amount of intravenous or inhalational agent used during the procedure. The intravenous administration of any narcotic, with the exception of those that are ultrashort-acting, must be limited in order to avoid postoperative respiratory depression. Local anesthetics or a combination of local anesthetic and narcotic delivered via the thoracic epidural catheter will allow the patient to emerge pain free and without respiratory depression. The absence of pain and respiratory depression are necessary to ensure successful extubation.

The management of intraoperative ventilation is based on the principles discussed earlier in the induction section. Peak inspiratory pressure must be limited to below 20 cm H_2O to avoid the development of air leaks and pneumothorax. Long expiratory times will prevent air trapping and the development of auto-positive-end-expiratory pressure (PEEP). This combination often leads to hypoventilation and a rise in an already elevated arterial concentration of carbon dioxide. Permissive hypercapnia is necessary to avoid the complications of more aggressive ventilatory management.

It is obviously difficult to maintain adequate ventilation under positive pressure in this severely compromised group of patients with end-stage pulmonary disease. One-lung ventilation compromises pulmonary function even further, as there is no ventilatory reserve. In addition, measures usually employed to treat hypoxemia and hypercarbia during one-lung ventilation may worsen the patient's status rather than improve it. Conventional therapy for the treatment of hypoxia during one-lung ventilation is the application of continuous positive airway pressure (CPAP) to the operative lung and/or PEEP to the ventilated lung. Continuous positive pressure applied to the emphysematous lung will result in significant air trapping, a rise in pulmonary artery pressure and decreased venous return resulting in worsening of both pulmonary and cardiovascular function. Hypoxia may worsen, air leaks may develop, hypercarbia may increase, and hypotension can result. For reasons aforementioned, application of positive-end expiratory pressure cannot be recommended in this population.

Hypoxia and hypercarbia must be tolerated to the greatest degree possible during one-lung ventilation. When treatment is necessary, gentle reinflation of the nonventilated lung with 100% oxygen will restore the oxygen saturation to its preincision value. The lung may be collapsed again and reinflated when hypoxia recurs. At the end of the procedure, the lung is reinflated gently, limiting peak inspiratory pressures to less than 20 cm H_2O in an effort to prevent the development of air leaks. During reinflation, it is helpful to clamp the tube serving the opposite lung in order to limit overall exposure to positive pressure.

The maintenance of normothermia will decrease both intraoperative and postoperative oxygen requirements. Warm air blankets and delivery of warm intravenous fluids will help maintain temperature at nearly normal values. The prevention of postoperative shivering and its early treatment, if it occurs, are key to limiting oxygen demand after extubation.

Emergence

The goal is to extubate the patient undergoing LVRS in the operating room at the conclusion of the surgical procedure. Extubation at this time will contribute to the success of the procedure by decreasing the development of airleaks and avoiding the deleterious hemodynamic effects of positive pressure ventilation. There are several therapeutic maneuvers that provide valuable assistance in extubating LVRS patients:

1. Pain relief;
2. Bronchodilation;
3. Pulmonary toilet;
4. Perioperative steroids;
5. Lowering the inspired concentration of oxygen to maintain saturation at about 90%.

Pain relief will prevent splinting, atelectasis, and the inability to clear secretions. The use of epidural local anesthetics and narcotics in the sternotomy patient or nerve blocks in the VATS patient should begin during wound closure in the operating room in order to ensure adequate respiratory efforts upon awakening. Although no protocol for emergence has been scientifically shown to be superior during these cases, the absence of pain is integral to the success of extubation.

Bronchodilation with intravenous agents such as aminophylline or inhaled agents prior to extubation and continuing postoperatively is crucial. The surgery is only palliative, and in the perioperative period, the remaining diseased lung tissue will require an armamentarium of medications similar to that preoperatively.

The work of breathing may be effectively reduced in the perioperative period by steroids (which reduce airway inflammation and edema) as well as vigorous pulmonary toilet (which improved air flow by clearing secretions). In addition, lowering the inspired oxygen concentration to maintain saturations at 90% will serve to maintain respiratory drive in the population of patients who are chronically hypoxemic and hypercarbic. Noninvasive BiPAP may be used postextubation if the $PaCO_2$ climbs to over 70 mmHg.

It is most important to recognize that the standard criteria employed in order to determine a patient's readiness for extubation are difficult, if not impossible, to utilize in this patient population. In LVRS patients, tidal volumes are often no greater than 300 mL, oxygen saturation may fall between 85–90%, and end tidal CO_2 is often greater than 60 mmHg. Accordingly, a key criterion for extubation in this high-risk group is the ability of the patient to remain awake and comfortable with the use of the supportive measures discussed earlier *(9)*.

POSTOPERATIVE PAIN MANAGEMENT

Postoperative management of incisional pain after LVRS is an integral part of the anesthetic management and is of particular importance in this patient population *(10,11)*. Thoracotomy or sternotomy result in severe pain and significant changes in pulmonary physiology. The pain is a result of the chest wall incision, periosteal irritation of the ribs, pleural and parenchymal resection, and chest tube irritation *(12,13)*. Inadequate control of pain in the early postoperative period will result in poor respiratory effort, inadequate ventilation, and impaired ability to cough and clear airway secretions *(10,14,15)*. The high-risk patients presenting for LVRS are predisposed to the development of atelectasis, hypoxemia, ventilation-perfusion mismatching, and pneumonitis, with alterations in postoperative breathing patterns. Effective pain management is vital to the success of this operative procedure and will improve comfort, decrease complications, and shorten hospital stay.

Traditionally, either systemic or regional medications have been used in the management of postoperative pain. The postoperative analgesic regimen must be tailored to the goals of early postoperative care, which include early ambulation, use of incentive spirometry, breathing techniques, and chest physiotherapy. The use of thoracic epidural analgesia has been widely recommended for LVRS performed by median sternotomy *(9)*. The data for postoperative analgesia for the patient group undergoing the procedure by VATS is less clear and systemic opioids or intercostal nerve blocks have been found to provide satisfactory pain relief *(11)*.

Systemic opioids are often difficult to manage because of their narrow therapeutic margin and the large degree of preoperative cardiopulmonary dysfunction in this patient population. Ideally, the drug should be administered by continuous infusion, have a short duration of action and few side effects. In general, the somnolence and respiratory depression caused by morphine and meperidine preclude their use in this population *(16)*. Fentanyl administered via patient-controlled analgesia (PCA) provides a reasonable alternative with its short duration of action and fewer side effects. NSAIDS are often used as adjuncts to systemic narcotics as they are potent and safe if used for a short period of time *(17–19)*. Prolonged use can result in platelet dysfunction, gastrointestinal bleeding, and reversible renal failure.

Intercostal neuronal blockade techniques can provide significant postoperative analgesia by interruption of the anterior rami of the spinal root *(20)*. The block is easy to perform, reliable and has the advantage of having few central nervous system or cardiovascular side effects. Although high levels of systemic absorption have been a concern, clinical studies of patients undergoing thoracotomy have documented safe plasma levels of local anesthetic. Single preclosure injections seem to have little value. Indwelling catheters permit either bolus injection or continuous infusion of local anesthetic, narcotic or a combination of the two *(21,22)*. There have been no clinical studies evaluating the use of intercostal blockade in patients undergoing LVRS via a thoracotomy technique. The blocks obviously have no place in pain relief after sternotomy or VATS. Clinical studies evaluating these blocks as an adjunct to systemic opioids have found the blocks to be highly effective and a valuable alternative to thoracic epidural analgesia when conditions preclude its use. The existing literature recommends the use of bupivacaine 0.5% with epinephrine by bolus or continuous infusion or 0.25% bupivacaine by continuous infusion *(23,24)*.

Thoracic epidural analgesia remains the most highly recommended technique for the relief of thoracotomy or sternotomy pain post LVRS *(9,11)*. The administration of a combination of opioids and local anesthetics will enhance the effect of both drugs at a lower dosage thereby avoiding side effects *(25)*. The catheter is placed and tested prior to the induction of anesthesia in the T4-5 or T5-6 interspace. At some institutions catheter position is confirmed by fluoroscopy prior to surgical incision. Adequate analgesia is crucial during emergence in order to ensure successful extubation at the conclusion of surgery. Early extubation may reduce the incidence and severity of airleaks and reduce the hemodynamic problems associated with mechanical ventilation in this patient population. Pulmonary and physical rehabilitation and early ambulation required to prevent respiratory complications cannot occur without adequate pain relief in the postoperative period. The LVRS patient continues to have chronic hypoxemia and hypercarbia postoperatively and is often extremely sensitive to either epidural local anesthetic or opioid administration. Low concentrations of bupivacaine (0.0625%) delivered by continuous infusion will spare motor function, provide analgesia, and preserve hemodynamics *(26)*. If sympathetic blockade produces hypotension, volume infusion may be necessary. In the fluid-restricted patient, the use of vasoconstrictors, such as phenylephrine, may be required. The lipophilic short-acting narcotic, fentanyl, can be added to the bupivacaine solution. Bupivacaine causes a dose-dependent decrease in the narcotic requirement to achieve pain control. The combination of bupivacaine (0.0625%) with fentanyl (2 mcg/mL) has been used extensively in LVRS patients postoperatively with excellent analgesia, no respiratory depression, and hemodynamic stability. These are the crucial elements of successful pain control in the immediate postoperative period.

REFERENCES

1. Cottrell JJ, Ferson PF (1992) Preoperative assessment of the thoracic surgical patient. *Clin Chest Med* 13: 47–53.
2. Preoperative pulmonary function testing. American College of Physicians. (1990) *Ann Intern Med* 112: 793–794.
3. Yusen RD, Lefrak SS, Trulock EP (1997) Evaluation and preoperative management of lung volume reduction surgery candidates. *Clin Chest Med* 18:199–224.
4. McKenna RJ Jr, Brenner M, Fischel RJ, Singh N, Yoong B, Gelb AF, Osann KE (1997) Patient selection criteria for lung volume reduction surgery. *J Thorac Cardiovasc Surg* 114: 957–967.
5. Thurnheer R, Muntwyler J, Stammberger U, Bloch KE, Zollinger A, Weder W, Russi EW (1997) Coronary artery disease in patients undergoing lung volume reduction surgery for emphysema. *Chest* 112: 122–128.
6. Bossone E, Martinez FJ, Whyte RI, Iannettoni MD, Armstrong WF, Bach DS (1999) Dobutamine stress echocardiography for the preoperative evaluation of patients undergoing lung volume reduction surgery. *J Thorac Cardiovasc Surg* 118: 542–546.
7. Krucylak PE, Naunheim KS, Keller CA, Baudendistel LJ (1996) Anesthetic management of patients undergoing unilateral video-assisted lung reduction for treatment of end-stage emphysema. *J Cardiothorac Vasc Anesth* 10: 850–853.
8. Zollinger A, Zaugg M, Weder W, Russi EW, Blumenthal S, Zalunardo MP, Stoehr S, Thurnheer R, Stammberger U, Spahn DR, Pasch T (1997) Video-assisted thoracoscopic volume reduction surgery in patients with diffuse pulmonary emphysema: gas exchange and anesthesiological management. *Anesth Analg* 84: 845–851.
9. Triantafillou AN (1996) Anesthetic management for bilateral volume reduction surgery. *Semin Thorac Cardiovasc Surg* 8: 94–98.
10. Kalso E, Perttunen K, Kaasinen S (1992) Pain after thoracic surgery. *Acta Anaesthesiol Scand* 36: 96–100.
11. Mulder DS (1993) Pain management principles and anesthesia techniques for thoracoscopy. *Ann Thorac Surg* 56: 630–632.
12. Richardson J, Sabanathan S, Mearns AJ, Evans CS, Bembridge J, Fairbrass M (1994) Efficacy of pre-emptive analgesia and continuous extrapleural intercostal nerve block on post-thoracotomy pain and pulmonary mechanics. *J Cardiovasc Surg* (Torino) 35: 219–228.
13. Stevens DS, Edwards WT (1991) Management of pain after thoracic surgery. In Kaplan SA, Ed. *Thoracic Anesthesia, 2nd Edition*, New York: Churchill Livingstone, pp. 563–591.
14. Johnson WC (1975) Postoperative ventilatory performance: dependence upon surgical incision. *Am Surg* 41: 615–619.
15. Shulman M, Sandler AN, Bradley JW, Young PS, Brebner J (1984) Postthoracotomy pain and pulmonary function following epidural and systemic morphine. *Anesthesiology* 61: 569–575.
16. Kavanagh BP, Katz J, Sandler AN (1994) Pain control after thoracic surgery. A review of current techniques. *Anesthesiology* 81: 737–759.
17. Dahl JB, Kehlet H (1991) Non-steroidal anti-inflammatory drugs: rationale for use in severe postoperative pain. *Br J Anaesth* 66: 703–712.

18. Pavy T, Medley C, Murphy DF (1990) Effect of indomethacin on pain relief after thoracotomy. *Br J Anaesth* 65: 624–627.
19. Rhodes M, Conacher I, Morritt G, Hilton C (1992) Nonsteroidal antiinflammatory drugs for postthoracotomy pain. A prospective controlled trial after lateral thoracotomy. *J Thorac Cardiovasc Surg* 103: 17–20.
20. Sabanathan S, Smith PJ, Pradhan GN, Hashimi H, Eng JB, Mearns AJ (1988) Continuous intercostal nerve block for pain relief after thoracotomy. *Ann Thorac Surg* 46: 425–426.
21. Eng J, Sabanathan S (1991) Site of action of continuous extrapleural intercostal nerve block. *Ann Thorac Surg* 51: 387–389.
22. Richardson J, Sabanathan S, Eng J, Mearns AJ, Rogers C, Evans CS, Bembridge J, Majid MR (1993) Continuous intercostal nerve block versus epidural morphine for postthoracotomy analgesia. *Ann Thorac Surg* 55: 377–380.
23. Majid AA, Hamzah H (1992) Pain control after thoracotomy. An extrapleural tunnel to provide a continuous bupivacaine infusion for intercostal nerve blockade. *Chest* 101: 981–984.
24. Deneuville M, Bisserier A, Regnard JF, Chevalier M, Levasseur P, Herve P (1993) Continuous intercostal analgesia with 0.5% bupivacaine after thoracotomy: a randomized study. *Ann Thorac Surg* 55:381–385.
25. Burgess FW, Anderson DM, Colonna D, Cavanaugh DG (1994) Thoracic epidural analgesia with bupivacaine and fentanyl for postoperative thoracotomy pain. *J Cardiothorac Vasc Anesth* 8: 420–424.
26. Liu S, Angel JM, Owens BD, Carpenter RL, Isabel L (1995) Effects of epidural bupivacaine after thoracotomy. *Reg Anesth* 20: 303–310.

11 Perioperative and Nursing Care of the LVRS Patient

Patricia A. Jellen, MSN, RN
and Frances Brogan, MSN, RN

CONTENTS

INTRODUCTION

The care of the lung volume reduction surgery (LVRS) patient relies on the expertise and skills of a multidisciplinary team consisting of nurses, physical therapists, respiratory therapists, social workers, nutritionists, and psychiatrists as well as physicians from the surgical, pulmonary, and anesthesia teams. The care of these patients can be challenging even to the most experienced health care provider. Education about the surgical procedure and postoperative care begins at the time of initial evaluation and is reinforced by all members of the team. Preparation for surgery should include discussions with the patient and family members about the risks and potential complications of the procedure, postoperative care, issues surrounding the health care proxy, the pulmonary rehabilitation program, and discharge planning.

From: *Lung Volume Reduction Surgery*
Edited by: M. Argenziano and M. E. Ginsburg © Humana Press Inc., Totowa, NJ

Before discussing the postoperative care of the LVRS patient, it is imperative to review the preoperative rehabilitation program. All surgical candidates are required to complete at least 6 wk of a comprehensive outpatient pulmonary rehabilitation program prior to surgery. Multiple studies have demonstrated that patients suffering from emphysema have decreased levels of physical activity and are very deconditioned (1). It is the goal of rehabilitation to increase exercise endurance and strength, optimizing the preoperative physical condition in order to reduce postoperative complications and hasten recovery. The program should include endurance training, muscle strengthening, airway clearance techniques, breathing retraining, relaxation techniques, and correct use of bronchodilator medications. It is during these sessions that the preoperative teaching is initiated and reinforced. The patient is evaluated for his or her commitment to the exercise program and potential for compliance with the postoperative protocol. It is clearly explained to the patient and family that the postoperative course will be intense and require a significant amount of work by the patient.

PERIOPERATIVE CARE

The patient is admitted the morning of surgery through the ambulatory surgery unit and escorted to the operating room with one family member. The preoperative preparation requires that the patient be NPO since midnight the night before surgery and that they shower the morning of surgery. Patients are instructed to take all medications as directed and to bring their bronchodilators to the hospital in case they need a treatment while being prepared for surgery.

Once in the holding area, the patient is attended to by an anesthesiologist who routinely inserts a large bore peripheral intravenous line and an arterial line, which is used for monitoring arterial blood pressure and arterial blood gases (ABG). A thoracic epidural catheter is placed to assist in intraoperative and postoperative pain management. To ensure accurate assessment of intake and output, a Foley catheter is inserted using sterile technique. Once moved to the operating room, the patient is intubated with a double-lumen endotracheal tube (1,2).

Positioning on the operating room table is dependent on the type of incision that will be utilized by the surgeon. Approaches used for LVRS include median sternotomy, transternal bilateral thoracotomy (clamshell), thoracotomy, or video-assisted thoracoscopic surgery (VATS).

Median Sternotomy

The patient is positioned by the operating room staff in the supine position on the table with the arms either abducted and placed on side boards or safely secured at the patient's side *(3)*. The incision generally extends in the midline from the suprasternal notch to a point just below the xyphoid process.

Transternal Bilateral Thoracotomy (Clamshell)

The patient is positioned supine with the arms abducted on arm boards. The incision generally extends from one midaxillary line to the other, across the anterior aspect of the chest at the level of the fourth intercostal space *(3)*.

Thoracotomy

The patient is positioned in the lateral decubitus position. The legs are separated by a pillow with the lower leg flexed at the knee and hip; the upper leg lies straight on top of the pillow *(3)*. The lower arm is either placed on an arm board at a right angle to the table or flexed at the elbow and placed beside the head. The upper arm is rotated forward and allowed to rest on an armboard or to hang over the operating room table, provided that it is supported by adequate padding.

Thorascopic Approach

For sequential unilateral VATS, the patient is placed in the lateral decubitus position. Once the procedure on the first side is complete, the patient is repositioned in the contralateral decubitus position for the second part of the procedure. For simultaneous bilateral VATS, the patient is positioned supine with the arms raised above the head in a flexed position. This approach usually requires three to five small incisions, which are made over each hemithorax for the entry of the thoracoscope and operating instruments. The specific number and the exact location of incision sites are modified as needed to provide maximal access for the best possible resection. For a more detailed discussion of these issues, *see* Chapter 9.

Regardless of the surgical approach, special attention must be paid to the care of the bony prominences when positioning the patient. The staff should pad the elbows, hips, knees, heels, and shoulders as needed. The operating room staff also needs to utilize body warming techniques in order to avoid postoperative hypothermia or shivering.

After the incision is closed, the anesthesiologist begins to awaken the patient in preparation for extubation. Treatment should be focused on maintaining adequate pain control while maximizing the patient's respiratory capacity. This period is considered by many to be most critical in postoperative management of these patients. Once extubated, the postoperative patient is transferred to the intensive care unit. A portable X-ray is performed prior to transfer to the intensive care unit (ICU) to evaluate the degree of lung expansion and to assess mediastinal position.

A small percentage of postoperative LVRS patients require ventilation during the early period after transfer to the ICU. If a specific patient cannot be extubated immediately postoperatively, the goal remains to aggressively wean ventilatory support, with the highest priority being early extubation.

POSTOPERATIVE NURSING CARE

When considering the postoperative care of the chronic obstructive pulmonary disease (COPD) patient, it is imperative to recognize the major causes of death following any pulmonary resection. Ginsberg et al. documented the causes of death after pulmonary resection: pneumonia and respiratory failure; bronchopleural fistula and empyema; myocardial infarction; and pulmonary embolism *(4)*. Recognition of these facts (coupled with research that documents patients with poor pulmonary reserve are at increased risk for complications) guides the care that the staff must render to patients undergoing LVRS. Emphysema patients undergoing LVRS approach the operating room at significant risk for postoperative complications. In order to properly care for the patient, it is imperative that the nursing staff recognizes the potential risk of each of these complications (*see* Table 1) *(5–13)*. In the following sections, system-specific protocols for management of the LVRS patient will be discussed individually.

Cardiopulmonary System

The patient is monitored continually in the ICU with blood pressure, oxygen saturation and telemetry readings for the first 24 h or until stable. For patient comfort and easy access, it is recommended that arterial line be maintained for frequent arterial blood gas analysis and pressure monitoring. It is usually recommended that the blood gases be monitored closely until the pCO_2 is less than 60 mmHg *(1)*. Vital signs should be initially monitored at least hourly. Hypotension is commonly seen in these patients. It should be treated appropriately with fluids or vasopressors. Further assessment for bleeding should include daily monitoring of the CBC until the chest tube output has decreased and the hematocrit is stable. Telemetry monitoring should be employed until the patient is transferred out of the step-down unit, with close attention paid to any changes in cardiac rhythm, since atrial fibrillation is a common complication in these patients. All changes in pulse rate and reported palpitations should be evaluated with an EKG and followed by the medical staff. Routinely, LVRS patients are treated preoperatively with digoxin 0.125 mg daily to help minimize the occurrence of these events. Pneu-

Table 1
Potential Complications of LVRS

System	Complication
Respiratory	Prolonged air leak
	Pneumonia
	Reintubation
	Prolonged ventilator support with tracheostomy
	Bleeding resulting in a pleural tent
	Diaphragmatic paralysis
	Pulmonary embolism
	Empyema
Neurological	CVA
	TIA
Gastrointestinal	GI Bleed
	Cecal perforation
Cardiac	Arrthymia
	Myocardial infarction
Genitourinary	Urinary retention
	Urinary tract infection
Integumentary	Infection
	-Wound
	-Epidural site
	-Phlebitis

matic compression or other antiembolic stockings should be utilized to help prevent deep vein thrombosis.

Respiratory System

The patient is usually admitted to the ICU with four chest tubes on waterseal. In the first 24 h, chest X-rays are performed every 4 h and as needed. After this time, the patient receives a daily chest X-ray to evaluate lung reexpansion. Chest tubes are discontinued sequentially based on the chest films. Chest tube output and the presence of air leaks and crepitus should be evaluated every hour in the immediate postoperative period and at least every 8 h thereafter. Excessive output (>100 cm^3/h) or presence of a new air leak or crepitus should be reported to the medical staff immediately. The patient's respiratory status should be monitored if a new air leak is noted, with particular attention paid to the oxygen saturation and chest X-ray. Suction (-10 cm H_2O) is only applied if the following criteria are met: $> 30\%$ pneumothorax; inability to maintain an oxygen saturation $> 90\%$ after adequate pain control, chest physical therapy and bronchodilation therapy; or significant subcutaneous emphysema (1). Chest tube dressings are changed every 48–72 h.

Each time a change occurs involving the chest tube system (i.e., discontinuance of a chest tube, change to/from suction/water seal) the staff needs to make more frequent assessments of the patient's respiratory status. Reports of increased dyspnea with increased oxygen requirements necessitate immediate nursing intervention and notification of the medical staff. These patients are very sensitive to changes in pleural pressure and can exhibit respiratory distress in various ways. A significant increase in the amount of oxygen needed to maintain an oxygen saturation >90% should trigger a complete physical exam focused on the respiratory system. Changes in the air leak status or the occurrence of crepitus should be followed closely with notification of the medical staff.

Breath sounds should be auscultated every hour immediately postoperatively, then every 4 h once the patient is deemed stable. Assessment of the patient's ability to cough and ability to clear secretions should be made. The amount, color, and frequency of the sputum need to be assessed on a continual basis. Significant changes need to be communicated expeditiously to the medical staff. Short-acting bronchodilators are administered every 4 h. Immediately postoperatively, the patient uses an acorn nebulizer. This treatment should be followed by chest physical therapy.

Intensive chest physical therapy is necessary to assist the patient in maintaining adequate oxygenation postoperatively. The nursing staff and pulmonary physical therapists need to collaborate to provide the patient with percussion and vibration, coughing and deep breathing exercises, and early ambulation. Instruction on incentive spirometry should be reiterated and a return demonstration provided to assure proper use. It is imperative that the patient be encouraged to use the incentive spirometer frequently (10 repetitions every hour) followed by coughing and deep breathing. Splinting with a pillow or similar device will provide support to the surgical incision. Patients need constant reinforcement in the use of diaphragmatic and pursed lip breathing as instructed preoperatively in the pulmonary rehabilitation program.

Early mobilization is critical to the care of the postoperative LVRS patient. On the first postoperative day, the team ensures that the hemodynamically stable patient is transferred out of bed to the chair. The patient is progressed to stepping and ambulating at the bedside on the first postoperative afternoon. The postoperative LVRS patient is routinely walked, even though attached to chest tubes, epidural and foley catheters, oxygen, and a pulse oximeter. Oxygen is titrated to keep the saturation above 90%. It needs to be reinforced that these patients routinely desaturate with activity and oxygen delivery should be adjusted accordingly. The patient is progressed to walking on the treadmill, leg exercises, and unweighted arm exercises while in the hospital.

Despite the use of bovine pericardium and pleural tents, persistent air leaks continue to complicate the postoperative course of many LVRS patients. Because the chest tube collection system is cumbersome (especially as the patient's activity level increases), we routinely utilize the Heimlich flutter valve in the management of persistent air leaks. The Heimlich valve is a one-way valve that allows air to exit from the pleural space without allowing air re-entry during inhalation *(14)*. The valve attaches directly to the chest tube. Because blood or pleural fluid may obstruct the ends of the valve, it is not recommended for use in patients with substantial pleural drainage. Assessments should include checks for patency. The walls of the patent Heimlich valve should open with exhalation, allowing air to escape, and close with inhalation, preventing the inflow of air *(15)*. The phasic fluttering of the valve usually stops when the airleak/pneumothorax resolve, but until the chest X-ray confirms this and rules out valve dysfunction, the staff needs to properly assess the patient for respiratory distress. If the patient's clinical status or chest X-ray suggest a worsening air leak of pneumothorax, the staff should assess the valve for possible obstruction and replace it as needed. If drainage and obstruction continue to be a problem, the chest tube may have to be reconnected to a standard collection system.

Although prolonged ventilator use is not routine, the staff needs to be aware that the LVRS patient is at significant risk for ventilator dependence. The staff must be cognizant of the potential need for chronic weaning, tracheostomy, or placement in a chronic care facility. These potential outcomes need to be addressed when the patient is considering the potential risks and benefits of surgery. It is imperative that the LVRS staff address the issues of Health Care Proxy and Advance Directives, because these patients are at significantly higher risk for ventilator dependence and chronic illness requiring advanced care.

PAIN CONTROL

Paramount to early mobilization is adequate pain control. LVRS patients are managed with an epidural catheter. On average, the catheter remains in place for 3–5 d, and is utilized to deliver a bupivacaine/fentanyl solution. The medical staff also administers NSAIDs to appropriate patients for the first five postoperative days. These medications should be used cautiously in patients with impaired renal function. Careful monitoring of the blood urea nitrogen (BUN) and creatinine is necessary to avoid renal complications. Management is focused on maximizing comfort, minimizing side effects, and managing potential, but uncommon, complications. Special attention needs to be paid to assessing the patient for side effects (see Table 2).

Table 2
Epidural Side Effects

Local Anesthetic	Opioids
Sensory losses	Nausea and vomiting
Motor weakness	Pruritus
Postural decrease in blood pressure	Respiratory depression
Urinary retention	Urinary retention

As noted above, one of the most common side effects of epidural pain control is urinary retention. To alleviate this symptom, a foley catheter is inserted in the operating room. Urine output should be monitored every 2 h progressing to every shift. The foley catheter, placed in the operating room, should not be removed until the epidural catheter is out and the patient is ambulating.

Assessment of adequate pain control should be performed utilizing standardized tools such as the Analgesia Scale, Sedation Scale, and Bromage Scale (see Table 3). It is very important that adequate pain control is maintained in order for the patient to progress in their postoperative recuperation. If malfunction of the epidural catheter occurs, adequate pain control should be maintained by either intravenous patient-controlled analgesia (PCA) or with oral pain medication. Careful assessment is required to monitor for signs and symptoms of respiratory depression. Once the PCA is discontinued, the patient is placed on oral pain medication (oxycodone/acetaminophen or acetaminophen/codeine). In addition to pain medication use, the patient should be reminded to utilize relaxation techniques to decrease anxiety and thus assist in pain control.

GASTROINTESTINAL

A common side effect of narcotic and opiod analgesics is constipation and decreased bowel function. Assessment of bowel function is imperative in the postoperative management of these patients. The nursing staff needs to auscultate bowel sounds every shift. It is important to avoid constipation. The patient routinely receives stool softeners unless contraindicated. The diet is progressed from clear liquid diet the first postoperative night to a regular diet, as tolerated.

Because of chronic steroid use and the frequent use of steroids postoperatively, these patients are at increased risk from GI discomfort, ulceration, and hemorrhage. It is thus recommended that the postoperative LVRS patient receive prophylactic agents, such as H2-blockers or proton pump inhibitors, to reduce gastric acidity. The nursing staff

Table 3
Pain Assessment

Analgesia Scale	Ask patient to rate pain 0–10
	0 = no pain
	10 = worst possible pain
Sedation Scale	0 = None–Awake and Alert
	1 = Mild–occasionally drowsy, easy to arouse
	2 = Moderate–frequently drowsy, easy to arouse
	3 = Severe–somnolent, difficult to arouse
Bromage Scale	0 = No block (0%)–full flexion of knees and feet possible
	1 = Partial (33%)–just able to flex knees, still full flexion of feet
	2 = Almost complete (66%)–unable to flex knees, still flexion of feet
	3 = Complete (100%)–unable to move feet or legs

should ensure that oral steroids are taken on a full stomach. The patient should be encouraged to report any gastrointestinal discomfort as promptly as possible.

INTEGUMENTARY

The surgical incisions, intravenous sites, epidural sites, chest tube sites, and foley catheter are all potential sites for infection. Assessments every shift should include evaluation of these areas for signs and symptoms of infection. Erythema, swelling, increased pain, or temperature above 101° Fahrenheit should alert the nursing staff to a potential postoperative infection. Special attention needs to be paid to the complete blood count and any cultures that are obtained.

Many postoperative patients are treated with steroids, and are subsequently at increased risk for clinically inapparent infections. Steroids also contribute to a delay in wound healing. Special attention should be paid to those patients who had a median sternotomy or clamshell because of the potential risk of wound dehiscence. Daily assessment of the sternal incision for the presence of a click is routine. The medical staff should be notified immediately if sternal instability is detected.

As with all postoperative patients, LVRS patients need to be placed on skin precautions to prevent pressure sores. Patients should be encouraged to turn and change position every 2 h when in bed. Pressure-relieving devices should be utilized as needed in these and all postoperative patients. The patient should be encouraged to eat a well-balanced diet to promote wound healing and good skin integrity. Small frequent feedings often work best with emphysema patients and should be used with the LVRS group.

PSYCHOSOCIAL

Studies of patients with COPD reveal a high incidence of depression, anxiety, and preoccupation with bodily functions (16). This can become a significant problem in the postoperative management of the emphysema patient. Hopefully, the preoperative rehabilitation program and teaching will have adequately prepared the patient and family for the postoperative course. The staff needs to recognize the signs of a panic attack and work to help the patient regain focus and work through the attack with coaching. All patients should receive instruction in pursed-lip breathing and other relaxation techniques preoperatively. The staff who care for the postoperative emphysema patient must reinforce the preoperative teaching and help the patient focus in order to interrupt an anxiety attack. These patients require support and encouragement from the staff in order to participate fully in daily physical therapy and to eventually assume responsibility for self-care. Patients may be disappointed with their initial results because of increased exhaustion, pain, decreased exercise tolerance, and general malaise. The staff needs to convey to the patient that all of these feelings are normal in the early postoperative course. It also should be reiterated that LVRS patients usually do not feel significant improvement for at least 6–8 wk postoperatively. Persistent problems with panic attacks, anxiety, or depression, which seem to impede the patient's participation with his or her activities of daily living need to be discussed with the medical staff. Intervention by a psychiatrist should be considered earlier rather than later in order not to waste valuable rehabilitation time postoperatively.

DISCHARGE PLANS

Discharge planning starts with preoperative teaching. The patients are informed that the average length of stay in the hospital is 7–14 d. Most patients are discharged home with outpatient pulmonary rehabilitation at the same center they utilized preoperatively. Almost all patients require some oxygen therapy postoperatively while they are reconditioning. This includes many patients who did not require it at all preoperatively. It is imperative that this issue be communicated to all patients before surgery so that there are no surprises when the patient is discharged with oxygen support.

Discharge instructions include monitoring for signs and symptoms of infection such as increased sputum production, erythema, swelling, or discharge from surgical or chest tube incision sites, or temperature > 101°F. The staff routinely instructs patients on activity restrictions postoperatively, such as limits for upper body strengthening. In general, in patients undergoing a median sternotomy or clamshell incision, we recommend delaying upper extremity range of motion exercises with weights for 4–6 wk postoperatively. Driving an automobile is generally restricted for at least 4 wk postoperatively or until the surgeon clears the patient at the first outpatient postoperative visit. This visit is usually scheduled for 10–14 d after the patient is discharged from the hospital with a chest X-ray done prior to the visit.

The patient is usually discharged home on the same medication regimen that they were on preoperatively. In addition, the patient is instructed to take analgesics every 4–6 h to help with pain control. If the patient is being discharged on a prednisone taper, it is very important that the staff adequately address the details of the tapering regimen in the discharge instructions.

Some patients require referral to an inpatient pulmonary rehabilitation facility if they are too debilitated to be discharged home safely. This group generally requires anywhere from a 2–4 wk stay in an inpatient facility which provides both physical and occupational therapy. The decision regarding inpatient vs outpatient rehabilitation is made individually with input from the medical, nursing, and physical therapy staff as well as the patient and family. (Please see Chapter 6 for a more detailed discussion of this and other issues related to pulmonary rehabilitation.)

ACKNOWLEDGMENT

The authors wish to thank to Kimberly Stavrolakes, MS and Jacqueline Pfeffer, MS for their input related to the physical therapy of the LVRS patient.

REFERENCES

1. Cooper JD, Patterson GA (1996) Lung volume reduction for sever emphysema. *Semin Thorac Cardiovasc Surg* 8: 52–60.
2. Allen GM (1996) Surgical treatment of emphysema using bovine pericardium strips. *AORN J* 63: 373–388.
3. Moores DW, Foster ED, McKneally MF (1995) Incisions. In: Pearson FG, et al., Eds. *Thoracic Surgery*, New York: Churchill Livingston, pp. 113–131.
4. Ginsberg RJ, Hill LD, Eagan RT, et al. (1983) Modern thirty-day operative mortality for surgical resections in lung cancer. *J Thorac Cardiovasc Surg* 86: 656.
5. Argenziano M, Moazami N, Thomashow B, Jellen PA, Gorenstein LA, Rose EA, Weinberg AD, Steinglass KM, Ginsburg ME (1996) Extended indications for lung volume reduction surgery in advanced emphysema. *Ann Thorac Surg* 62:1588–1597.
6. Cooper JD, Patterson GA, Sundaresan RS, Trulock EP, Yusen RD, Pohl MS, Lefrak SS (1996) Results of 150 consecutive bilateral lung volume reduction procedures in patients with sever emphysema. *J Thorac Cardiovasc Surg* 112: 1319–1330.

7. Eugene J, Dajee A, Kayaleh R, Gogia HS, Dos Santos C, Gazzangia AB Reduction pneumonoplasty for patients with a forced expiratory volume in one second of 500 millimeters for less. (1996) *Ann Thor Surg* 63: 186–192.

8. Gelb AF, Brenner M, McKenna RJ, Zamel N, Fischel R, Epstein JD (1996) Lung function 12 months following emphysema resection. *Chest* 110: 1407–1415.

9. Gelb AF, Zamel N, McKenna RJ, Brenner M (1996) Mechanism of short-term improvement in lung function after emphysema resection. *Am J Respir Crit Care Med* 154:945–951.

10. McKenna RJ, Fishel RJ, Brenner M, Gelb AF (1996) Combined operations for lung volume reduction surgery and lung cancer. *Chest* 110: 885–888.

11. Miller JI, Lee RB, Mansour KA (1996) Lung volume reduction surgery lessons learned. *Ann Thorac Surg* 61: 1464–1469.

12. O'Donnel DE, Webb KA, Bertley JC, Chau LK, Conlan AA (1996) Mechanisms of relief of exertional breathlessness following unilateral bullectomy and lung volume reduction surgery in emphysema. *Chest* 110:18–27.

13. Yusen RD, Trulock EP, Pohl MS, Biggar DG, The Washington University Emphysema Surgery Group (1996) Results of lung volume reduction surgery in patients with emphysema. *Semen Thorac Cardiovasc Surg* 112:1319–1330.

14. Connor PA (1997) When & how do you use a Heimlich flutter valve. *Am J Nursing* 288–290.

15. Mchugh JM (1985) Chest tube management. In Millar S, et al. Eds. *ACCN Procedure Manual for Critical Care*, 2nd ed., Philadelphia: WB Saunders, pp. 258–274.

16. Petty TL, Nett LM (1995) *Enjoying Life with Chronic Obstructive Lung Disease*, 3rd ed. New Jersey: Laennec, pp. 111–115.

12 Selection of Candidates for Lung Volume Reduction Surgery

Byron Thomashow, MD

CONTENTS

INTRODUCTION

Chronic obstructive pulmonary disease (COPD) is now the fourth leading cause of death in this country and the only major disease continuing to increase in prevalence and mortality (1). There are more than 20 million people in the United States with COPD (2,3). Most of these have the asthmatic or chronic bronchitic forms of the disease, but more than two million are believed to suffer from the predominantly emphysematous type. Although asthma and chronic bronchitis tend to be medically treatable, medically controllable diseases, there is no good medical therapy for emphysema (4). Disability is the exception in asthma and chronic bronchitis. It is the rule in progressive emphysema. Finally, in studies comparing mortality risks, 10-yr mortality is far higher in emphysema than in the asthmatic or chronic bronchitic groups (5). Because medical therapy has been so limited in emphysema, surgical options have been sought for over 100 yr. Over those years, many procedures have been attempted; most initially appeared promising, only to be abandoned because of ineffectiveness, morbidity, or mortality risks (6–9). See Chapter 7 for a more detailed review of this interesting history.

In 1993, Cooper reintroduced a surgical procedure initially performed by Otto Brantigan in the 1950s (10,11) in which the worst areas of

From: *Lung Volume Reduction Surgery*
Edited by: M. Argenziano and M. E. Ginsburg © Humana Press Inc., Totowa, NJ

emphysematous lung were removed. Within a few years, Cooper et al. published some very encouraging initial results *(12)*. Subsequently, lung volume reduction surgery (LVRS) was performed in a number of centers around the country. Published reports from numerous centers suggested that LVRS might be beneficial in selected emphysema patients *(13–16)*. Notwithstanding early enthusiasm for this novel procedure, early investigators recognized that the operation did carry significant morbidity and mortality risks, without certainty regarding longevity of any benefits that might be apparent after surgery. Because of these concerns, the procedure is now the subject of a multicenter, randomized, 7-yr National Institutes of Health study, the National Emphysema Treatment Trial (NETT). This study should determine relative risks and benefits of the procedure and outline selection criteria. Ultimately, these selection criteria will allow better definition of the evaluation process for potential LVRS candidates.

EARLY SELECTION CRITERIA

Part of the problem in evaluating early studies of surgery for emphysema involves the variability of selection criteria and variation in preoperative evaluations in different studies. In Brantigan's initial discussion of LVRS, one of the major criteria for inclusion appears to be that before surgery "every patient for a long time had been unable to work" *(10)*. Preoperative radiographic studies were performed and bronchoscopy and bronchography were used to identify (and eliminate) associated diseases, particularly bronchiectasis. Brantigan admitted that "unfortunately" pulmonary function studies were not performed in many of the patients. Despite the lack of pulmonary function data, Brantigan did conclude that "it is obvious that pulmonary function studies cannot measure the potential lung function that may be restored" with surgery.

In 1991, Wakabayashi et al. described the results of thoracoscopic carbon dioxide laser treatment of bullous emphysema *(17)*. Inclusion criteria included respiratory symptoms sufficient to cause major impairment of activity and lifestyle. Radiographic studies, including computerized tomographic (CT) scanning, were used to define the extent and location of bullous disease, "preferably" revealing evidence of crowding of adjacent lung tissue. Preoperative functional evaluation included physical examination, routine laboratory studies, and for most patients, pre- and postbronchodilator pulmonary function testing. Most patients also underwent maximal exercise testing using a modified low-level protocol. Lewis et al. in 1993 *(18)* and Little et al. in 1995 *(19)* used dyspnea scales, CAT scans, and pulmonary function studies including lung volume measurements to select their patients.

In Cooper's 1995 publication, the standard for future evaluation of patients for LVRS was established *(12)*. Patients in this series underwent standard spirometry (pre- and postbronchodilator), lung volume measurement by body plethysmography and nitrogen washout, standardized 6-min walk testing, and arterial blood gas (ABG) analysis. Radiographic evaluation included inspiratory and expiratory chest radiographs (CXR), CAT scans, and quantitative nuclear perfusion and ventilation lung scanning. Patients completed quality-of-life and dyspnea assessments. All patients underwent right-heart catheterization. It is to Cooper's credit that more than 5 yr after completing this initial study, the evaluation of patients for LVRS has remained basically unchanged. Of the screening described in his initial report, only nitrogen washout, ventilatory radionuclear scanning, and right-heart catheterization are no longer routinely included in LVRS evaluations.

EVALUATION OF CANDIDATES FOR LVRS

The evaluation of patients for LVRS can be broadly divided into three areas: clinical status, pulmonary function evaluation, and radiographic assessment.

Clinical Status

The evaluation of potential LVRS candidates starts with a complete history, physical examination, and routine laboratory studies. Important clinical issues include patient age, smoking history, bronchitic disease component, nutritional status, level of disability, extent of systemic steroid requirements, cardiac status, presence of pulmonary hypertension, presence of other significant lung diseases, and presence of other significant medical diseases.

The age of the patient appears to be an important prognostic factor. While at Columbia Presbyterian Medical Center (CPMC) and other centers, patients over age 80 have successfully undergone LVRS, most studies suggest that patients over the age of 70 face increased perioperative risks, and higher mortality *(20,21)*. In the CPMC experience, patients over age 70 have a predicted 4-yr mortality of more than 60% compared with a 40% mortality under age 70. Most centers do not view age over 70 yr as an absolute contraindication to LVRS, although most suggest that only the most ideal of these elderly patients should be considered for surgery. In this regard, in order to be enrolled in the NETT, patients over age 70 must have an FEV_1 greater than 15% of predicted.

Most patients with emphysema are elderly. However, younger patients (under age 55) occasionally present with significant emphysema. Many of these patients have the α-1 antitrypsin deficiency variant. Most of these have a lower lobe predominance of disease, as opposed to the upper lobe predominance seen in most cases of emphysema. Patients with α-1 antitrypsin deficiency have undergone LVRS. Results in these patients have been less impressive, with benefits of shorter duration than in other patients. In these younger patients, LVRS may simply be a "bridge" to transplantation, as Cooper initially suggested.

The link between cigarette smoking and development of emphysema has been well documented *(22,23)*. Active cigarette smokers have a much more marked yearly reduction in FEV_1 than nonsmokers or former smokers *(24)*. In addition, cigarette smokers face higher postoperative risks of bronchitic exacerbation, atelectasis, or pneumonia *(25)*. Most centers require that potential LVRS candidates stop smoking at least 4 mo prior to evaluation. Patients in the NETT undergo regular serum cotinine testing. If not using nicotine-preventive products, plasma cotinine levels must be less than 31.7 ng/mL. If using nicotine preventive products arterial carboxyhemoglobin levels must be less than 2.5%.

Most patients with COPD have the bronchitic form of the disease *(26)*. LVRS is not appropriate for these patients. Many patients with emphysema have a bronchitic component. The greater the bronchitic component, the less likely LVRS will be of benefit. In addition, the greater the bronchitic component, the higher the risk of postoperative complications, including atelectasis, pneumonia, and respiratory failure. For these reasons, a history of recurrent bronchial infections or significant daily sputum production is viewed as a contraindication to LVRS.

Nutritional status is a concern in patients with advanced emphysema *(27)*. Studies suggest that more than 20% of outpatients with significant COPD, andmore than 50% of hospitalized COPD patients are malnourished *(28,29)*. Nutritional status also correlates with mortality risk. Emphysema patients below 80% of ideal body weight face 3-yr mortality rates over 30%. Despite enteral and parenteral modalities aimed at improving nutritional parameters, these patients remain severely functionally limited. In the CPMC experience, malnourished patients undergoing LVRS have had significantly higher morbidity and mortality. Most centers exclude patients with unplanned weight loss over 10% of usual weight in the 90 d prior to evaluation. Whereas patients with significant emphysema are rarely overweight, obesity also confers a higher postoperative risk of morbidity and mortality. Therefore, NETT patients must have a body mass index (BMI) < 31.1 kg/m$_2$ in men or < 32.3 kg/m$_2$ in women.

Level of disability and degree of limitation are critically important issues. Because results of LVRS are impossible to guarantee, and benefits of LVRS vary and are not permanent, and also because the procedure carries major risks, candidates for LVRS must be severely limited. Although severity of limitation usually correlates with the severity of reduction in FEV_1, there is considerable variability *(30)*. Different patients with the same level of FEV_1 can have very different degrees of limitation and very different degrees of dyspnea. Therefore, there is general agreement that dyspnea indices and quality-of-life assessments are important parts of any LVRS evaluation. Some potential LVRS candidates may be too limited to undergo the procedure. If, after completing pulmonary rehabilitation, patients are still unable to walk more than 140 m in 6 min, most investigators do not believe they are appropriate LVRS candidates.

Patients with severe emphysema are at risk of developing pulmonary hypertension from a combination of loss of the pulmonary capillary bed and disturbances in gas exchange *(31,32)*. Some authors have suggested that in certain patients, LVRS can actually improve pulmonary hemodynamics *(33)*. However, this is an area of major concern to pulmonolgists and thoracic surgeons caring for these patients *(34–36)*. Whereas surgeons aim to resect areas of lung with decreased vascular perfusion on CAT scan or perfusion lung scan, a certain amount of capillary bed is invariably removed. Thus, the potential of worsening pulmonary hypertension exists, especially if too much functioning lung is removed. If peak systolic pulmonary artery pressure (PAP) on echocardiogram evaluation is equal to or over 45 mmHg, right-heart catheterization is suggested. If this degree of systolic pulmonary hypertension (or mean PAP $\geq$ 35 mmHg) is found on catheterization, the patient is not a candidate for LVRS. Screening echocardiograms may also give information about left-ventricular function and valvular problems that could require cardiac consultation before making decisions regarding LVRS eligibility.

Most patients with emphysema are former cigarette smokers and are also at risk for coronary artery disease *(31)*. Because of their respiratory limitations, typical anginal symptoms may not be present. A clinical history suggesting unstable angina, a myocardial infarction within 6 mo, an S3 gallop or a history of CHF within 6 mo, a left-ventricular ejection fraction < 45%, syncope, or significant ventricular ectopy may be viewed as possible contraindications for the procedure and require cardiac clearance before proceeding. Many of these patients may not be able to complete a treadmill exercise study. Therefore, most centers suggest performing dobutamine radionuclide cardiac scanning in these patients. A positive study would require cardiac consultation before deciding whether LVRS remains an option.

Cardiopulmonary exercise testing helps delineate cardiac, pulmonary, and deconditioning components of a patient's generalized disability *(37,38)*. It plays a role in outlining the degree of limitation, and helps set up an appropriate pulmonary rehabilitation program (*see* Chapter 2). In the NETT, one of the main study outcomes is maximum exercise performance, and repeat cardiopulmonary exercise studies are the crucial part of that evaluation. There is no question about the importance of these tests in ongoing research studies of LVRS. However, at present, the ultimate role of cardiopulmonary exercise testing in clinical LVRS evaluations remains somewhat unclear.

Patients facing LVRS obviously are severely limited. Any other pulmonary or medical problems could adversely effect surgical and long-term results. Significant kyphoscoliosis, bronchiectasis, or pleural or interstitial lung disease would preclude surgery. Evidence of a systemic disease or malignancy that is expected to compromise survival would be a contraindication to the procedure. Uncontrolled hypertension with systolic blood pressure > 200 mmHg or diastolic blood pressure >110 mmHg could significantly increase operative risks, and would have to be better controlled before proceeding with LVRS. Dependence on high-dose systemic steroids raises additional concerns, including the risk of osteoporosis, which could compromise postoperative recovery *(39)*. In addition, because emphysema is not a steroid-responsive disease, significant systemic steroid dosing may suggest a greater asthmatic or bronchitic component. The NETT eliminates patients using more than 20 mg of prednisone daily.

At this time, prior lung resection surgery, including prior LVRS, is viewed as a contraindication because procedures performed in this setting have been complicated and usually poorly tolerated. Adhesions from prior procedures can dramatically increase air leak and bleeding risks. At CPMC and other centers, unilateral LVRS has been performed in patients with old pleural disease on the contralateral side, and in patients status post prior contralateral lung resection including prior unilateral LVRS. Whereas the procedure can be safely performed in this setting, results are generally not as good as with the bilateral LVRS procedure *(40,41)*.

Pulmonary Function Evaluation

Pulmonary function studies are an important part of the evaluation of potential LVRS candidates *(42)*. Routine spirometry measured both before and after bronchodilator administration serve to eliminate many COPD patients from consideration. A significant bronchodilator response suggests a significant airways disease component. Most centers eliminate patients with a postbronchodilator response of greater than 30% or greater than 300 mL. Recognizing that this procedure should only be considered in severely limited patients, most centers also require an FEV_1 less than or equal to 45% predicted. The lower limit of FEV_1 greater than 15% of predicted is, as aforementioned, reserved for patients over age 70.

Loss of lung elasticity with associated increase in pulmonary compliance are major pathophysiologic determinants in emphysema. Indeed, recent data suggests that improvement in lung elasticity may play a major role when this operation is successful *(43)*. Pulmonary compliance studies are being used in research protocols, but are not indicated in clinical screening. Evaluation of lung volumes, however, is required *(44)*. Body plethysmography gives much more accurate data than nitrogen washout techniques. Initially, both studies were performed in the hope that an estimation of "trapped gas" volume could be determined by calculating the difference between the volumes measured by the two techniques. Subsequent work has suggested that nitrogen washout adds little to the evaluation. Most centers suggest that patients have a total lung capacity equal to or over 100% predicted and that residual volume be equal to or over 150% predicted to be considered candidates.

ABGs remain an important part of the LVRS evaluation. In the CPMC experience, patients with a preoperative partial pressure of oxygen (PaO_2) > 60 mmHg have had significantly greater 4-yr survival than patients starting with lower PaO_2. The NETT requires a room air resting $PaO_2 \geq 45$ mmHg and oxygen requirements during rest or with oxygen titration not exceeding 6 L/min to keep saturation over 90%. Higher oxygen requirements either reflect the severity of underlying emphysema (suggesting little remaining functional lung tissue), or the presence of another lung problem in addition to emphysema. In either case, LVRS would likely be of little benefit, and operative risks could be high. Significant $PaCO_2$ elevations are also of concern, again reflecting the severity of disease. Numerous studies have suggested that patients with significant $PaCO_2$ elevations have increased operative risks, poorer results, and decreased survival *(45,46)*. The NETT requires a $PaCO_2$ no higher than 60 mmHg. The role of diffusing capacity (DLCO) monitoring remains unclear. Although there is data suggesting that the severity of emphysema can be gaged by the severity of DLCO reduction *(47)*, DLCO monitoring has not been found to be helpful in LVRS evaluations. The NETT no longer uses DLCO as part of inclusion or exclusion criteria.

Radiographic Assessment

Inspiratory and expiratory CXR can act as simple screen for emphysema. These studies can provide evidence of air trapping, large lung fields, flattened diaphragms, and decreased diaphragmatic movement. High-resolution CT scanning, however, has clearly become the radiographic study of choice in evaluating potential LVRS candidates *(48)*. This study not only allows an estimation of extent and severity of emphysema, it also allows judgment of the heterogeneity or homogeneity of the process *(49)*. Cooper et al. have shown that this procedure is potentially beneficial in patients with the heterogeneous pattern with so-called target areas of worse emphysema potentially amenable to resection. Most centers have

Table 1
Assessment of Patients for LVRS

Complete history
Physical examination Routine laboratory tests
Serum cotinine level
α-1 antrypsin level
Inspiratory/expiratory CXR
High-resolution CAT scan
Perfusion lung scan
Spirometry pre- and postbronchodilator
Lung volumes by plethysmography
Arterial blood gasses
Dyspnea index
Quality-of-life evaluation
Echocardiogram
Dobutamine radionuclide cardiac scanning
Possibly cardiopulmonary exercise testing

avoided patients with homogeneous disease fearing that there is little "good lung" to expand in this group. If LVRS works by downsizing the lungs and improving lung elasticity, presumably some of these patients with the homogeneous pattern may benefit as well. At this point, the role of LVRS in homogeneous emphysema remains unclear.

CT scanning is also of value in elucidating other pulmonary problems. CAT scanning can define the extent of bronchiectasis or the presence of unexpected interstitial or pleural parenchymal disease. It may also reveal potentially malignant lung nodules. The incidence of lung nodules in patients screened for LVRS has ranged from 7% to more than 30%. Suspicious lung nodules are not necessarily a contraindication to LVRS. At CPMC and other centers, lung nodules have been successfully resected concomitantly during an LVRS procedure (50). At CPMC, almost half of the resected nodules have been malignant. Although many of these patients would not have been candidates for nodule resection prior to the availability of LVRS, it is too early to determine whether this is a reasonable lung cancer operation in patients with severe emphysema (see Chapter 15).

Ventilation/perfusion lung scans were used routinely in early LVRS studies (51). Data suggest that the ventilation scan results added little, and this procedure is now rarely performed. Perfusion lung scanning continues to have a role, but is not as helpful as the CAT scan. In patients with homogeneous disease on CAT scanning, perfusion scans could pick up "target areas" of heterogeneous perfusion, suggesting that these patients might benefit from LVRS. Most surgeons still prefer to see perfusion scan

Table 2
LVRS Inclusion Criteria

History and physical examination consistent with emphysema
CAT scan evidence of bilateral emphysema
Nonsmoker for 4 mo prior to evaluation
FEV_1 < 45% predicted
FEV_1 post bronchodilator increase < 30% or < 300 mL
FEV_1 > 15% predicted if over age 70
Total lung capacity > 100% predicted
Residual volume > 150% predicted
Room air $PaCO_2$ < 60 mmHG
Room air PaO_2 >45 mmHG
BMI < 31.1 kg/m$_2$ in men or < 32.3 kg/m$_2$ in women
Cardiac clearance required for angina, S3 gallop, left-ventricular ejection
    fraction <45%, positive dobutamine radionuclide cardiac scan,
    ventricular ectopy

Table 3
LVRS Exclusion Criteria

CAT scan evidence of diffuse emphysema felt unsuitable for LVRS
Pleural or interstitial disease which precludes LVRS
Significant bronchiectasis
Significant kyphoscoliosis
History of recurrent infections with significant daily sputum production
Myocardial infarction within 6 mo and ejection fraction < 45%
Congestive heart failure within 6 mo and ejection fraction < 45%
Uncontrolled hypertension: systolic > 200 mmHg, diastolic >110 mmHg
Pulmonary hypertension: mean pulmonary pressure>35 mmHg or peak>45 mmHg
Unplanned weight loss > 10% normal weight within 90 d prior to evaluation
Daily use of 20 mg or more Prednisone or equivalent steroid dosing
Oxygen requirements during rest or oxygen titration exceeding 6 L/min to keep
    sat > 90%
Significant systemic illness or malignancy expected to compromise survival
6-min walk distance < 140 m postrehabilitation

results prior to LVRS in hope of better defining regions to be removed. Cooper et al. have used dynamic MRI scans, but there seems little role for this procedure at this time. (Please see Chapter 4 for a more detailed discussion of radiographic evaluation of LVRS candidates.)

SUMMARY

A summary of the basic assessment for potential LVRS candidates is listed in Table 1. An algorithm for COPD patient evaluation is shown in

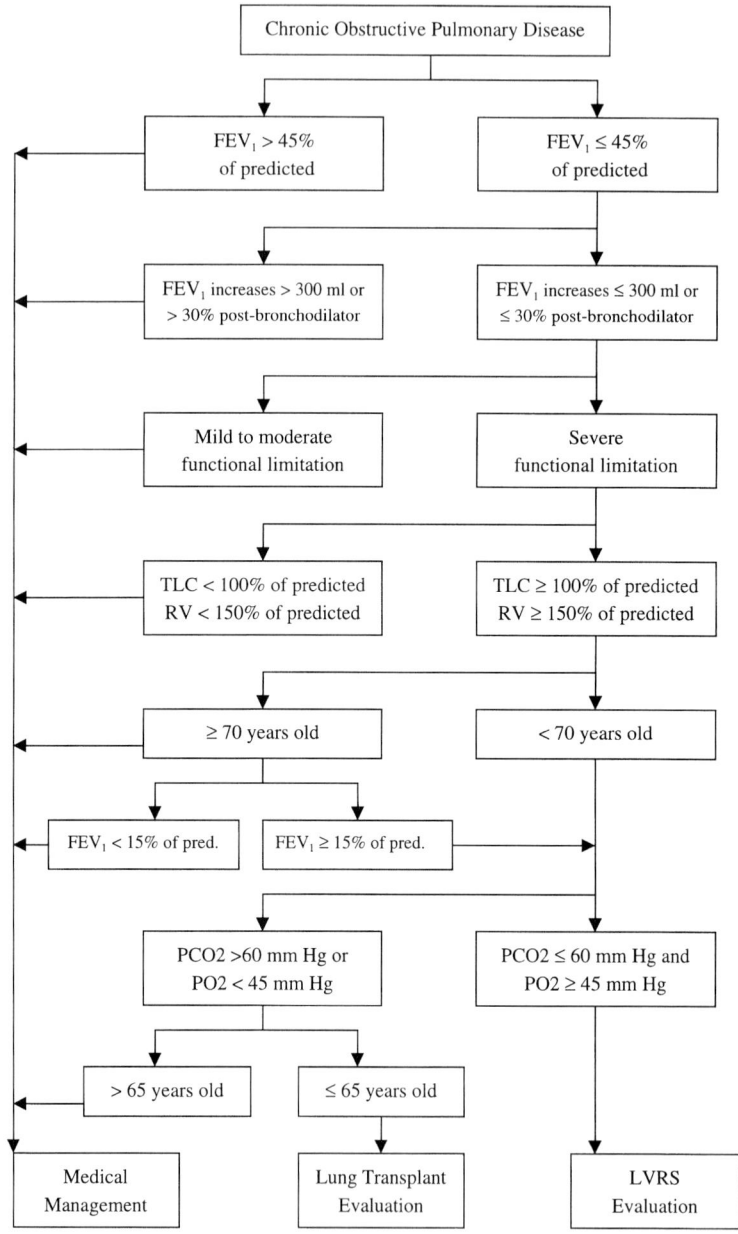

Fig. 1. A follow-up algorithm for patients felt to be LVRS candidates is shown in Fig. 2. Inclusion and exclusion criteria for LVRS are shown in Tables 2 and 3.

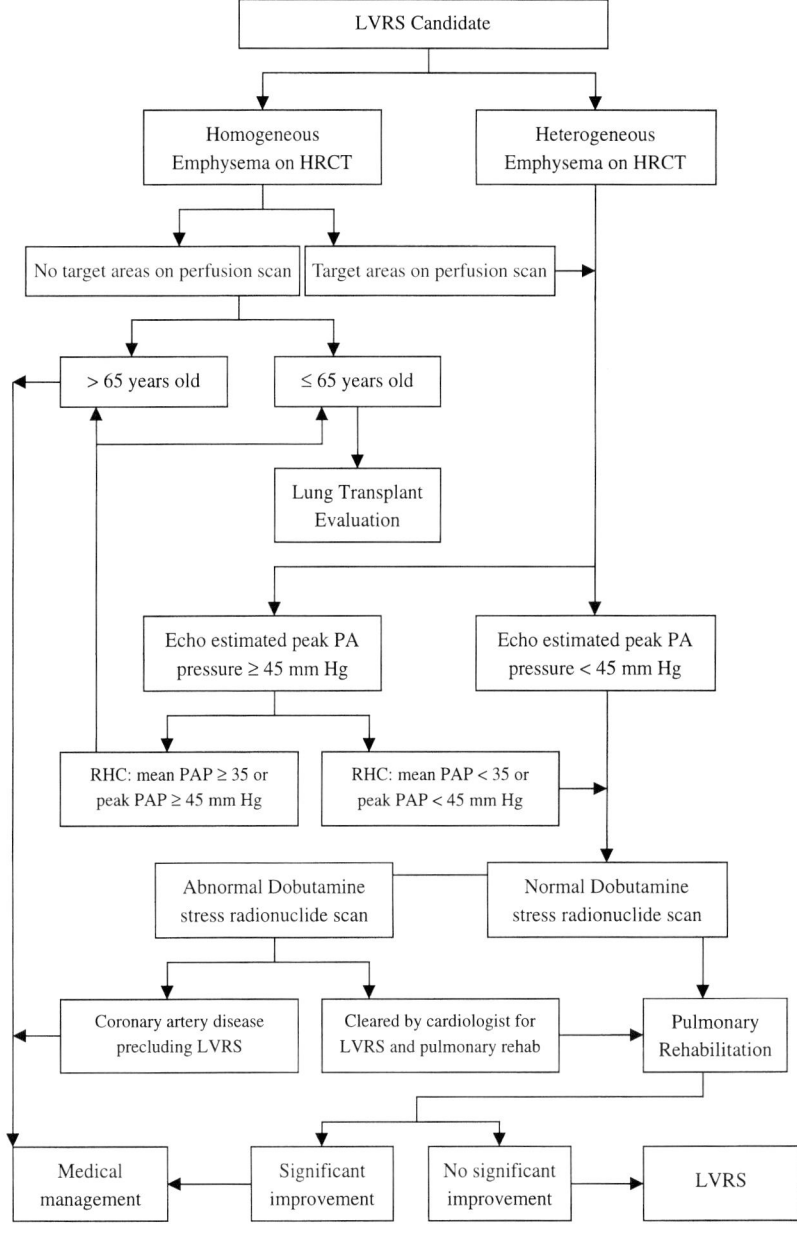

Fig. 2.

The evaluation of potential LVRS candidates remains complicated, time-consuming, and expensive. It is hoped that the NETT
will provide a better understanding of how LVRS works and in whom

it works best, and that this information will allow streamlining of the
evaluation process.

REFERENCES

1. National Center for Health Statistics (1993) Advance report of final mortality statistics 1991. *Monthly Vital Statistics Report* 42.
2. Celli BR, Snider GL, Heffner J, et al. (1995) Standards for the diagnosis and care of patients with COPD. *Am J Respir Crit Care Med* 152:S78–121.
3. Adam RF, Benson V (1992) Current estimates from the National Health Interview Survey, 1991. National Center for Health Statistics. *Vital Health Stat* 10.
4. Burrows, B, Bloom JW, Traver GA, et al. (1987) The course and prognosis of different forms of chronic airways obstruction in a sample from the general population. *N Engl J Med* 317: 1309–1314 .
5. Hodgkin J (1990) Prognosis in chronic obstructive pulmonary disease. *Clin Chest Med* 11:3:555–569.
6. Knudson R, Gaensler E (1965) Surgery for emphysema. *Ann Thorac Surg* 1:332–362.
7. Foreman S, Weil H, Duke R, et al. (1968) Bullous disease of the lungs: physiologic improvement after surgery. *Ann Intern Med* 69:757–767.
8. American Thoracic Society (1968) Current status of the surgical treatment of pulmonary emphysema and asthma. *Am Rev Respir Dis* 97:486–489.
9. Fitzgerald M, Keelan P, Cagell D, et al. (1974) Long-term results of surgery for bullous emphysema. *J Thorac Cardiovasc Surg* 65:566–587.
10. Brantigan O, Mueller E (1957) Surgical treatment of pulmonary emphysema. *Am Surg* 23:789–804.
11. Brantigan O, Mueller E, Kress M (1959) A surgical approach to pulmonary emphysema. *Am Rev Respir Dis* 80:194–202.
12. Cooper J, Trulock E, Triantafillou A, et al. (1995) Bilateral pneumectomy (volume reduction) for chronic obstructive pulmonary disease. *J Thorac Cardiovasc Surg* 109:106–119.
13. Argenziano M, Mozami, N, Thomashow B, et al. (1996) Extended indications for volume reduction pneumectomy in advanced emphysema. *J Thorac Cardiovasc Surg* 62:1588–1597.
14. Yusen R, Trulock E, Pohl M, et al. (1996) Results of lung volume reduction surgery in patients with emphysema. *Semin Thorac Cardiovasc Surg* 8:99–109.
15. Mc Kenna RJ, Brenner M, Gelb AF, et al. (1996) A randomized prospective trial of stapled lung reduction versus laser bullectomy for diffuse emphysema. *J Thorac Cardiovasc Surg* 111:317–311.
16. Bingisser R, Zollinger A, Hauser M, et al. (1996) Bilateral volume reduction surgery for diffuse pulmonary emphysema by video assisted thoracoscopy. *J Thorac Cardiovasc Surg* 112: 875–882.
17. Wakabayashi A, Brenner A, Kagaleh R, et al. (1991) Thoracoscopic carbon dioxide laser treatment of bullous emphysema. *Lancet* 337:881–883.
18. Lewi A, Caccavale R, Sisler G (1993) VATS- argon beam coagulation treatment of diffuse end stage bilateral bullous disease of the lung. *Ann Thorac Surg* 55: 1394–1399.
19. Little A, Swain T, Nino J, et al. (1995) Reduction pneumoplasty for emphysema: early results. *Ann Surg* 222: 365–374.
20. Brenner M, Yusen R, Mc Kenna R (1996) Lung volume reduction surgery for emphysema. *Chest* 110:205–218.

21. Brenner M, McKenna R, Chen J, et al. (1999) Survival following bilateral staple lung volume reduction surgery for emphysema. *Chest* 115:390–396.
22. Snider G (1992) Emphysema: the first two centuries- and beyond. A historical overview, with suggestions for future research. *Am Rev Respir Dis* 146:1334–1344.
23. Sherill D, Lebowitz M, Burrows B (1990) Epidimiology of chronic obstructive pulmonary disease. *Clin Chest Med* 11: 375–387.
24. Anthonisen NR, Cennett JE, Kiley JP, et al. (1994) Effects of smoking intervention and the use of inhaled anticholinergic bronchodilators on the rate of decline of FEV1: the Lung Health Study. *JAMA* 272: 1497–1505.
25. Stokes J, Rigotti NA (1988) The health consequences of cigarette smoking and the internist's role in smoking cessation. *Adv Intern Med* 33: 431–460.
26. Wilson R, Wilson C (1997) Defining subsets of patients with chronic bronchitis. *Chest* 112: 303–310.
27. Gray- Donald K, Gibbons L, Shapiro S, et al. (1996) Nutritional status and mortality in chronic obstructive pulmonary disease. *Am J Respir Crit Care Med* 153: 961–966.
28. Wilson DO, Rogers RM, Wright E, et al. (1989) Body weight in chronic obstructive pulmonary disease: the National Institute of Health intermittent positive pressure breathing trial. *Am Rev Resp Dis* 139: 1435–1438.
29. Myers MF, Green JH (1993) Weight loss in chronic obstuctive pilmonary disease. *Eur Respir J* 6:729–734.
30. Sweer L, Zuillich C (1990) Dyspnea in the patient with chronic obstructive pulmonary disease. *Clin Chest Med* 11:417–437.
31. Burrows B, Kittel NJ, Niden AG, et al. (1972) Patterns of cardiovascular dysfunction in chronic obstructive lung disease. *N Engl J Med* 286: 912–918.
32. Schulman L, Lennon P, Wood J, et al. (1994) Pulmonary vascular resistance in emphysema. *Chest* 105:798–805.
33. Wex P, Ebner H, Dragojevic D (1983) Functional surgery of bullous emphysema. *Thorac Cardiovasc Surg* 31: 346–351.
34. Kubo K, Koizami T, Fujimoto K, et al. (114) Effects of lung volume reduction surgery on exercise pulmonary hemodynamics in severe emphysema. *Chest* 114: 1575–1582.
35. Oswald- Mammoser M, Kessler R, Massard G, et al. (1998) Effect of lung volume reduction surgery on gas exchange and pulmonary hemodynamics at rest and during exercise. *Am J Resp Crit Care Med* 158: 1020–1025.
36. Weg I, Rossoff L, Mc Keon K, et al. (1999) Development of pilmonary hypertension after lung volume reduction surgery. *Am J Resp Crit Care Med* 159: 552–556.
37. Wasserman K (1997) Diagnosing cardiovascular and lung pathophysiology from exercise gas exchange. *Chest* 112: 1091–1101.
38. Nosed A, Carpiaux JP, Prigogine T, et al. (1989) Lung function, maximum and submaximum exercise testing in COPD patients: reproducibility over a long interval. *Lung* 67: 247–257.
39. Mc Evoy C, Niewoener D (1997) Adverse effects of corticosteroid therapy for COPD. *Chest* 111: 732–743.
40. McKenna R, Brenner M, Fischal R, et al. (1996) Should lung volume reduction be unilateral or bilateral? *J Thorac Cardiovasc Surg* 112: 1331–1339.
41. Argenziano M, Thomashow B, Jellen P, et al. (1997) A functional comparison of unilateral vs bilateral lung volume reduction surgery. *Ann Thorac Surg* 64: 321–327.
42. Szekely L, Oelberg D, Wright C, et al. (1997) Preoperative predictors of operative morbidity and mortality in COPD patients undergoing bilateral lung volume reduction surgery. *Chest* 11: 550–558.

43. Gelb A, Brenner M, McKeon R, et al. (1997) Serial lung function and elastic recoil two years after lung volume reduction surgery for emphysema. *Chest* 111: 550–558.

44. Cooper J, Patterson GA (1995) Lung volume reduction surgery for emphysema. *Chest Surg Clin North Am* 5: 815–831.

45. Keenan R, Landreneau R, Sciurba F, et al. (1996) Unilateral thoracoscopic surgical approach for diffuse emphysema. *J Thorac Cardiovasc Surg* 112:208–216.

46. Yusen R, Lefrak S (1996) Evaluation of patients with emphysema for lung volume reduction surgery. *Semin Thorac Cardiovasc Surg* 8: 83–93.

47. Morrison NJ, Abboud RT, Ramadon F, et al. (1989) Comparison of single breath carbon monoxide diffusing capacity and pressure volume curves in detecting emphysema. *Am Rev Respir Dis* 139:1179–1187.

48. Becker M, Berkman Y, Austin J, et al. (1998) Lung volumes before and after lung volume reduction surgery. Quantitative CT analysis. *Am J Resp Crit Care Med* 157:1593–1599.

49. Slone R, Gierada D (1996) Radiology of pulmonary emphysema and lung volume reduction surgery. *Semin Thorac Cardiovasc Surg* 8: 61–82.

50. De Rose J, Argenziano M, El- Amer M, et al. (1998) Lung reduction operation and resection of pulmonary nodules inpatients with severe emphysema. *Ann Thorac Surg* 65: 314–318.

51. Thurnheer R, Engel H, Weder W, et al. (1999) The role of lung perfusion scintigraphy in relation to chest CT and pulmonary function in the evaluation of candidates for lung volume reduction surgery. *Am J Resp Crit Care Med* 159: 301–310.

13 Clinical Results and Clinical Trials in Lung Volume Reduction Surgery

Charles W. Hoopes, MD
and Mark D. Iannettoni, MD

CONTENTS

INTRODUCTION

Early recognition of the anatomic changes characteristic of chronic emphysema resulted in a number of operative interventions designed to restore normal thoracic anatomy, improve pulmonary mechanics, and treat perceived physiologic abnormalities *(1)*. These included attempts at thoracoplasty to reduce chest volume, disruption of the phrenic nerve *(2)*, or pneumoperitoneum *(3)* to elevate the diaphragm, mechanical pleurodesis to create ancillary systemic to pulmonary blood flow *(4)*, denervation of the lung via pulmonary plexectomy *(5)*, and excision of the carotid body (glomectomy) as originally reported by Nakayama *(6)*. Despite anecdotal reports of clinical success and subjective improvement in patient symptoms, none of these historical procedures has been demonstrated by objective postoperative criteria to produce significant improvement in pulmonary function or patient survival (see Chapter 7 for a more detailed discussion of these and other historical operations

From: *Lung Volume Reduction Surgery*
Edited by: M. Argenziano and M. E. Ginsburg © Humana Press Inc., Totowa, NJ

for emphysema). In this chapter, we will review the available clinical data reported in the modern era of lung volume reduction surgery (LVRS), summarize the areas of agreement as to the method and efficacy of LVRS from nonrandomized studies, and critically analyze the utility and limitations of randomized controlled trials in LVRS in the context of the National Emphysema Treatment Trial (NETT).

CLINICAL RESULTS

The original report of lung volume reduction was published in October 1954 by Brantigan *(7)*, who described 26 patients (24 males and 2females, 16–64 yr of age) in whom operation was designed to "reduce the volume of lung by removing the least functioning areas." Five in-hospital postoperative deaths were recorded — four from respiratory insufficiency "because too much lung volume was removed, a mistake in judgement," and another death from "acute suppurative bronchitis." Fourteen patients returned to work with an "obvious increase in the ventilation of the lung as shown...by increased exercise tolerance." The original operation was combined with radical hilar stripping to create an extensive autonomic denervation, thereby reducing bronchospasm and bronchial secretions and furthering the procedure's stated goal of restoring the impaired physiological mechanism of circumferential pull upon the smaller airways. Given a mortality of 19% with no objective demonstration of improvement in pulmonary function, the procedure was not widely embraced as it was "difficult to believe that a disease characterized by extensive loss of lung parenchyma can be effectively treated by further resection of lung" *(8)*.

Brantigan's original work was largely ignored until 1995 when Cooper et al. *(9)*, noting that the thoracic distention of patients with severe COPD returned to normal following transplantation, published the results of bilateral lung volume reduction in 20 patients. Preliminary analysis suggested that a reduction in lung volume resulted in a significant increase in FEV_1 (from 25% to 44% of predicted), a reduction in total lung capacity (from 140% to 110% of predicted), and an improvement in quality of life (QOL) as measured by the Medical Research Council Dyspnea Scale, the Nottingham Health Profile, and the Medical Outcomes Study 36-Item Health Survey (MOS SF-36). These observations were subsequently extended to 150 patients under age 75 yr with emphysema characterized by hyperinflation, a heterogeneous distribution of disease, and an $FEV_1 < 35\%$ predicted (10). Nearly 80% of patients evaluated for LVRS were excluded secondary to diffuse patterns of disease with no definable target areas (30%), minimal thoracic hyperinflation as documented by inspiratory and expiratory chest radiographs (16%), significant medical comorbidity (16%), associated pleural disease (8%), or $PCO_2 > 55$ mmHg (7%).

Patients who met inclusion criteria underwent at least 6 wk of pulmonary rehabilitation prior to bilateral reduction of 20–30% of each lung via a median sternotomy approach. Target areas were identified by the distribution of function as defined by quantitative ventilation and perfusion scans and the relative degree of parenchymal destruction as defined by computed tomography (CT). Operative mortality (< 90 d) was 4% (6 patients) with 4 additional late deaths: 2 from pneumonia, 1 from stroke, and another from respiratory failure more than 1 yr after surgery. At 6 mo, FEV_1 increased by an average of 51% (from 0.7 L to 1.06 L), residual volume decreased by an average of 28% (from 6.0 L to 4.3 L), and mean PaO_2 increased from 62 mmHg to 70 mmHg. The mean distance for the 6-min walk was 856 ft before pulmonary rehabilitation, 1110 ft following rehabilitation, 1280 ft 3 mo postoperatively, and 1316 ft at 6 mo after surgery with a nearly 50% reduction in the number of patients requiring supplemental O_2. QOL assessments demonstrated that 78% of patients considered their health much better after the operation, 20% somewhat better, and only 1 patient somewhat worse.

Initial studies from Emory University (11) paralleled the research design initially described by the Washington University group (9), with the exception that rather than viewing participation in preoperative pulmonary rehabilitation as a prerequisite for LVRS, admission to the operating room required specific standards of exercise tolerance (e.g., 30 min of cycling at 1.5 mph and 30 min of treadmill walking at 1 mph). Patients were excluded for age > 75 yr, predominantly bullous emphysema, active tobacco use, significant coronary artery disease (>70% luminal occlusion not amenable to angioplasty), mean pulmonary artery pressure (PAP) > 35 mmHg or peak systolic PAP > 45 mmHg, prednisone dose > 15 mg/d, multiple psychiatric drugs, and active bronchitis or asthma. Additional inclusion criteria included FEV_1 < 30% predicted, $PaCO_2$ < 50 mmHg, and a room air PaO_2 > 40 mmHg. Forty-six patients underwent median sternotomy with bilateral reduction of between 50–75 g of tissue per lung. An additional seven patients underwent unilateral LVRS via a thoracotomy secondary to a history of previous lung surgery on the opposite side, pleural sclerosis, or unfavorable anatomy (e.g., excavatum). Eighty percent of the 53 patients operated on had specific target areas as defined by preoperative CT and quantitative lung perfusion scans. Significant improvement was noted 6 mo postoperatively in FEV_1 (from 0.56 L to 1.1 L), FVC (from 57% to 85% of predicted), MVV (from 18% to 40% of predicted), PO_2 (from 62 mmHg to 70 mmHg) and 6-min walk distance (from 785 ft to 1600 ft). All postoperative patients were subjected to at least 2 mo of supervised pulmonary rehabilitation prior to 6-mo testing.

A significant aspect of the Miller study was the identification of previously unrecognized complications of LVRS: panic attacks occurred in 15 patients and were the precipitating event in all three hospital deaths, 8 patients had significant colonic distention (right side) with 2 requiring abdominal exploration and colostomy, and 1 patient died from progressive, delayed onset (POD 7) pulmonary hypertension (see Table 1). Overall mortality was 9% with 1 early (< 30 d) and 4 late deaths (from pneumonia, SVT, or respiratory failure). Morbidity was concentrated in patients over 70 yr of age, with preoperative $PaCO_2$ > 50 mmHg (50% mortality), a preoperative FEV_1 < 0.5 L after rehabilitation, preoperative MVV < 15% predicted, or preoperative DLCO < 10% predicted. Interestingly, the most significant factor contributing to postoperative complications and poor outcome was a history of panic attacks, particularly if preoperative symptoms were not controlled with minimal doses of benzodiazepines (0.5 mg lorazepam po BID). Overall, recommendations were for extremely strict and selective criteria in evaluating patients for LVRS. However, early observations from the group at Columbia University *(12)* suggested that certain, generally accepted exclusionary criteria not be regarded as absolute.

Argenziano et. al. *(12)* operated on 85 emphysematous patients selected on the basis of hyperinflation with poor diaphragmatic excursion, pulmonary perfusion and ventilation deficits (indicating disease heterogeneity), and significant functional disability. The study population included nine patients with severe hypercapnia ($PaCO_2$ > 55 mmHg), 26 patients with significant steroid dependence (prednisone dose > 10 mg/d), 34 patients with a preoperative FEV_1 < 0.5 L, and 35 patients who were unable to complete preoperative pulmonary rehabilitation. The preoperative Medical Research Council dyspnea index was greater than four (housebound/breathless while dressing) for all patients. There were a total of 6 deaths within 30 d of operation, including 4 from respiratory failure, 1 from perforation of a duodenal ulcer, and another from complications of a cerebrovascular accident. Overall, all patients demonstrated a significant postoperative improvement by 3 mo with respect to FEV_1 (from 0.52 L to 0.8 L), FVC (from 1.6 L to 2.1 L), 6-min walk distance (from 598 ft to 919 ft), and dyspnea index (from 4.1 to 1.8:stops for breath while walking on the level). High-risk hypercapnic patients (mean preoperative $PaCO_2$ = 66.9 mmHg) demonstrated the most marked degree of improvement in dyspnea index and significant improvement in all other measured parameters. Steroid-dependent patients had equivalent functional results with the exception of 6-min walk distance. High-risk patients with profound pulmonary dysfunction as measured by FEV_1 exhibited greater increases in FVC than the lower risk group, equivalent improvement in all other parameters, and comparable actuarial survival at 12 mo.

Table 1
Reported Complications of LVRS in 564 Patients
Described in 8 Clinical Series Described in the Text
(see Table 2)

Air leak > 7 d	247
Pneumonia	33
Reoperation	22
Tracheostomy	21
Reintubation	21
Arrhythmia	11
GI (nonoperative)	9
Cardiac event/MI	5
CVA	5
"Infection"	5
Wound infection	3
Duodenal perforation	3
Hemorrhage	3
Acute abdomen	2
Cecal perforation	2
Cholecystitis	1
Empyema	1

Only a very limited number of studies have compared unilateral to bilateral lung volume reduction with respect to patient selection, efficacy, and morbidity. Nonetheless, there is a consensus opinion that the majority of patients with heterogeneous emphysema benefit most from a bilateral procedure (see *12a*). McKenna et al. *(13)* studied 116 patients in a nonrandomized trial with sequential assignment to either unilateral or bilateral thoracoscopic LVRS. Patients were excluded for active tobacco use, age greater than 80 yr, $PaCO_2 > 55$ mmHg, coronary artery disease, malignancy within 5 yr, or a history of previous thoracic procedure. Mean FEV_1 was 0.67 (25% of predicted) and all patients demonstrated heterogeneous disease by CT scan, hyperinflation, and specific target areas defined by quantitative lung perfusion. No patient underwent preoperative pulmonary rehabilitation. There were no statistically significant differences in baseline characteristics between the two study groups preoperatively.

Overall, patients subjected to the bilateral procedure were more likely to be independent of supplemental oxygen (68% vs 35%) and steroids (86% vs 56%) postoperatively. Postoperatively, bilateral LVRS patients had a 57% improvement in FEV_1 after 3 mo as opposed to only 31% in the unilateral LVRS group, and just 12% of bilateral LVRS patients reported grade 3 or 4 dyspnea postoperatively, compared to 44% of the unilateral LVRS patients. However, although perioperative mortality (< 30 d) did not differ between groups (approx 3%), 1-yr mortality was 17% for unilateral patients vs 2.5% in the bilateral population. More importantly, the 1-yr mortality for the sickest patients undergoing unilateral reduction (e.g., age > 75 yr, $FEV_1 > 0.5$ L, $PaO_2 < 50$ mmHg) was 30% with all deaths resulting from respiratory failure. The authors suggest that bilateral lung reduction is the treatment of choice for all patients. This may be particularly true in the highest risk group where the functional results of best possible operation might offset some of the morbidity associated with severe debility, as suggested by the cited Columbia study. Although multivariate analysis of McKenna's data did not identify any group of patients which benefited from unilateral LVRS, unilateral LVRS did produce comparable results to bilateral reduction in patients with unilateral disease. Nonetheless, the authors concluded that previous unilateral thoracic surgery, pleural disease or sclerosis remain relative contraindications to effective bilateral lung volume reduction and may require a unilateral approach in the symptomatic patient.

In a separate analysis of the Columbia data, Argenziano et al. *(14)* studied the functional differences between unilateral and bilateral LVRS in a total cohort of 92 patients. Of these, 28 patients underwent unilateral LVRS for a number of indications, including asymmetric disease distribution, prior thoracotomy, or concomitant tumor resection. In their analysis, the authors found that unilateral and bilateral LVRS resulted in comparable improvements in exercise capacity and dyspnea severity at short-term follow-up, but that patients with a bilateral procedure demonstrated greater improvements in spirometric indices of pulmonary function. Perioperative mortality was 7.4% for bilateral LVRS and 3.6% for unilateral LVRS, but there was no significant difference between the groups with respect to 24-mo actuarial survival. The authors concluded that although the bilateral procedure appeared superior, the unilateral approach conferred sufficient subjective benefit to be justified in patients with contraindications for bilateral surgery or markedly asymmetric disease distribution.

Additional case series include the Daniel et al. *(15)* study of 26 patients with 3-mo follow-up demonstrating a 49% improvement in FEV_1 (from 0.75 L to 1.02 L), a 14% reduction in total lung capacity (from 8.39 L to 7.19 L), and a significant improvement in QOL in 71% of patients surveyed. A unique aspect of this study is the use of single positron emission CT scans (SPECT) to evaluate the 3-D distribution of lung perfusion and subsequent segmental localization of diseased target areas. Contrary to standard anatomical CT scans, SPECT analysis identified disease heterogeneity in every patient evaluated. Despite clinical presentations consistent with emphysematous COPD and centrilobar disease confined to the upper lobes, SPECT analysis identified lower lobe disease for segmental resection in 50% of patients. In another small study (20 patients) from Australia, Snell et al. *(16)* also demonstrated significant improvement in lung function (54% increase in FEV_1), exercise tolerance as measured by 6-min walk distance (from 306 m to 431 m), and symptoms (MRC Dyspnea Score from 3.4 to 2.1). Outcomes for LVRS clinical trials are summarized in Table 2.

The recent study of Criner et al. *(17)* represents the first prospective, randomized, controlled trial of pulmonary rehabilitation vs rehabilitation with subsequent LVRS. Of 200 patients with nonbullous emphysema initially recruited, only 37 met study criteria for randomization: NYHA Class III or IV disease, evidence of airflow obstruction and hyperinflation by pulmonary function testing (i.e., FEV_1 < 30% of predicted and FRC or TLC > 120% of predicted), and hyperinflated target areas defined by high-resolution CT scan with quantitative perfusion lung scans demonstrating decreased or absent perfusion. Patients with refractory hypoxemia (PaO_2/FIO_2 ratio < 150), hypercapnia requiring mechanical ventilation, severe pulmonary hypertension (mean PAP > 35 mmHg), severe debilitation (body weight < 70% of ideal weight), significant extrapulmonary comorbidity (cardiac, renal) with end-organ dysfunction expected to limit survival, psychosocial dysfunction, or continued tobacco use were excluded from participation. All patients meeting selection criteria underwent evaluation for functional status, gas exchange, symptom limited maximal exercise tolerance, and QOL assessment followed by 8 wk of outpatient pulmonary rehabilitation and repeat data collection. Patients were then randomized to medical therapy and 3 mo of additional maintenance rehabilitation or bilateral LVRS via a median sternotomy with the goal of removing 20–40% of the volume of each lung. Both randomized groups underwent repeat evaluation at 3 mo Study design allowed randomized patients completing the 3 mo of medical therapy to electively crossover to the lung volume reduction treatment group.

Overall, results of this study mirror those of nonrandomized trials. Patients undergoing pulmonary rehabilitation alone had no significant change in values for spirometry, lung volume, or diffusion capacity. Although there was a trend toward a higher 6-min walk distance (269 m to 285 m), only total time on maximal exercise test was significantly improved from baseline after 8-wk of pulmonary rehabilitation (from 5.8 min to 7.4 min). There was no significant improvement in oxygen consumption (VO_2), gas exchange ($PaCO_2$, PaO_2/FiO_2), or pattern of breathing (frequency, tidal volume, or maximum ventilation). In

Table 2
Summary of Pre- and Postoperative LVRS data for 8 Nonrandomized Clinical Trials Discussed in the Text

	Cronin	Miller	Argenziano	Daniel	McKenna	Bingisser	Cooper	Kotloff
Pro FEV1	0.69 L	0.56 L	0.52 L	0.73 L	0.64 L	0.80 L	0.70 L	0.73L
Post FEV1	0.85 L	1.08 L	0.80 L	1.02 L	0.97 L	1.09 L	1.06 L	1.02L
Pre TLC	7.0 L			8.39 L		8.78 L	8.4 L	
Post TLC	6.5 L			7.19 L		7.34 L	7.2 L	
Pre 6MW	260 m	785 ft	598 ft			495 m*	1125 ft	999 ft
Post 6MW	321 m	1250 ft	919 ft			688 m*	1311 ft	1181 ft
QOL/DS	Yes		Yes		Yes	Yes	Yes	
Mortality	9.4%	5.6%	7%	3.8%	2.5%	0%	4%	4.2%

QOL/DS Represents various QOL and dyspnea score indices. "Yes" indicates statistically significant improvement. Mortality reflects perioperative events variously defined as in-hospital deaths or death within 30 or 90 days. *12-min walk distance. **Represents data from median sternotomy patients only.

contrast, bilateral LVRS in addition to maximal medical therapy and pulmonary rehabilitation resulted in substantial improvement in FVC (from 2.3 L to 2.79 L) and FEV_1 (from 0.65 L to 0.85 L), a significant decrease in TLC (from 7.65 L to 6.53 L) and FRC (from 5.7 L to 4.5 L), a reduction in resting $PaCO_2$ (from 47 mmHg to 43 mmHg), and a statistically significant improvement in diffusion capacity (DLCO, from 1.8 to 2.1) and maximal ventilatory volume (from 26 L/min to 35 L/min).

TECHNICAL CONSIDERATIONS

Whereas there is a reasonable consensus as to the efficacy of bilateral LVRS in patients with severe COPD, controversy continues with respect to the surgical approach (sternotomy vs thoracotomy), the surgical timing (staged vs single procedure), and the surgical technique (thoracoscopic vs open) of volume reduction. Results of a bilateral thoracoscopic approach to LVRS published by Bingisser et al. *(18)* demonstrated outcomes comparable to those of median sternotomy with respect to pulmonary function (42% increase in FEV_1, from 0.8 L to 1.09 L), improvement in residual volume (from 5.8 L to 4.4 L), grading of dyspnea (from MRC Dyspnea Index 3.9 to 1.8), and exercise performance (increase in MVO_2 from 10 to 13 cc/kg/min). A unique aspect of this thoracoscopic series was the observation of immediate improvements in pulmonary function tests postoperatively, with similar functional characteristics at 3 mo. This is in contrast to the median sternotomy LVRS data, wherein maximal improvement in pulmonary function testing is consistently demonstrated only after 3–6 mo. It is unclear whether the more immediate improvement in pulmonary function after the thoracoscopic procedure is the result of the limited incisional injury with this approach.

The study of Kotloff et al. *(19)* currently represents the only direct comparison of median sternotomy (MS) and video-assisted thoracoscopy (VATS) for LVRS. In a nonrandomized trial of 120 patients undergoing volume reduction by either median sternotomy ($n = 80$) or bilateral VATS ($n = 40$), no significant differences between the groups were noted for postoperative FEV_1 (0.73 L to 1.02 L for median sternotomy vs 0.73 L to 1.00 L for VATS), FVC (2.28 L to 2.65 L for median sternotomy vs 3.13 L to 2.72 L for VATS), or 6-min walk distance (999 ft to 1181 ft for median sternotomy vs 969 ft to 1244 ft for VATS). Whereas functional results, duration of postoperative air leak, and mean length of stay were similar in the two groups, the median sternotomy approach was associated with a statistically significant increase in mortality. In-hospital mortality was 2.5% in the VATS group compared with 4.2% in the median sternotomy group at 30 d. An additional six patients died in the median sternotomy group prior to discharge from an in-patient facility, although there were no additional deaths in the VATS group. Mechanisms of death included respiratory failure in two patients, bowel perforation in two patients, sepsis in three patients, and cardiac arrest in one patient. Mortality was highest for older patients, with 21% of the median sternotomy patients greater than 65 yr of age dying prior to hospital discharge.

RANDOMIZED CONTROLLED TRIALS: THE NATIONAL EMPHYSEMA TREATMENT TRIAL

The role of randomized controlled trials (RCTs) in clinical surgery remains controversial and poorly understood. Recent reviews of the surgical literature have identified the case series as the most common investigative method of surgical evaluation (20) and found published surgical trials to be of poor quality with respect to methodological design, calculations of statistical power, and adequate definitions of outcome (21). Although this lack of randomization in surgical series has been explained by the inherent difficulty in standardization of surgical techniques (22), disagreement as to appropriate end points, and the inability to design study protocols that are acceptable to both surgeons and patients alike (23) effective surgical trials have been published for carotid artery disease (24) and breast cancer (25). In addition, surgical series that fail to meet the strict criteria currently established for reporting randomized trials (26) may have significant merit. As noted by Marquis (27), clinical evidence need not be conclusive to be valuable, nor does it need to be definitive to be suggestive. Nonetheless, the randomized controlled trial remains the standard for evidence-based medicine and the NETT represents a unique collaboration between the NHLBI and HCFA for funding a randomized protocol of LVRS (28).

NETT is a prospective, unblinded, randomized clinical trial comparing medical management of severe emphysema to a program of medical therapy and bilateral LVRS via either a median sternotomy or VATS approach (29). Based upon the historical experience with LVRS in 1741 patients, the NETT Coordinating Center was unable to establish convincing evidence for the efficacy of volume reduction surgery when evaluated by logistic regression analysis. In the context of the reportedly poor outcome for LVRS patients reported by HCFA after analysis of Medicare claims (23% 12-mo mortality), significant questions remained as to the risk/benefit ratio of surgical therapy. Consequently, the NETT study was designed to evaluate the efficacy of LVRS and to identify patients who might receive disproportionate benefit or inordinate risk from volume reduction surgery. The trial is to include patients with both heterogeneous and homogeneous emphysema with survival and maximum exercise capacity defined as the primary measures of outcome. Secondary outcome measures include QOL and disease-specific symptoms, pulmonary function testing with assessment of gas exchange, O_2 requirements, 6-min walk distance, ECHO evaluation of cardiovascular function, testing of psychomotor function, and cost analysis. All patients participate in 6–10 wk of preoperative pulmonary rehabilitation prior to randomization to medical therapy alone vs medical therapy and LVRS. Patients in the surgical arm undergo a second randomization to procedure by either VATS or median sternotomy. Detailed criteria for inclusion and exclusion from the NETT study have recently been published (29).

Despite the obvious merits of the NETT study, such randomized trials are not without controversy and technical limitations. Bauchner and Wise (30) have pointed out that clinical decision making is guided not only by empirical evidence—ideally derived from consensus among randomized controlled trials—but also by the professional experiences of referring and treating physicians and a patients' knowledge of treatment options and outcomes in the context of their personal values. Each of these domains may be in direct conflict and subsequently influence the perceived need for and use of randomized trials among both clinicians and the public at large.

Randomization may itself be considered unethical. Patients seek medical advice and reasonably expect physicians to offer therapeutic options based upon their interpretation of available empirical data and clinical experience. Physicians may feel a therapeutic obligation to recommend surgical intervention, particularly in patients who are already undergoing pulmonary rehabilitation with maximal medical therapy in the context of progressive disease. Likewise, such patients resent the personal costs in time and finance required to travel to designated NETT centers in an attempt to meet inclusion criteria, which may, at best, result in a 50% chance of randomization to surgery. This has resulted in legislative attempts to preclude randomization (e.g., The Coalition for Pulmonary Patient Care). Whether these issues will significantly influence enrollment in the NETT study is unclear.

Acceptable end points represent a second area of controversy. Patients with progressive chronic illnesses frequently pursue therapeutic modalities which promote a reduction in disease-specific symptoms and a perceived improvement in QOL independent of survival advantage or objective evidence of treatment efficacy. The NETT study is not a blinded trial and there is no allocation concealment of treatment groups—participants are readily aware of the treatment arm to which they are assigned. Accordingly, personal narrative of treatment outcome influences potential trial participants. Electronic databases of treatment experience (www.ctsnet.org) suggest that patients with end-stage lung disease seek trial enrollment as a therapeutic intervention to alleviate symptoms with an overwhelming interest in surgical therapy. Survival and performance may represent objective and quantifiable outcome variables that meet standards of research design, but more proximate therapeutic goals relating to symptom relief and QOL may represent the outcome variables most important to patients. This discrepancy could result in a health care policy that does not necessarily coincide with acceptable health care practice because it is unclear how the NETT study will be used to inform this public debate. If LVRS offers no statistically significant survival advantage, but only a transient improvement in QOL, will this be interpreted as a qualitative difference in treatment efficacy or as a treatment failure? This potential dichotomy between the well-intentioned goals of rigorous research design and the ethical concerns of providing patient care is not unique to trials of LVRS and has recently been explored in the controversial use of sham surgery for trials of fetal cell transplants in Parkinson's disease *(31)*.

Finally, much of the controversy among participants in randomized trials in general and LVRS trials in particular is a direct result of misinformation. Informed consent of patients being enrolled in clinical trials should strive to eliminate the misconception that participation in randomization is designed to be clinically therapeutic *(31)*. Although patients enrolled in clinical trials should not be considered nontherapeutic research subjects, clinical trials by definition are experimental and designed not to treat participants, but to establish the efficacy and scientific basis of a presumed clinically useful strategy. Efficacious therapeutic intervention is not a goal of clinical trials, but a fortunate accident of randomization, although there is some data to support the notion that participation in a randomized trial is a superior therapeutic alternative to nonparticipation when no consensus therapy exists *(32)*.

Criticisms of the NETT study should not be construed as nonsupport. The trial represents an exceptional collaboration between the National Heart, Lung, and Blood Institute and the Health Care Financing Administration. The study will undoubtedly produce much useful information. How this information will be used to construct public health policy for LVRS remains to be seen.

SUMMARY

There is consensus from nonrandomized clinical series that lung volume reduction results in significant improvement in measures of dyspnea and pulmonary mechanics as measured by pulmonary function testing. Less consensus exists with respect to the variable improvement in exercise performance. No consensus exists with respect to survival advantage. Although NETT is designed to address a number of these questions, several important clinical issues remain largely unexplored. These include the role of LVRS in COPD patients with malignancy who are currently considered unresectable by standard measures of pulmonary function (*see* Chapter 15); the role of combined LVRS with coronary artery bypass grafting in patients who are excluded from volume reduction by cardiac criteria and simultaneously precluded from surgical revascularization because of compromised pulmonary status; and the role of LVRS in the context of lung transplantation (*see* Chapter 16). Clinical trials designed to answer these questions will require the specific descriptive information currently being gathered in the NETT study with respect to patient selection and survival, relative procedural risk, and duration of measurable clinical improvement.

REFERENCES

1. Cooper JA (1997) The history of surgical procedures for emphysema. *Ann Thor Surg* 63:312–319.
2. Allison PR (1947) Giant bullous cysts of the lung. *Thorax* 2:169.
3. Carter MG, Gaensler EA, Kyllonen A (1950) Pneumoperitoneum in the treatment of pulmonary emphysema. N Engl J Med 243:549–558.
4. Crenshaw GL, Rowles DF (1952) Surgical management of pulmonary emphysema. *J Thoracic Surg* 24:398–410.
5. Abbott OA, Hopkins WA, Van Fleit W, Robinson JS (1953) A new approach to pulmonary emphysema. *Thorax* 8:115–132.
6. Nakayama K (1961) Surgical removal of the carotid body for bronchial asthma. *Dis Chest* 40:595–604.
7. Brantigan O (1954) Surgical treatment of pulmonary emphysema. *W Virg Med J* 50:283.
8. Knudsen RJ, Gaensler EA (1965) Surgery for emphysema. *Ann Thoracic Surg* 1:332–362.
9. Cooper JD, Trulock EP, Triantafillou AN, et al. (1995) Bilateral pneumectomy (volume reduction) for chronic obstructive pulmonary disease. J Thorac Cardiovasc Surg 109:106–119.
10. Cooper JD, Patterson GA, Sundaresan RS, Trulock EP, Yusen RD, Pohl MS, Lefrak SS (1996) Results of 150 consecutive bilateral lung volume reduction procedures in patients with severe emphysema. J Thorac Cardiovasc Surg 112:1319–1330.
11. Miller JI, Lee RB, Mansour KA (1996) Lung volume reduction surgery:lessons learned. *Ann Thor Surg* 61:464–469.
12. Argenziano M, Moazami N, Byron T, et al. (1996) Extended indications for lung volume reduction surgery in advanced emphysema. *Ann Thorac Surg* 62:1588–1597.
12a. Akaishi T, Kaneda I, Higuchi N (1996) Thorascopic en bloc total esophagectomy with radical mediastinal lymphadenectomy. *J Thorac Cardiovasc Surg* 112:1533–1540.

13. McKenna RJ, Brenner M, Fischel R, Gelb AF (1996) Should lung volume reduction for emphysema be unilateral or bilateral? *J Thorac Cardiovasc Surg* 112:1331–1339.

14. Argenziano M, Thomashow B, Jellen PA, Rose EA, Steinglass KM, Ginsburg ME, Gorenstein LA (1997) A functional comparison of unilateral versus bilateral lung volume reduction surgery. *Ann Thorac Surg* 64:321–326, discussion 326–327.

15. Daniel TM, Chan BBK, Bhaskar V, Parekh J, Walters PE, et al. (1996) Lung volume reduction surgery: Case selection, operative technique, and clinical results. *Ann Surg* 223:526–533.

16. Snell GI, Solin P, Chin W, Rabinov M, Williams TJ, et al. (1997) Lung volume reduction surgery for emphysema. *Med J Austral* 167:529–532.

17. Criner GJ, Cordova FC, Furukawa S, et al. (1999) Prospective ransdomized trial comparing bilateral lung volume reduction surgery to pulmonary rehabilitation in severe chronic obstructive pulmonary disease. *Am J Respir Crit Care Med* 160:2018–2027.

18. Bingisser R, Zollinger A, Hauser M, Bloch KE, Russi EW, Weder W (1996) Bilateral volume reduction surgery for diffuse pulmonary emphysema by video-assisted thoracoscopy. *J Thorac Cardiovasc Surg* 112:875–882.

19. Kotloff RM, Gregory T, Bavaria JE, Palevsky HI, Hansen-Flaschen J, Wahl PM, Kaiser LR (1996) Bilateral lung volume reduction surgery for advanced emphysema: A comparison of median sternotomy and thoracoscopic approaches. *Chest* 110:1399–1406.

20. Horton R (1996) Surgical research or comic opera: questions , but few answers. *Lancet* 347:984,985.

21. Solomon MJ, Laxamana A, Devore L, McLeod RS (1994) Randomized controlled trials in surgery. *Surgery* 115:707–712.

22. Majeed AW, Troy G, Nicholl JP, et al. (1996) Randomized, prospective, single blind comparison of laparoscopic versus small incision cholecsytectomy. *Lancet* 347:989–994.

23. Udelsman R, Lakatos E, Ladenson P (1996) Optimal surgery for papillary thyroid carcinoma. *World J Surg* 20:88–99.

24. ECST collaborative group (1998) Randomized trial of endarterectomy. *Lancet* 351:1379–1387.

25. Fisher B, Redmond C, Poisson R, et al. (1989) Eight year results of a randomized clinical trial comparing total mastectomy and lumpectomy with with or without irradiation in the treatment of breast cancer. N Engl J Med 320:822–828.

26. (1996) CONSORT: Consolidated Standards of Reporting Trials. *JAMA* 276:637.

27. Marquis D (1999) How to resolve an ethical dilemma concerning randomized clinical trials. N Engl J Med 341:691–693.

28. Utz JP, Hubmayr RD, Deschamps C (1998) Lung volume reduction surgery for emphysema: Out on a limb without a NETT. *Mayo Clin Proc* 73:552–566.

29. NETT Research Group (1999) Rationale and design of the National Emphysema Treatment Trial: A prospective randomized trial of lung volume reduction surgery. *Chest* 166:1750–1761.

30. Bauchner A, Wise PH (2000) Antibiotics without prescription: "bacterial or medical resistance." *Lancet* 355:1480.

31. Macklin R (1999) The ethical problems with sham surgery in clinical research. N Engl J Med 341:992–995.

32. Davis S, Wright PW, Schulman, et al. (1985) Participants in prospective, randomized clinical trials for resected non-small cell lung cancer have improved survival compared with nonparticipants in such trials. *Cancer* 56:1710.

14 Effects of Lung Volume Reduction Surgery on Survival in Patients with Advanced Emphysema

Michael Argenziano, MD,
Lyall A. Gorenstein, MD,
and Mark E. Ginsburg, MD

CONTENTS

INTRODUCTION

As detailed in Chapter 13, early reports have suggested that in many patients, lung volume reduction surgery (LVRS) could provide significant improvements in respiratory function and dyspnea with low perioperative morbidity and mortality *(1–7)*. More recent data from centers reporting their medium-term experiences confirm the functional and subjective benefits of LVRS in selected patient populations *(8–11)*. Some investigators, however, have raised questions about the durability

From: *Lung Volume Reduction Surgery*
Edited by: M. Argenziano and M. E. Ginsburg © Humana Press Inc., Totowa, NJ

of these benefits, which appear to be short-lived in many patients *(12,13)*. Only the analysis of longer-term data will clarify whether improvements in pulmonary function after LVRS will be long-lived or gradually be lost as the underlying disease process pursues its natural course.

Because emphysema is a progressive disease with no known cure, LVRS is currently regarded as a palliative, rather than curative, procedure. Although much has been written about the functional and subjective consequences of LVRS, less attention has been focused on the impact of LVRS on survival beyond the early postoperative period. The long-term effects of LVRS on the natural history of advanced emphysema are not known, because no clinical study to date has randomized patients to LVRS vs medical treatment. In addition, the identification of clinical predictors of short- and long-term survival after LVRS would be helpful in the selection of candidates for this procedure. We thus undertook a study, summarized in this chapter, of the determinants of medium-term survival in 136 patients undergoing LVRS for advanced emphysema at our institution over a 4-yr period *(14)*. We also analyzed the influence of a variety of demographic and clinical factors on survival, identifying several characteristics predictive of reduced longevity after LVRS.

PATIENT SELECTION AND PREOPERATIVE ASSESSMENT

Operative candidates were selected on the basis of hyperinflation, heterogeneity of disease, pulmonary perfusion and ventilation deficits, and significant functional disability. Patients with morbid obesity, chronic bronchitis and/or excessive sputum production, metastatic cancer, continued or recent cigarette smoking, or less-than-severe functional disability were excluded from consideration.

Preoperative evaluation included inspiratory and expiratory posteroanterior and lateral chest radiographs as well, and inspiratory and expiratory chest computed tomography (CT) scans. Quantitative ventilation-perfusion scans with xenon washout studies were obtained in all patients, and dobutamine stress thallium studies and/or left-heart catheterization were performed in patients with suspected coronary artery disease. Patients with suspected right-ventricular dysfunction underwent echocardiography and/or right-heart catheterization. All patients were offered preoperative rehabilitation therapy, and the majority participated in a rehabilitation program prior to operation.

Pulmonary function was assessed by standard spirometry, including measurement of forced expiratory volume in one second (FEV_1), forced vital capacity (FVC), total lung capacity (TLC), and residual volume (RV), as well as lung volume determination by helium dilution and body plethysmography. Arterial blood gas analysis, cardiopulmonary stress testing, and 6-min walk test were also performed. Finally, patients were asked to subjectively classify their degree of dyspnea according to the Modified Medical Research Council (MRC) Dyspnea Index *(15)*. This screening tool grades the degree of dyspnea on a scale ranging from 0 to 5. Grade 0 represents no functional impairment, and grade 5 represents dyspnea at rest.

Repeated spirometry, 6-min walk test, and dyspnea grading were requested from patients 3–6 mo postoperatively, and at 6-mo intervals thereafter. For purposes of the postoperative data analysis, measurements obtained closest to 6 mo postoperatively were used. Survival status was assessed by contacting all patients directly or through their primary physicians.

STATISTICAL ANALYSIS

Data were analyzed using SAS system software (SAS Institute, Inc., Cary, NC). The paired student's *t*-test was used for analyzing the relationship between preoperative and postoperative data. Survival data were first examined univariately by means of standard contingency tables and the Kaplan-Meier Product-Limit estimate. Any variable with a *p*-value less than 0.25 was next explored as a potential risk factor in multivariable analyses. Three separate multivariable analyses were conducted. The first analyzed the influence of preoperative and demographic variables listed in Table 1 on long-term survival. The second included both pre- and postoperative assessments of these variables. In each case, the Cox Proportional Hazard model was utilized. A third analysis applied multiple logistic regression to compute an equation predicting "early death" (death within three months of surgery). All *p*-values are reported without corrections for multiple comparisons, and $p < 0.05$ was considered significant. Next, utilizing Cox proportional hazard techniques, the preoperative characteristics found to be independently associated with survival (by multivariable analysis) were entered into a predictive statistical model, yielding the equation:

$$S(t) = S_o(t)e^{(\beta_1 x_1 + \beta_2 x_2 + \beta_3 x_3 + \beta_4 x_4 + \beta_5 x_5)}$$

where $S(t)$ is the survival probability at time t for an individual with covariate values x_1, x_2, x_3, x_4, and x_5, $So(t)$ is the baseline survivor function, and β_1 to β_5 are constants approximating the risk of death associated with the presence of each variable. The covariate values (x_1 to x_5) are numerical values corresponding to the presence or absence of each of the

Table 1
Baseline Demographics of 136 Patients
Undergoing LVRS

Characteristic	Value
Age, years	62.1 ± 7.7
Gender, no (%)	
Female	78 (57.4%)
Male	58 (42.6%)
Operation, no (%)	
Unilateral LVRS	50 (36.8%)
Bilateral LVRS	86 (63.2%)
Spirometry (mean ± SD)	
FEV_1, mL	590 ± 227
FEV_1, % predicted	23.4 ± 8.2
FVC, mL	1740 ± 650
FVC, % predicted	50.2 ± 15.5
RV, L	5.2 ± 1.5
RV, % predicted	257.3 ± 69.9
TLC, L	7.2 ± 1.7
TLC, % predicted	132.1 ± 25.6
RV/TLC ratio	0.72 ± 0.09
DLCO, mL/min/mmHg	7.1 ± 6.5
pO_2 (mmHg)	62.5 ± 10.7
pCO_2 (mmHg)	43.8 ± 8.6
Functional Indices	
Dyspnea Index	3.7 ± 0.9
6-min walk distance, ft	696 ± 399

five identified preoperative risk factors for death (age, gender, year of operation, and preoperative pO_2 and FEV_1). After substituting these five values into the equation for a particular patient, the survivor function yields a predicted actuarial survival curve specific to that patient.

OPERATIVE TECHNIQUE

LVRS was performed by thoractotomy in 54 cases, median sternotomy in 48 cases, bilateral thoracosternotomy (clamshell) in 46 cases, and thoracoscopy in 5 cases. With the aid of alternating lung deflation, resections were performed utilizing GIA stapling devices (U.S. Surgical, Inc., Ethicon, Inc.) lined with bovine pericardial strips (BioVascular, Inc.) to minimize air leakage. Extent of resection was guided by preoperative radiographic and physiologic studies.

RESULTS

Demographics and Early Postoperative Results

A total of 153 patients underwent LVRS over a 51-mo period. Advanced emphysema was the primary indication for surgery in 136 cases. Ten other patients underwent limited lung reduction in association with wedge resection or lobectomy for confirmed or suspected malignant disease, and seven had unilateral lung reduction after failed unilateral lung transplantation. For the purposes of the present analysis, only patients undergoing LVRS for emphysema as a primary indication ($n = 136$) were considered. Mean age was 62 ± 8 yr, 78 patients (58%) were female, and mean preoperative FEV_1 was 590 ± 227 mL ($23 \pm 8\%$ of predicted). Complete demographic and baseline clinical characteristics of the patient cohort are listed in Table 1. Seven deaths occurred perioperatively (in hospital or within 30 d of surgery), corresponding to an operative mortality of 5.1%. Because 14 patients did not survive to the first postoperative testing interval (6 mo) and another 6 were alive, but had not yet reached this interval at the time of this analysis, a total of 116 patients were eligible for early postoperative evaluation. Of these, pulmonary function data were complete for 114, or 98%, and dyspnea indices were available in 105, or 91%. Mean postoperative FEV_1 was 809 ± 363 mL ($31 \pm 12\%$ of predicted), representing an increase of $44 \pm 50\%$ over preoperative values ($p < 0.0001$). Likewise, the dyspnea index (DI) improved significantly, from 3.7 ± 0.9 preoperatively to 1.7 ± 1.1 postoperatively ($p < 0.0001$). Of interest, an analysis of the larger group of patients ($n = 153$) yielded similar results with respect to demographics and actuarial survival (data not shown).

Overall Survival

Survival information was complete for all 136 patients at the time of analysis. Mean postoperative followup time was 28 ± 16 mo (median 29.3 mo; range 3–54 mo). The number of patients who had achieved 1, 2, and 3 yr of follow-up were 108, 72, and 46, respectively. A total of 49 deaths occurred between 2 d and 49 mo after surgery, corresponding to a postoperative actuarial survival of 85%, 71%, and 60% at 1, 2, and 3 yr, respectively (see Fig. 1). By multivariable analysis, survival was significantly influenced by a number of preoperative and postoperative variables.

Preoperative predictors of decreased survival are listed in Table 2, and included increasing age, male gender, hypoxemia, and less-than-severe impairments in FEV_1. Univariate Kaplan-Meier survival curves

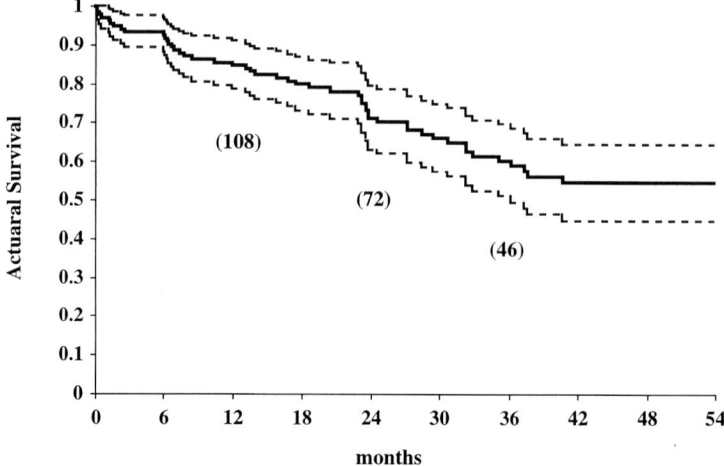

Fig. 1. Actuarial survival in 136 patients undergoing LVRS. Dashed lines indicate upper and lower 95% confidence limits.

Table 2
Multivariable Analysis of Risk Factors Influencing Actuarial Survival

Variable	Risk Factor	Odds Ratio	95% C.L.[*]	p value
Preoperative factors ($n = 136$)				
gender	male	3.3	1.7–6.2	0.0003
FEV_1, % predicted	> 25	2.8	1.5–5.5	0.002[**]
year of operation	before 1996	2.3	1.1–4.8	0.03
pO_2, mmHg	≤ 60	2.1	1.1–3.8	0.019
age	10-yr increase	1.9	1.2–3.0	0.009[**]
Postoperative factors ($n = 114$)				
% increase in FEV_1[†]	20% increase	0.83	0.69–0.97	0.05
Dyspnea index	each 1.0 on scale[††]	1.5	1.1–2.0	0.02
Preoperative predictors of early death (within 3 mo of surgery)				
Age (yr)	≥ 70	19.7	3.6–107.4	0.0006
FEV_1 (% predicted)	≥ 25	5.3	1.1–25.6	0.03

[*]C.L. = Confidence limit;
[**] These were also significant as continuous variables;
[†] Because odds ratio is less than 1.0, this is actually not a risk factor but a factor predictive of improved survival;
[††] For example, a patient with a postoperative DI = 4 has a 1.5-fold greater risk of death than a patient with a postoperative DI = 3, and a three-fold greater risk of death than a patient with a postoperative DI = 2.

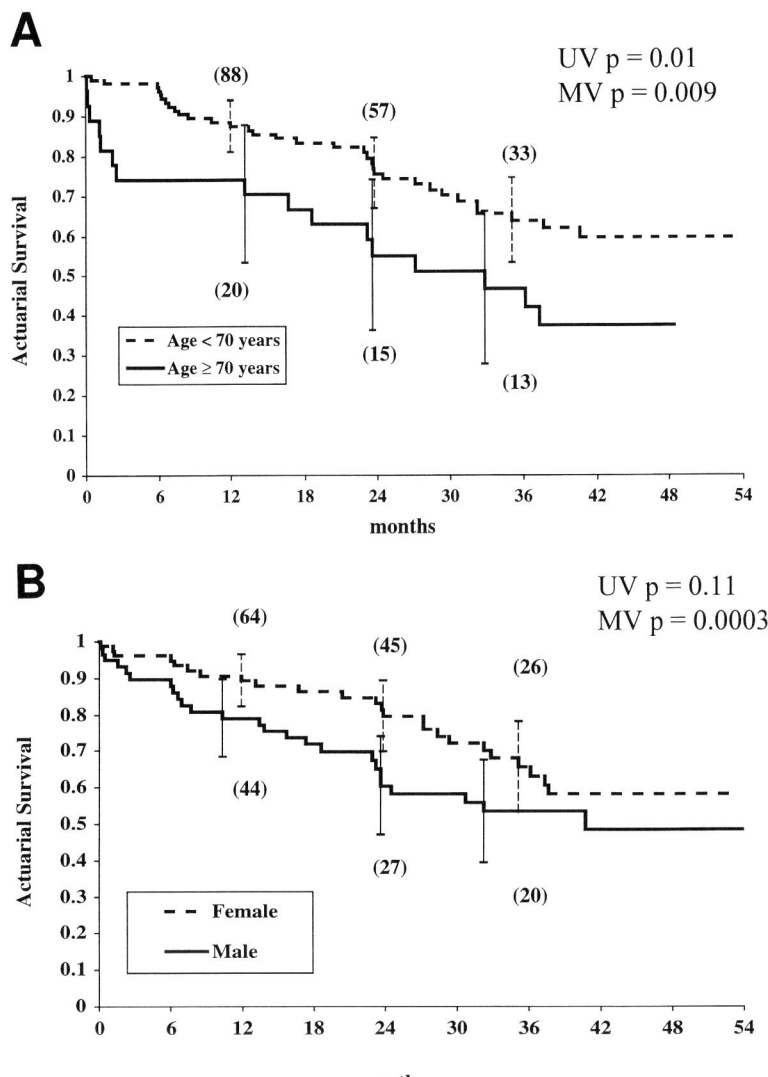

Fig. 2. Influence of (a) age; (b) gender; (c) preoperative pO_2 ; (d) preoperative FEV_1; (e) year of operation on actuarial survival in 136 patients undergoing LVRS. UV = univariate p-value; MV = multivariate p-value; error bars represent 95% confidence intervals at 12, 24, and 36 mo.

comparing each of these variables are represented in Figs. 2a–2e. Conversely, survival was not significantly influenced by preoperative pCO_2 or DI, or by extent of operation (unilateral vs bilateral).

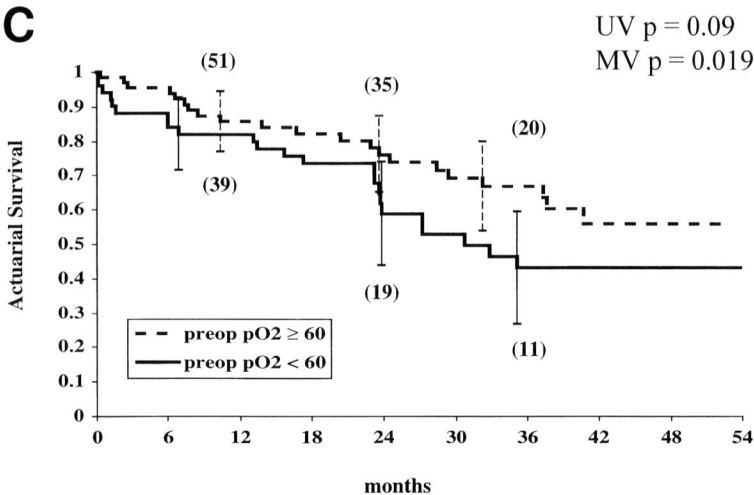

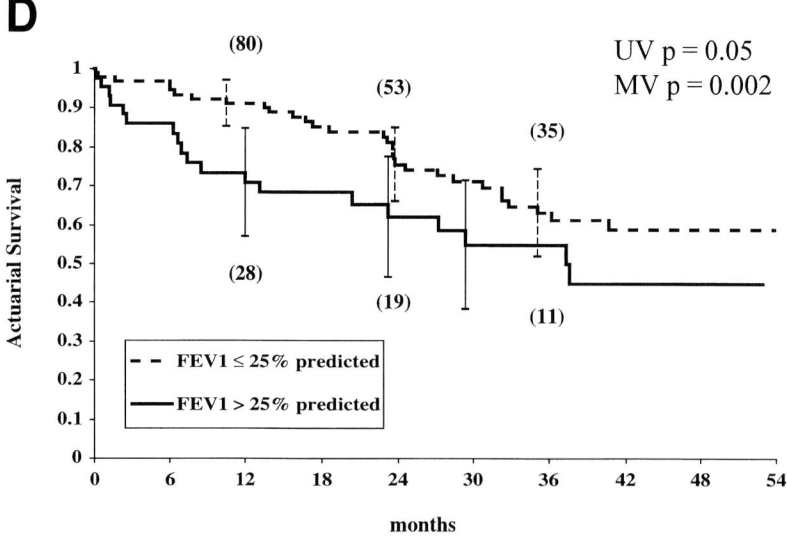

Fig. 2. (cont.)

In the second multivariable analysis, 114 patients surviving to their first postoperative evaluation were studied. Although both preoperative and early postoperative data were included in this model, the only two factors identified as independent predictors of subsequent survival were postoperative improvement in FEV$_1$ and postoperative DI (Figs. 3a,b). As summarized in Table 2, the risk of death was decreased by 17% for

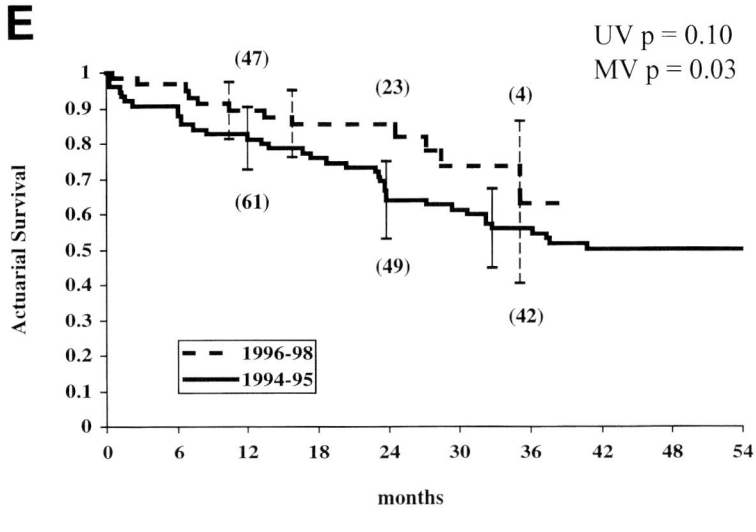

Fig. 2. (cont.)

every 20% increase in FEV_1 over baseline, and increased by a factor of 1.5 for every one-point increase in the postoperative DI.

Predictive Model of Survival

Utilizing Cox proportional hazard techniques, the five preoperative characteristics found to be independently associated with survival (age, gender, year of operation, and preoperative pO_2 and FEV_1) were entered into a predictive statistical model (see Methods section). In Fig. 4, this predictive model is utilized to project 3-yr actuarial survival curves for four hypothetical patients undergoing LVRS.

Incidence and Predictors of Early Postoperative Death

Although the standard definition of operative mortality (death in hospital or within 30 d of operation) was applied in the present analysis, it is our belief that any death occurring within 3 mo of LVRS should be considered a failure of the operation and receive particular attention. We termed these "early deaths," and performed a separate analysis of the incidence and predictors of this outcome after LVRS. Of 136 patients, nine (6.6%) died within 3 mo of surgery. Multivariate analysis identified two characteristics that were strongly and independently predictive of early death: age greater than 70 yr (odds ratio = 19.7) and preoperative $FEV_1 > 25\%$ of predicted (odds ratio = 5.3) (*see* Table 2). The strong association between advanced age and early death is illustrated by the

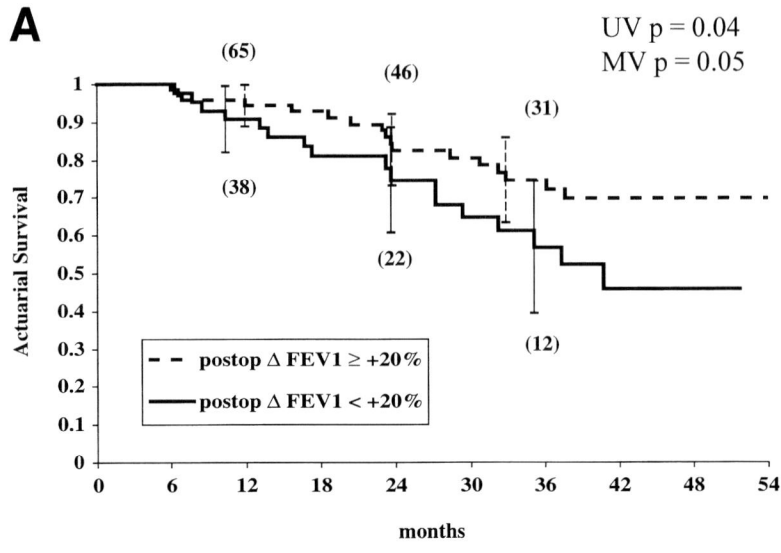

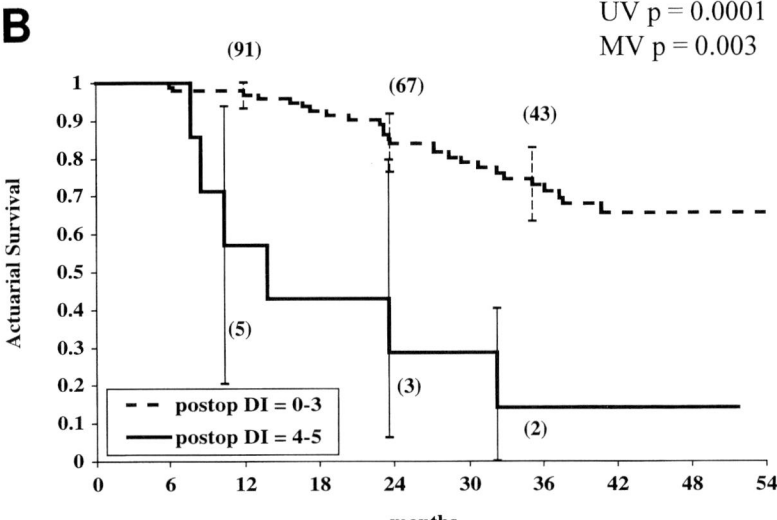

Fig. 3. Influence of postoperative improvement in (a) FEV₁ and (b) DI on actuarial survival in 136 patients undergoing LVRS. UV = univariate p-value; MV = multivariate p-value.

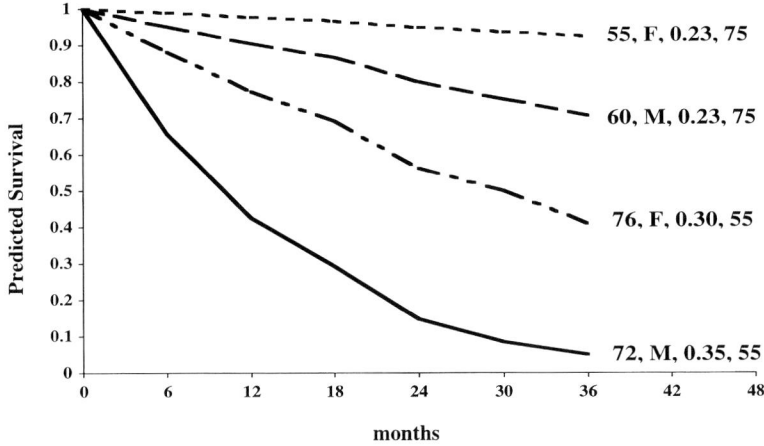

Fig. 4. Application of Cox proportional hazard model in the prediction of 3-yr survival for four hypothetical patients. Risk factors are summarized in the legend adjacent to each curve, in the following sequence: age, gender, preoperative FEV$_1$ (% predicted), and preoperative pO$_2$ (mmHg).

fact that seven of nine patients (78%) who died within 3 mo of surgery in our series were over 70 yr of age.

DOES LVRS IMPROVE SURVIVAL IN PATIENTS WITH SEVERE EMPHYSEMA?

Since its modern reintroduction a few years ago, LVRS has emerged as a promising, but controversial, option in the treatment of advanced emphysema. Short-term results have been encouraging, with several groups reporting early improvements in symptoms and pulmonary function in patients refractory to other available therapies *(3,12)*. However, concerns about data quality and completeness have tempered the enthusiasm generated by many of these studies. Furthermore, although most early studies have reported operative mortality rates, little attention has been paid to the impact of LVRS on survival beyond the early postoperative period. In the only study of its kind, Meyers et al. *(16)* compared a small group of patients who were denied funding for LVRS to a similar group undergoing LVRS. Whereas the cohort undergoing LVRS demonstrated superior pulmonary function postoperatively, significant differences could not be shown in 1- and 3-yr survival rates, likely because of small sample size.

Because emphysema is a progressive disease without a known cure, LVRS is considered a palliative procedure, intended to improve quality of life by alleviating the subjective sensation of dyspnea and increasing functional capacity. An additional benefit of LVRS may be prolongation of life in selected patients with emphysema. Even if LVRS is not expected to extend survival, an understanding of postoperative life expectancy, as well as predictors of mortality, would be clinically important for several reasons. First, a clearer understanding of the demographic and clinical determinants of long-term survival will greatly simplify the evaluation of patients referred for LVRS, focusing the diagnostic workup on factors relevant to the prediction of operative success or failure. Second, such knowledge will facilitate selection of patients for LVRS, allowing the procedure to be offered preferentially to patients in whom the expected functional and symptomatic benefits outweigh the predicted risk of mortality. Third, awareness of factors likely to influence survival will aid in the planning and execution of randomized trials, facilitating risk group stratification. Finally, because many functional variables, including dyspnea measurement scales, quality of life indices, and even pulmonary function tests can be difficult to standardize and meaningfully interpret, long-term survival may emerge as an unambiguous measure which further validates the efficacy of LVRS.

In our study of 136 patients undergoing LVRS at a single institution over 4 yr, operative mortality was 5.1% and actuarial survival at 1, 2, and 3 yr was 85%, 71%, and 60%, respectively. In addition to confirming an acceptable operative risk in this chronically ill patient population, these data suggest that a significant proportion of LVRS patients will survive at least several years. Although these figures compare favorably with historical survival estimates in medically treated patients with similar degrees of pulmonary impairment *(17)*, the absence of prospective randomization of patients to operative vs nonoperative management precludes the formulation of any conclusions regarding the survival benefit of LVRS. To this end, the National Emphysema Treatment Trial (NETT), an NIH-sponsored, randomized, prospective trial of LVRS in patients with advanced emphysema, is currently underway.

PREDICTORS OF DECREASED SURVIVAL AFTER LVRS
Preoperative Factors

Our analysis of preoperative variables identified five factors predictive of decreased survival after LVRS. The identification of advanced age as a risk factor for mortality was consistent with the findings of others *(5)*, although the degree to which advanced age increased the risk of early and late death in our study was noteworthy. Improved survival in patients operated on after 1995 was consistent with a learning curve phenomenon, both with respect to selection of patients and clinical management. Hypoxemia also portended a lower long-term survival. Because pure emphysema is characterized by ventilation/perfusion inequality with a predominance of high V/Q lung zones, hypoxemia is an inconsistent pathophysiogic consequence with poor correlation to the severity of outflow obstruction. In fact, severe hypoxemia in the emphysemic patient suggests the coexistence of reactive airway disease or the presence of extensive parenchymal destruction *(18)*. Thus, a lower survival in hypoxemic patients may have been related to disease states less suited to lung volume reduction.

Our analysis also found an inverse relationship between preoperative FEV_1 and survival. Although this observation appears counterintuitive upon initial consideration, there are at least two potential explanations for this finding. First, because fixed, severe impairments in FEV_1 are more characteristic of pure advanced emphysema than chronic bronchitis *(19)*, patients with higher FEV_1 might represent a subgroup of patients with mixed disease (with a significant bronchitic component) which might not benefit as much from LVRS. Second, it is possible that this finding represents a degree of selection bias, because the most severely compromised patients (with the lowest FEV_1) might have been subjected to stricter selection criteria, although those with higher FEV_1 might have been accepted for LVRS despite lesser degrees of disease heterogeneity. Whatever the explanation, our findings support the continued use of significantly reduced FEV_1 as an absolute requirement in the selection of patients for LVRS, without exclusion of patients with severely depressed values ($< 20\%$ of predicted). Our analysis also identified male gender as a predictor of poor survival. Whether this reflects true gender-related differences in the natural history of emphysema or simply a higher incidence of confounding comorbid characteristics in males is a matter of speculation.

Preoperative Factors

The multivariable analysis of patients surviving to the first postoperative evaluation interval identified two postoperative factors predictive of improved survival: degree of improvement in FEV_1 and postoperative DI. The observed correlation between improvement in FEV_1 and survival is not surprising, because FEV_1 has long been known to correlate with survival in medically managed patients *(20,21)*. Perhaps more notably, the relationship between postoperative DI and survival raises the possibility that a palliative operation designed to relieve dyspnea may also ultimately be shown to improve long-term survival. Furthermore, the fact that these two factors did correlate with enhanced survival tends to validate their continued use in assessing the efficacy of LVRS. Finally, the diminished significance of preoperative variables in the analysis of patients surviving to their first postoperative evaluation suggests that preoperative characteristics were important predictors of early survival, but that postoperative functional measures were more important determinants of subsequent survival. This conclusion is supported by our "early death" analysis, which suggests that advanced age and higher preoperative FEV_1 exert their influence on survival primarily by increasing early postoperative mortality. Although these data suggest that certain patients may be at high risk for mortality after LVRS, it does not necessarily follow that these patients should be denied the procedure, because their prognosis with medical therapy might be even worse than after LVRS. Ultimately, accurate risk-benefit assessments in patients considered to be at high operative risk can only be made utilizing data from a randomized trial.

LIMITATIONS

Apart from its nonrandomized nature, this study has several limitations. Although many clinical variables were considered in our analysis, several factors with potential impact on the outcome of LVRS were not analyzed. The results of radiologic studies, utilized clinically to estimate the extent and heterogeneity of disease, were not analyzed because the degree, pattern, and location of emphysema could not be quantified in a meaningful way. Hemodynamic data were difficult to record in all patients because of the invasive procedures required to obtain this information. Finally, the extent and location of lung resection was not quantified intraoperatively. For these and other reasons, variables other than those chosen for inclusion in this study may ultimately have greater importance in determining long-term survival after LVRS.

SUMMARY

Our study identified several pre- and postoperative variables that were predictive of medium-term survival in a selected group of patients undergoing LVRS at a single institution. We believe that the impact of LVRS on survival is of clinical importance, both with respect to evaluation of treatment efficacy, as well as patient selection and timing of intervention. The application of LVRS to a highly selected group of patients makes comparison of survival data to historical controls inappropriate. For this reason, results of a prospective, randomized clinical trial will likely be required to fully define the effects of LVRS on long-term survival.

REFERENCES

1. Cooper JD, Trulock EP, Triantafillou AN, et al. (1995) Bilateral pneumectomy (volume reduction) for chronic obstructive pulmonary disease. *J Thorac Cardiovasc Surg* 109:106–119.

2. Cooper JD, Patterson GA, Sundaresan RS, et al. (1996) Results of 150 consecutive bilateral lung volume reduction procedures in patients with severe emphysema (see comments). *J Thorac Cardiovasc Surg* 112:1319–1329; discussion 1329,1330.
3. Argenziano M, Moazami N, Thomashow B, et al. (1996) Extended indications for lung volume reduction surgery in advanced emphysema. *Ann Thorac Surg* 62:251–257.
4. Yusen RD, Trulock EP, Pohl MS, Biggar DG (1996) Results of lung volume reduction surgery in patients with emphysema. *Semin Thor Cardiovasc Surg* 8:99–109.
5. Daniel TM, Chan BB, Bhaskar V, et al. (1996) Lung volume reduction surgery: case selection, operative technique, and clinical results. *Ann Surg* 223:526–531; discussion 532,533.
6. Sciurba FC, Rogers RM, Keenen RJ, et al. (1996) Improvement in pulmonary function and elastic recoil after lung reduction surgery for diffuse emphysema (see comments). *N Engl J Med* 334:1095–1099.
7. Gelb AF, Brenner M, McKenna RJ, et al. (1996) Lung function 12 months following emphysema resection. *Chest* 100:1407–1415.
8. Brenner M, McKenna R, Gelb A, et al. (1997)Objective predictors of response for staple versus laser emphysematous lung reduction. *Am J Respir Crit Care Med* 155:1295–1301.
9. Argenziano M, Thomashow B, Jellen PA, et al. (1997) Functional comparison of unilateral versus bilateral lung volume reduction surgery. *Ann Thorac Surg* 64:321–326; discussion 326,327.
10. Keller CA, Ruppel G, Hibbett A, et al. (1997) Thoracoscopic lung volume reduction surgery reduces dyspnea and improved exercise capacity in patients with emphysema. *Am J Respir Crit Care Med* 156:60–67.
11. Martinez FJ, de Oca MM, Whyte RI, et al. (1997) Lung volume reduction improved dyspnea, dynamic hyperinflation, and respiratory muscle function. *Am J Respir Crit Care Med* 155:1984–1990.
12. Brenner M, McKenna RJ, Gelb AF, et al. (1998) Rate of FEV_1 change following lung volume reduction surgery. *Chest* 113:652–660.
13. Kesten S, Elpern E, Warren W, Szidon P. (1999) Loss of pulmonary function gains after lung volume reduction surgery. *J Heart Lung Transplant* 18:266–268.
14. Argenziano M, Thomashow B, Jellen PA, Gorenstein LA, Rose EA, Steinglass KM, Weinberg AD, Ginsburg ME. Effects of lung volume reduction surgery on survival in patients with end-stage emphysema. *Ann Thorac Surg 2001*, in press.
15. Sweer L, Zwillich CW (1990) Dyspnea in the patient with chronic obstructive pulmonary disease. *Clin Chest Med* 11:417–445.
16. Meyers BF, Yusen RD, Lefrak SS, et al. (1998) Outcome of medicare patients with emphysema selected for, but denied, a lung volume reduction operation. *Ann Thorac Surg* 66:331–336.
17. Anthonisen N, Wright E, Hodgkin J, et al. (1986) Prognosis in chronic obstructive pulmonary disease. *Am Rev Respir Dis* 133:14–20.
18. Morell NW, Wignall BK, Biggs T, Seed WA (1994) Collateral circulation and gas exchange in emphysema. *Am J Respir Crit Care Med* 150:635–641.
19. Mead J, Turner J, Macklem P, et al. (1966) Significance of the relationship between lung recoil and maximum expiratory flow. *J Appl Physiol* 22:95–108.
20. Nocturnal Oxygen Therapy Trial Group (1980) Continuous or nocturnal oxygen therapy in hypoxemic chronic obstructive lung disease: a clinical trial. *Ann Intern Med* 93:391–398.
21. Intermittent Positive Pressure Breathing Trial Group (1983) Intermittent positive pressure breathing therapy of chronic obstructive pulmonary disease. *Intern Med* 99:612–620.

15 Management of the Patient with Lung Cancer and Severe Emphysema

Joseph J. DeRose, Jr., MD,
Michael Argenziano, MD,
and Mark E. Ginsburg, MD

INTRODUCTION

Patients with chronic obstructive pulmonary disease (COPD) have an increased risk of developing bronchogenic carcinoma as a result of common etiologic factors. Surgical resection provides the best chance for cure. However, even some patients with early stage peripheral tumors are considered inoperable because of inadequate pulmonary reserve because of severe emphysema.

The resurgence of lung volume reduction surgery (LVRS) has allowed for new surgical approaches to patients with severe pulmonary disability. In properly selected patients, significant improvements in dyspnea, exercise capacity, and pulmonary function have been demonstrated following bilateral and unilateral LVRS *(1–8)*. By applying the rationale and techniques of LVRS, it has been possible to resect pulmonary neoplasms in patients otherwise considered inoperable by traditional preoperative respiratory function criteria.

From: *Lung Volume Reduction Surgery*
Edited by: M. Argenziano and M. E. Ginsburg © Humana Press Inc., Totowa, NJ

INCIDENCE

The coexistence of severe emphysema and lung cancer is not uncommon. In clinical practice, severe emphysema may be discovered during the preoperative work-up of a lung tumor; alternatively, a patient with known emphysema may be diagnosed with a lung tumor during LVRS evaluation. The incidence of lung nodules detected during LVRS work-up is fairly well documented. Hazelrigg et al. detected 142 lung nodules in 281 patients (39.5%) undergoing LVRS surgery *(9)*. Although the majority of these nodules were detected by preoperative chest CT, 14 nodules were identified only at the time of surgery. There were also an additional 14 nodules that were discovered only in the pathology specimen, escaping both radiologic and intraoperative identification. Seventy-eight nodules were felt to be suspicious and were resected, of which 61 (78.2%) were benign and 17 (21.8%) malignant. The overall incidence of lung cancer in the screened population was 6.4%. Of the neoplastic lesions resected, three were identified by CT scan only, five by chest X-ray and CT, four in the operating room only, and five found incidentally in the pathology specimen.

Pigula et al. found a similar incidence of unsuspected neoplasms in a series of 128 patients undergoing LVRS at the University of Pittsburgh *(10)*. Of the 10 patients (7.8%) found to have neoplasms, 6 were detected on preoperative radiologic evaluation and 4 were found only on routine pathologic examination of the resected lung tissue. Rozenshtein et al. likewise found suspicious nodules in 17 of 148 patients (11%) during preoperative evaluation for LVRS at the Columbia-Presbyterian Medical Center *(11)*. Of these, 16 were removed surgically; 9 (6% of screened population) were nonsmall cell cancers and 7 were benign.

The incidence of severe COPD precluding safe resectional surgery in patients with lung cancer is much more difficult to define. Epidemiological studies demonstrate a linear relationship between the rise in cases of both COPD and lung cancer with increasing cigarette consumption over the past decade (see Fig. 1). It has been estimated that 90% of lung cancer patients have signs and symptoms of COPD at the time of diagnosis. Marshall and Olsen estimated that at least 20% of patients with lung cancer have a forced expiratory volume in one second (FEV_1) less than or equal to 1.2 L *(12)*.

CONVENTIONAL PREOPERATIVE PULMONARY ASSESSMENT

Physiologic assessment of the lung resection candidate aims to estimate the postoperative pulmonary function associated with the removal

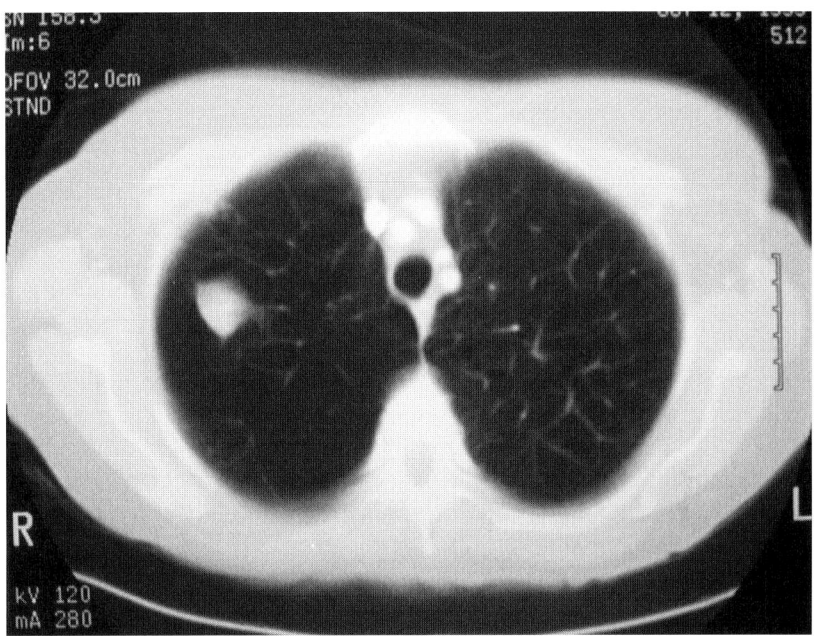

Fig. 1. CT scan showing right upper-lobe lung cancer in setting of significant upper-lobe bullous emphysema.

of normal and/or diseased lung tissue. Two undesirable effects occur following resection of lung tissue. The first is a reduction in the pulmonary capillary bed. This has little effect on the postoperative pulmonary vascular resistance in patients with normal lungs, even after pneumonectomy. However, in patients with pre-existing pulmonary vascular disease, excessive lung resection can lead to postoperative pulmonary hypertension, cor pulmonale, and death. The second undesirable effect of lung resection is a reduction in ventilatory function. This can lead to both acute and chronic respiratory failure with impairments ranging from severe exercise intolerance to ventilator dependence.

The challenge, then, is to perform the best curative resection while leaving the patient with the smallest physiologic deficit. In the classic evaluation, each resectable patient is evaluated as a possible pneumonectomy candidate. If the patient is physiologically acceptable for pneumonectomy, then a smaller resection will be even less detrimental. Likewise, if intraoperative finding necessitate pneumonectomy than a curative resection can safely be performed.

Routine Pulmonary Function Tests

Routine spirometric studies are used to assess airflow, lung volume, lung mechanics, and gas exchange. Routine pulmonary function tests

(PFT) are used to rule out or quantify underlying COPD. Severe impairments in PFT warrant further investigations of pulmonary function but do not necessarily render a patient inoperable. The reason for this is that PFT measure the function of both lungs working together at rest. However, anatomic and pathologic considerations can make the function of each lung quite different and therefore greatly affect the postoperative outcome of resectional surgery. Table 1 includes some of the classic pulmonary function criteria for lung resection as adapted from the early work of Gaensler and others *(13–15)*.

Split-Lung Function Studies

Standard ventilation scanning with xenon 133 and perfusion scanning with technetium 99m-labeled albumin microaggregates can be modified to estimate regional lung function. The addition of a computer to the gamma camera allows quantification of each lung region and expression of regional ventilation and perfusion as a percentage of the total. By using these split-lung function calculations, a predicted postoperative (ppo) FEV_1 can be calculated following pneumonectomy. Further refinements of the technique can also allow an assessment of segmental lung perfusion, and therefore a calculation of ppo FEV_1 following lobectomy. A ppo FEV_1 of less than 35% of normal has been associated with an unacceptably high risk in several prospective studies *(16,17)*.

Exercise Testing

Maximal oxygen consumption (VO_2max) is the highest oxygen uptake measured during intense incremental workload exercise. In the earliest study of VO_2max as a predictor of postoperative mortality, Eugene et al. demonstrated that 75% of patients with a preoperative VO_2 max less than 1 L died after lung resection *(18)*. No patients with a VO_2max greater than 1 L died in the postoperative period. Both groups in this study had similar preoperative spirometry values. Subsequent studies have documented that a VO_2max less than 15mL/kg/min is associated not only with an increased mortality, but also with an increase in postoperative complications *(19)*. Other investigators have attempted to refine measurements of VO_2max by using split-lung function studies to determine a postoperative predicted VO_2max. In a study of 25 patients with severe pulmonary dysfunction, all three patients with a postoperative predicted VO_2max less than 10 mL/kg/min died postoperatively *(20)*.

PATIENT SELECTION FOR LVRS WITH CONCOMITANT TUMOR RESECTION

In order for the techniques of LVRS to be successfully applied to resectional lung surgery, selection criteria for both LVRS and cancer

Table 1
Pulmonary Function Criteria for Pneumonectomy

Study	Operable	Further Studies Warranted
FEV$_1$	>60% predicted	<60% predicted
FVC	>60% predicted	<60% predicted
FEV$_1$/FVC	>50%	<50%
MVV	>60% predicted	<60% predicted
CO diffusing capacity	>60% predicted	<60% predicted
Room air pCO$_2$	<45 mmHg	>45 mmHg

(FVC-forced vital capacity, FEV$_1$-forced expiratory volume in 1 s,
MVV,-maximum voluntary ventilation, CO-carbon monoxide)

surgery must be respected (see Table 2). An exception to this statement
relates to the traditional use of preoperative lung function as a predictor
of postoperative survival after lung resection. Because LVRS in appropriately selected patients is expected to result in improvements in lung
function, the addition of LVRS to a lung cancer resection might allow
successful tumor extirpation in patients that would not traditionally not
be expected to tolerate these resections. In this respect, the location of
the lesion in relation to LVRS target areas is an important determinant
of both operability and extent of resection. Clearly, resection of masses
that are located within LVRS target areas are expected to result in less
loss of lung function than removal of masses located within relatively
normal lung parenchyma.

The initial evaluation of a solitary pulmonary nodule in a patient with
severe emphysema aims at establishing a diagnosis prior to proceeding
with surgery. It must be remembered that despite an increased incidence
of carcinoma among patients with emphysema, the majority of pulmonary nodules detected on chest CT are benign. The CT radiologic
features of most of these lesions can characterize them as benign or
malignant. However, noncalcified nodules warrant a tissue diagnosis in
this population. Although CT-guided needle biopsy can be performed
on peripheral nodules in patients with severe emphysema, it should be
understood that the risk of postprocedural pneumothorax is substantially higher. The use of PET scanning may be helpful in evaluating the
primary lesion and determining its likelihood of malignancy.

Once a diagnosis of malignancy has been suggested by either pathologic or radiologic criteria, it is the responsibility of the surgeon to exclude
distant and/or unresectable locoregional disease. Routine work-up in our
practice includes a brain imaging study (MRI or CT), abdominal CT, bone
scan, and a whole body PET scan. The use of mediastinoscopy should be

Table 2
Inclusion and Exclusion Criteria for LVRS and Tumor Resection

Inclusion Criteria

Severe dyspnea
Localized or diffuse disease
Hyperinflation with air trapping
Diaphragmatic dysfunction
Regional heterogeneity of disease with appropriate target areas for resection
Pulmonary nodule $\leq$ 3.0 cm

Exclusion Criteria

Predominant airway disease such as asthma, bronchiectasis or chronic
   bronchitis with excessive purulent secretions
Obliteration of pleural space by previous disease or surgery
Inappropriate emphysematous target areas for resection
Evidence of unresectable locoregional neoplastic disease
Evidence of metastatic disease
Anatomic location of tumor necessitates resection of an unacceptable amount
   of functional lung parenchyma

applied aggressively to rule out stage III disease prior to embarking on thoracotomy in this high-risk group of patients.

If a patient with severe emphysema is deemed a surgical candidate based on preoperative staging, then LVRS criteria should be rigidly applied. Routine preoperative assessment of these patients should include a careful history of prior pulmonary infections, bronchitic symptoms or thoracic surgery, as well as a detailed review of old radiologic studies. Physiologic evaluation should include a room air arterial blood gas, standard spirometry studies, lung volume measurements by both plethysmography and nitrogen washout, 6-min walk distance, and selective use of dobutamine thallium stress test/ stress echocardiogram. Radiologic studies routinely include inspiratory and expiratory chest films, chest CT scans with cuts beyond the adrenal glands, and quantitative ventilation and perfusion scans. Regions of hyperinflation on chest CT and/or hypoperfusion on perfusion scan are identified as appropriate resectional target areas.

It should be emphasized that patients with severe emphysema who meet criteria for both curative lung cancer resection and LVRS are operated on under the assumption that postoperative increases in pulmonary function conferred by LVRS will allow tumor resections that would not otherwise be tolerated. Thus, patients with severe emphysema who meet criteria for curative lung resection (localized disease, negative mediastinal lymph nodes) but not LVRS are expected to fare poorly if a combined procedure is undertaken.

TECHNIQUE OF OPERATION

Combined LVRS and tumor resection can be performed through a number of incisions including a thoracoscopic approach. The extent of resection is based on the location of the lesion in relation to emphysematous target areas (*see* Fig. 2). Wedge resections can commonly be accomplished whether the lesion exists within a target area or not. Lung reduction surgery is aimed at target areas of hyperinflation and may be performed as part of or in combination with nodule resection. When an entire lobe is affected with hyperinflated airway disease, a formal lobectomy can sometimes be performed. Although the friability of emphysematous lung parenchyma frequently limits extensive nodal dissection within the hilum and fissures, a representative nodal sampling is possible. Postoperative care is identical to that employed during routine lung reduction and includes epidural analgesia, minimal chest tube suction, and aggressive pulmonary toilet, including frequent bronchoscopy.

RESULTS OF COMBINED LVRS AND TUMOR RESECTION

There have been several reports of combined LVRS and pulmonary nodule resection in the literature dating back to the resurgence of LVRS a few years ago (*see* Table 3). We reported our early experience with LVRS and tumor resection at Columbia-Presbyterian Medical Center in 1998 *(21)*. In this series, 13 lesions were resected in 11 patients and included nonsmall cell carcinoma *(7)*, caseating granuloma *(3)*, hamartoma *(2)*, and aspergilloma *(1)*. One formal lobectomy and 10 wedge resections were performed. There was one postoperative death from a large bronchopleural fistula in a patient who had previously undergone ipsilateral lung surgery. All other patients survived with no evidence of recurrent or metastatic disease through a mean follow-up of 11.3 ± 6.4 months (1–19.3 mo). Furthermore, significant improvements in dyspnea index (DI), FEV_1, forced vital capacity (FVC), and 6-min walk distance were noted at both 3- and 6-mo follow-up.

McKenna et al. reported a similar experience of 53 nodules including 11 nonsmall cell lung cancers resected in combination with LVRS *(22)*. Seven wedge resections and four lobectomies were performed with no postoperative mortality and an average length of stay of 8.7 d. Significant improvements in FEV_1 and dyspnea were noted over a short follow-up of 3 mo.

The largest experience of nodule resection and LVRS comes from Hazelrigg et al. who reported 78 resected nodules, including 17 neoplasms *(9)*. Of these neoplasms there were 13 primary lung cancers (of which four were detected only in the pathology specimen). All resections were wedge resections and there were no postoperative deaths. There were five deaths among the patients with neoplastic disease over a 12-mo follow-up: 1 of metastatic renal cell carcinoma, 1 of unresectable mesthelioma, 2 of progression of primary lung cancer, and 1 of a cerebrovascular accident. No report was made regarding functional improvement following operation in this series.

CONCLUSION

Without therapy lung cancer is 100% fatal. Although some authors have found 5-yr survival rates of up to 35% for patients with stage I disease who are treated with radiation therapy alone *(23)*, overall survival rates in most series are low *(24,25)*. To date, surgery remains the only significant chance for cure in patients with early stage lesions. After lobectomy, patients with T1 N0 nonsmall cell lung cancer experience up to an 80% 5-yr cancer-free survival *(26)*.

With the advent of LVRS, many of the classic criteria for determining operability in lung cancer must be reassessed. Most of the patients reported in the above series would have historically been excluded from surgical resection based on preoperative indices of pulmonary function. However, morbidity and mortality has been acceptable following LVRS and tumor resection in all published reports. Furthermore, the accompanying improvement in dyspnea and pulmonary spirometry has translated into an improved quality of life for many of these lung cancer patients.

The degree of resection remains an unresolved issue. The majority of resections performed in the setting of severe emphysema are wide wedge resections. The Lung Cancer Study Group has shown lobectomy to be superior to wedge resection in terms of early locoregional recurrence without a significant difference in overall survival for stage I lung cancer *(13)*. However, it should be noted that the behavior of a lung cancer arising in emphysematous lung tissue with severely damaged regional lymphatic channels is not entirely known. In these select cases, wide wedge resection may provide adequate excision of both the primary lesion and the poorly preserved surrounding lymphatic basin. Long-term follow-up of combined wedge resection and LVRS will be needed to determine if adequate local control and/or a survival advantage is conferred by this operation.

In conclusion, by employing the techniques of LVRS, emphysematous patients with suspicious pulmonary nodules and severe pulmonary dysfunction can be offered resection aimed at both cure of tumor and improvement in quality of life. The currently employed predictors of perioperative risk in lung resection do not accurately apply to LVRS candidates. As such, new criteria based on LVRS risk factors and tumor location will continue to be developed in order to accurately assess the operability and curative resectability of patients with severe emphysema and pulmonary nodules.

Table 3
Results of Combined Lung Cancer Resection and LVRS

Author	Date	No. of Nodules Resected	No. of Lung Cancers	Wedge Resection	Lobectomy	F/U (mos)	Mortality	Pre-op FEV$_1$	Post-op FEV$_1$
McKenna, Los Angeles, CA	1996	53	11	7	4	3	0%	22% predicted	49% predicted
Ojo, Ann Arbor, MI	1997	11	3	11	0	3	0%	26% predicted	39% predicted
Hazelrigg, Springfield, IL	1997	78	14	14	0	12	0%	not reported	not reported
DeRose, New York, NY	1998	11	7	10	1	6	9%	26% predicted	40% predicted

REFERENCES

1. Cooper JD, Trulock EP, Triantafillou, et al. (1995) Bilateral pneumectomy (volume reduction) for chronic obstructive pulmonary disease. *J Thorac Cardiovasc Surg* 109: 106–119.
2. Little AG, Swain JA, Nino JJ, et al. (1995) Reduction pneumoplasty for emphysema. Early results. *Ann Surg* 222(3): 365–374.
3. Argenziano M, Moazami N, Thomashow B, et al. (1996) Extended indications for lung volume reduction surgery in advanced emphysema. *Ann Thorac Surg* 62: 1588–1597.
4. Yusen RD, Trulock EP, Pohl MS, et al. (1996) Results of lung volume reduction surgery in patients with emphysema. *Semin Thorac Cardiovasc Surg* 8: 99–109.
5. Naunheim KS, Keller CA, Krucylak PE, et al. (1996) Unilateral video-assisted thoracic surgical lung reduction. *Ann Thorac Surg* 61: 1092–1098.
6. Keenan RJ, Landreneau RJ, Sciurba FC (1996) Unilateral thoracoscopic surgical approach for diffuse emphysema. *J Cardiovasc Surg* 111: 308–316.
7. Naunheim KS. Kaiser LR. Bavaria JE, et al. (1999) Long-term survival after thoracoscopic lung volume reduction: a multiinstitutional review. *Ann Thorac Surg* 68: 2026–2031.
8. Argenziano M, Thomashow B, Jellen PA, et al. (1997) Functional comparison of unilateral versus bilateral lung volume reduction surgery. *Ann Thorac Surg* 64: 321–326.
9. Hazelrigg SR, Boley TM, Webee D, Magee M J, Naunheim KS (1997) Incidence of lung nodules found in patients undergoing lung volume reduction. *Ann Thorac Surg* 64: 305,306.
10. Pigula FA, Keenan RJ, Ferson PF, Landreneau RJ (1996) Unsuspected lung cancer found in work-up for lung reduction operation. *Ann Thorac Surg* 61: 174–176.
11. Rozenshtein A, White CS, Austin JHM, Romney BM, Protopapas Z, Krasna M (1998) Incidental lung carcinoma detected at CT in patients selected for lung volume reduction surgery to treat severe pulmonary emphysema. *Radiology* 207: 487–490.
12. Marshall MC, Olsen GN (1993) The physiologic evaluation of the lung resection candidate. *Clin Chest Med* 14: 305–320.
13. Gaensler EA, Cugell DW, Lindgren I, et al. (1955) The role of pulmonary insufficiency in mortality and invalidism following surgery for pulmonary tuberculosis. *J Thorac Surg* 29: 163–187.
14. Olsen GN, Block AJ, Swenson EW, et al. (1975) Pulmonary function evaluation of the lung resection candidate: a prospective study. *Am Rev Respir Dis* 111: 379–387.
15. Reilly JJ, Mentzer SJ, Sugarbaker DJ (1993) Preoperative assessment of patients undergoing pulmonary resection. *Chest* 103: 342S–345S.
16. Wernly JA, DeMeester TR, Kirchner PT, Myerowitz PD, Oxford DE, Golomb HM (1980) Clinical value of quantitative ventilation-perfusion lung scans in the surgical management of bronchogenic carcinoma. *J Thorac Cardiovasc Surg* 80: 535–543.
17. Markos J, Mullan BP, Hillman DR, et al. (1989) Preoperative assessment as a predictor of mortality and morbidity after lung resection. *Am Rev Resp Dis* 139: 902–910.
18. Eugene J, et al. (1982) Maximum oxygen consumption: a physiologic guide to pulmonary resection. *Surg Forum* 33: 260–266.
19. Smith TP, Kinasewitz GT, Tucker WY, Spillers WP, George RB (1984) Exercise capacity as a predictor of post-thoracotomy morbidity. *Am Rev Resp Dis* 129: 730–734.

20. Bolliger CT, Wyser C, Roser H, Soler M, Perruchoud AP (1995) Lung scanning and exercise testing for the prediction of postoperative performance in lung resection candidates at increased risk for complications. *Chest* 108: 341–348.
21. DeRose JJ, Jr, Argenziano M, El-Amir N, et al. (1998) Lung reduction surgery and resection of pulmonary nodules in patients with severe emphysema. *Ann Thorac Surg* 65: 314–318.
22. McKenna RJ Jr, Fischel RJ, Brenner M, Gelb AF (1996) Combined operations for lung volume reduction surgery and lung cancer. *Chest* 110: 885–888.
23. Zhang HX, Yin WB, Zhang LJ, et al. (1989) Curative radiotherapy of early operable non small cell lung cancer. *Radiother Oncol* 14: 89–94.
24. Dosoretz DE, Katin MJ, Blitzer PH, et al. (1992) Radiation therapy in the management of medically inoperable carcinoma of the lung: results and implications for future treatment strategies. *Int J Radiat Oncol Biol Phys* 24: 3–9.
25. Cooper JD, Pearson FG, Todd TRJ, et al. (1985) Radiotherapy alone for patients with operable carcinoma of the lung. *Chest* 87: 289–292.
26. Ginsberg RJ, Rubinstein LV (1995) Randomized trial of lobectomy versus limited resection for T1 N0 non-small cell lung cancer. Lung Cancer Study Group. *Ann Thorac Surg* 60: 615–622.

16 Lung Transplantation and LVRS in the Treatment of Advanced Emphysema

Larry L. Schulman, MD

INTRODUCTION

Lung transplantation and lung volume reduction surgery (LVRS) have become intimately related as clinical experience with each procedure has increased. Revitalization of LVRS was a direct consequence of single-lung transplantation when it was observed that even when the single lung allograft functioned poorly after transplantation there was improvement in hemithoracic diaphragmatic position, reduction of chest hyperinflation, and diminution in patient sensation of dyspnea *(1)*. This clinical "success" despite the apparent "failure" of the single-lung allograft provided the insight to thoracic surgeons to revisit the question of surgically reducing the thoracic hyperinflation characteristic of pulmonary emphysema. The subsequent early success of lung volume reduction has fostered a productive and continually evolving relationship between lung transplantation and LVRS for the treatment of advanced pulmonary emphysema.

The interrelationship between lung transplantation and LVRS can be divided into five broad categories, each of which will be dealt with as follows:

From: *Lung Volume Reduction Surgery*
Edited by: M. Argenziano and M. E. Ginsburg © Humana Press Inc., Totowa, NJ

1. Lung transplantation vs LVRS;
2. LVRS as a "bridge" to lung transplantation;
3. LVRS and single-lung transplantation as simultaneous procedures;
4. LVRS after single-lung transplantation to reduce native lung hyperinflation; and
5. LVRS after single-lung transplantation to salvage chronic allograft rejection.

LUNG TRANSPLANTATION VS LVRS

This section discusses the issues surrounding the decision to offer lung transplantation or LVRS to patients with end-stage lung disease. This discussion will include consideration of a number of factors that play a role in these decisions, including candidate selection, as well as postoperative pulmonary function, utilization of resources, and mortality and morbidity associated with each procedure.

CANDIDATE SELECTION

The ideal candidate for lung transplantation or LVRS fits the original description of patients with emphysema (type A chronic obstructive pulmonary disease [COPD]). This includes individuals with little cough, occasional and scanty sputum, fixed dyspnea, thin body habitus, large translucent lungs with low diaphragms and a small cardiothoracic ratio, absence of right ventricular enlargement, and a normal hematocrit *(2)*. Optimal candidates for lung transplantation or LVRS should not manifest reversible airflow obstruction, copious sputum production, respiratory infection, obesity, or respiratory muscle weakness. By these criteria, optimal candidates tend to manifest less severe derangements of gas exchange (hypoxemia and hypercarbia) and less severe elevations of pulmonary arterial pressures *(3,4)*. Experience indicates that even in the majority of patients with a "mixed" clinical picture, one of the types usually dominates to allow appropriate selection of patients for lung transplantation or LVRS.

These criteria, especially regarding sputum production and respiratory infection, may be relaxed for patients who are being considered for bilateral lung transplantation. Under these circumstances, sputum production and respiratory infection may be eradicated by the transplant surgery, as occurs following bilateral lung transplantation for patients with idiopathic bronchiectasis or cystic fibrosis. By these expanded criteria, candidates for bilateral lung transplantation may manifest more severe derangements of gas exchange and elevation of pulmonary arterial pressures *(5)*.

Patients should be referred for lung transplantation when FEV_1 falls below 25–30% of predicted levels *(6)*. Candidates for lung transplantation should meet general criteria, which have been published recently as

Table 1
Preoperative Considerations for Lung Transplantation for Advanced Pulmonary Emphysema

Requirements:

- Age ≤ 65 yr for single lung transplant; ≤ 60 yr for bilateral-lung transplant
- Ambulatory in supervised rehabilitation program
- 70% ≤ Ideal body weight ≤ 130%
- Social support network
- Prescription medication coverage
- Motivation
- Compliance

Contraindications:

- Unresolved substance abuse
- Uncontrolled psychiatric illness
- Coronary artery disease
- Left ventricular dysfunction
- Renal insufficiency
- Hepatic dysfunction
- Active or recent cancer (except skin)
- Infection with HIV, hepatitis B, hepatitis C (biopsy)
- Acute or critical illness
- Mechanical ventilation

an international consensus statement *(6)*. Requirements for lung transplantation, as well as contraindications to lung transplantation, are summarized in Table 1. Several excellent general reviews of lung transplantation have been published recently *(7,8)*. For the purposes of this chapter, the discussion will focus on criteria specific for patients with advanced pulmonary emphysema.

Optimal candidates for single-lung transplantation should be ≤ 65 yr of age; candidates for bilateral lung transplantation should be ≤ 60 yr of age (*see* Table 1). All candidates must be ambulatory. One study has indicated that a 6-minute walk distance less than 300 m is predictive of poor outcome *(9)*. All candidates must participate in a supervised pulmonary rehabilitation program *(10)*. Patients' weight should not be below 70% of ideal body weight, nor exceed 130% of ideal body weight. All patients should have adequate social support and prescription medication coverage. All patients should demonstrate motivation, willingness, and ability to adhere to an intensive medical regimen after surgery. Global assessment of psychosocial "risk" before transplant has been predictive of noncompliance with medication regimen, diet, exercise, and smoking abstinence after transplantation *(11)*.

Table 2
Postoperative Complications After Lung Transplantation For Advanced Pulmonary Emphysema

Respiratory Complications

- Perioperative
  - ischemia-reperfusion injury
  - acute mediastinal shift
  - pneumothorax
  - bronchial anastomotic complications (ischemia, dehiscence, stenosis)
  - pulmonary vein thrombosis
  - pneumonia
- Acute rejection
- Opportunistic infection
- Chronic rejection
- Native lung hyperinflation
- Native lung diseases
  - pneumothorax
  - bronchogenic carcinoma
  - bacterial, fungal, mycobacterial infections

Nonrespiratory Complications

- Hypertension
- Renal insufficiency
- Diabetes mellitus
- Hyperlipidemia
- Gastroparesis
- Seizures
- Osteoporosis
- Post-transplant lymphoproliferative disorder (PTLD)

Candidates for lung transplantation should not have coronary artery disease or left-ventricular dysfunction (*see* Table 1). Because many candidates are former smokers, transplant centers frequently require preoperative coronary arteriography *(12,13)*. Candidates for lung transplantation should not be acutely or critically ill at the time of transplant. Mechanically ventilated patients have been demonstrated to have poor postoperative outcomes related to infection and respiratory muscle weakness *(14,15)*. Ambulatory patients who have a chronic tracheostomy for nocturnal ventilation may be eligible for transplantation. Noninvasive mechanical ventilation such as BIPAP mask is acceptable for transplantation.

The impact of previous thoracic surgery on transplant eligibility should be individualized for each potential lung transplant recipient. In general, in patients with previous unilateral thoracic surgery, single transplantation of the contralateral lung is acceptable. Bilateral lung transplantation is acceptable in patients with previous minor thoracic procedures, including open lung biopsy, thoracostomy tube placement, tetracycline or bleomycin pleurodesis, and mechanical abrasion of the pleural surface *(16,17)*. Previous lung volume reduction via sternotomy or clamshell incision is also acceptable. Caution should be exercised in patients with previous talc instillation, pleurectomy, or lobar resection. These thoracic surgical procedures confer an increased risk of bleeding at the time of transplant, especially when performed on cardiopulmonary bypass *(17)*.

Patients with active or recent lung cancer are generally not considered eligible for lung transplantation. Although it has been proposed that patients with bronchoalveolar carcinoma limited to the lung may be transplantable, because the disease characteristically remains confined to the thorax *(18,19)*, a recent report documenting several cases of recurrent disease in donor lungs suggests a limited role for transplantation in these patients *(19)*. Tobacco usage should not be tolerated *(6)*. Many centers test potential candidates repeatedly for nicotine metabolites, and reserve the right to remove patients from the list if there is evidence of tobacco usage. Most centers have detected a return to smoking in a small percentage of patients after successful lung transplantation.

Optimal candidates for lung transplantation should not take chronic systemic corticosteroids, or if clinically needed, the lowest dose possible should be prescribed. Candidates for lung transplantation should be screened for skeletal muscle weakness and osteoporosis. Muscle weakness is most often related to steroid-induced myopathy, but hypoxemia, malnutrition, inactivity, and even testosterone deficiency may play a contributory role *(20,21)*. Osteoporosis is extremely common in end-stage pulmonary disease *(22,23)*. In one study of 70 patients awaiting lung transplantation, only 34% of patients had normal bone density at the lumbar spine and 22% had normal bone density at the hip *(22)* (*see* Fig. 1). The average femoral neck T score of patients with emphysema (-2.7 ± 0.3) fell into the osteoporotic range, was similar to that in cystic fibrosis, and was significantly lower that of patients with other lung diseases (-1.5 ± 0.3) *(22)*. Duration of exposure to glucocorticoids correlated negatively with lumbar spine bone density. Disturbingly, very few patients in this study were on sufficient regimens to prevent bone loss, and up to 20% of patients with emphysema were deficient in vitamin D. Osteoporosis should be treated aggressively before transplantation to minimize risk of subsequent fracture *(24)*.

In contrast to lung transplantation, inclusion and exclusion criteria for LVRS are less restrictive *(25)*. Common eligiblity criteria for LVRS

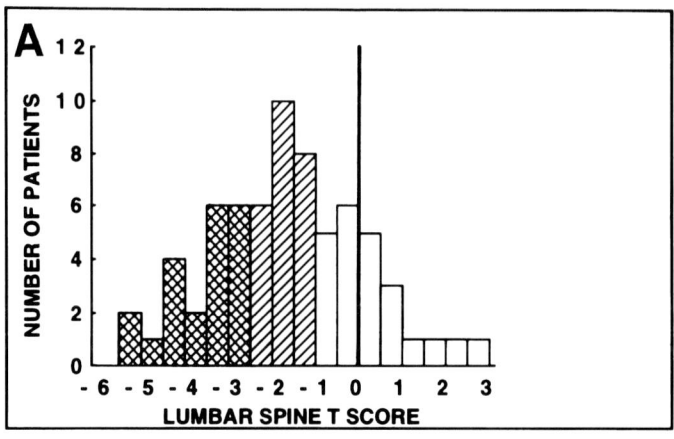

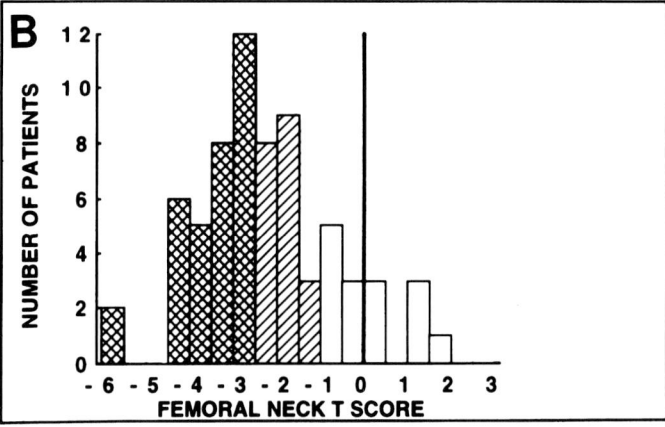

Fig. 1. Frequency distribution of bone mineral density of the lumber spine (A) and femoral neck (B) in patients with end-stage lung disease awaiting transplation. From (22) with permission.

include age < 75 yr, advanced pulmonary emphysema, severe dyspnea, FEV_1 < 35% predicted, thoracic hyperinflation, and the ability to complete a preoperative pulmonary rehabilitation program *(25)*. Exclusionary criteria include recent cigarette smoking, obesity or cachexia, severe comorbid illness, severe hypercapnia or pulmonary hypertension, ventilator dependence, or inability to participate in rehabilitation *(25)*. Nonrespiratory issues such as osteoporosis, renal insufficiency, and coronary artery disease must be individualized for each LVRS candidate, but may be acceptable if the conditions are of mild-moderate severity, and deemed unlikely to affect postoperative recovery.

Accordingly, LVRS is especially useful for patients with advanced pulmonary emphysema who are not suitable candidates for lung transplantation. Such patients are usually older than age 60–65, or have contraindications to lung transplantation as outlined in Table 1 *(6)*. Conversely, lung transplantation is the only surgical option for patients with advanced pulmonary emphysema who are not suitable candidates for LVRS. Such patients usually have diffuse anatomic pulmonary emphysema without specific "target" areas for LVRS *(26)*. Most patients with α-1 antitrypsin deficiency fall into this category. Unfortunately, a large proportion of patients with advanced pulmonary emphysema are not eligible for either lung transplantation or LVRS. Therefore, the debate about whether lung transplantation or LVRS is the more appropriate surgical procedure for patients with advanced pulmonary emphysema really centers on patients who are eligible and suitable candidates for either procedure.

PULMONARY FUNCTION AFTER LUNG TRANSPLANTATION AND LVRS

A general review of the physiology of the transplanted lung, including pulmonary denervation, impaired cough and mucociliary clearance, lymphatic interruption, vascular tone, and right ventricular function, has been published recently *(27)*. This section will limit discussion to aspects of lung transplantation specific to pulmonary emphysema.

Most bilateral lung transplant recipients achieve normal spirometry, normal static and dynamic lung volumes, and resolution of thoracic hyperinflation *(28–31)*. By 1 yr after transplantation, lung volumes return to values predicted by the patient's sex, age, and height, even though there may have been considerable disparities between the donor lung size and the recipient's preoperative TLC *(32)*. For donor-recipient matching, therefore, it is most appropriate to use the recipient's predicted lung volumes as the normal values after transplantation, and the best method of matching donor and recipient volumes is to use their respective predicted TLC values *(32)*.

Aside from spirometry and lung volumes, other parameters of respiratory function after bilateral lung transplantation for pulmonary emphysema are remarkably intact. There is no evidence of airflow obstruction (normal FEV_1/FVC, normal airway resistance) *(29–31,33)*, and a number of other parameters, including distribution of alveolar ventilation (measured by single breath N2 washout) *(34)*, muscle pressures *(33,35)*; pulmonary arterial pressures *(36,37)*, gas exchange at rest and with exercise *(29)*, and the resting breathing pattern are normal *(29)*.

In contrast, pulmonary function in single-lung transplant recipients is highly dependent on physiologic interactions between the transplanted and the emphysematous (native) lung. In the immediate postoperative period, there may be acute mediastinal shift secondary to overdistention of the native emphysematous lung with impaired gas exchange and even impaired hemodynamics (*see* Fig. 2A) *(38)*. To minimize mediastinal shift in patients with pulmonary emphysema, transplant surgeons prefer to implant an "oversized" lung. Later in the postoperative course, the transplant lung usually appears radiographically "smaller" than the native, hyperinflated lung (*see* Fig. 2B). In one study, the volume of the transplant lung was only 33% of TLC, whereas the volume of the native emphysema lung was as high as 75–80% of TLC *(39)*.

Despite these volume discrepancies after single–lung transplantation, there is marked clinical improvement *(30,40–42)*. Spirometry and arterial oxygen tension rapidly improve (*see* Fig. 3). Typically, FEV_1 increases by 1.0–1.5 L, whereas FVC increases somewhat less than 1.0 L *(30,40–42)*. Lung function continues to improve during the first postoperative year. In one study, at 12 mo after single-lung transplantation, mean FEV_1 increased from 0.49 (16% of predicted) to 1.6 (54% of predicted), FVC increased from 1.7 (43% of predicted) to 2.4 (62% of predicted), and FEV_1/FVC rose from 0.3 to 0.62 *(42)*. Mean PaO_2 increased from 58 mmHg to 90 mmHg, and no patient required supplemental oxygen at rest or exercise. Quantitative ventilation and perfusion to the transplanted lung were 84% and 80%, respectively. These improvements were sustained during the second year after transplant *(42)*.

There do not appear to be significant differences in physiologic parameters in patients undergoing right vs left single-lung transplantation for emphysema *(42)*. A biphasic pattern of expiratory flow is often observed in the flow-volume curve *(43)*. The initial high-flow phase of the flow-volume curve derives from the transplanted lung, and the terminal low flow from the native, emphysematous lung. In the absence of anastomotic stenosis, the flow-limiting segment is located in the native bronchus, immediately proximal to the anastomosis *(43)*.

Despite the improvement in airflow obstruction after single-lung transplantation, however, the thorax remains hyperinflated, with TLC ranging from 110–120% predicted *(39,44)*. Measurement of diaphragmatic dimensions after single-lung transplantation demonstrate that total diaphragm surface area and dome surface area are smaller on the transplant side compared to the native lung, and that the curvature of the diaphragm on the transplant side returns to normal *(45)*.

Results of exercise testing after lung transplantation have been disappointing. Despite satisfactory allograft function, most transplant recipients, including bilateral lung transplants, are unable to achieve maximal levels of work and O_2 consumption *(29,46–48)*. In one study, bilateral lung recipients with normal spirometry achieved lower work

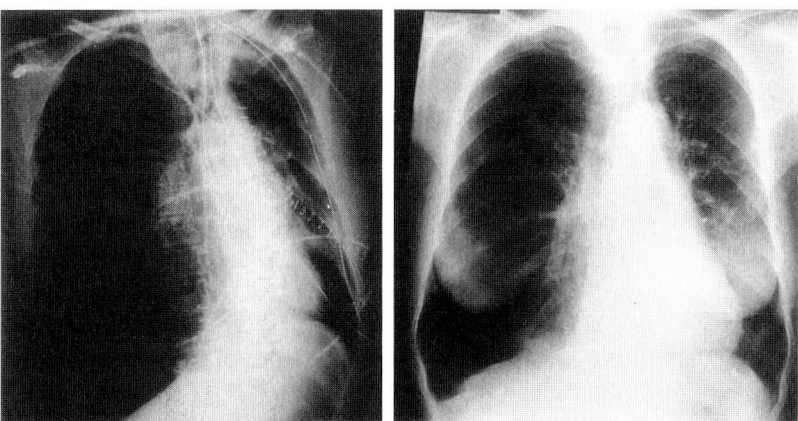

Fig. 2. A. Postoperative mediastinal shift in a 50-yr-old woman after left single-lung transplantation for severe pulmonary emphysema. The native right lung has massively overinflated across the midline, displacing both heart and transplanted left lung to the left. B. Chest radiograph in the same patient 6 mo after left single transplantation. The native right lung remains hyperinflated compared to the transplanted left lung, but there is no mediastinal shift. From:*(45a)* with permission.

(62 vs 155 W) and O_2 consumption (0.88 vs 2.26 L/min) than control subjects *(46)*. Within their limited range of exercise, however, ventilatory responses were normal *(46)*. In all studies, poor exercise performance seems related to limited limb muscle endurance associated with deconditioning, but also possibly to the effects of corticosteroids (myopathy) and cyclosporine (impaired muscle vasodilation). Transplant recipients invariably report leg fatigue and pain as the reason they stop exercising during testing *(49)*. Abnormal skeletal muscle oxidative capacity after lung transplantation has been elegantly demonstrated by ^{31}P-magnetic resonance spectroscopy *(47)*. During exercise, transplant recipients demonstrated a lower pH and greater release of potassium ion than control subjects *(47,48)*.

Aerobic exercise training after transplant increases peak oxygen uptake. In one study, a 6-wk aerobic exercise training program improved peak work (from 66 to 81 W) and O_2 consumption (from 1.1 to 1.3 L/min) *(49)*. Nevertheless, these improved values were still only 55–65% compared to control subjects, and all transplant recipients still terminated exercise because of leg pain.

Remarkably, single-lung transplant recipients perform as well as bilateral recipients in exercise capacity, despite marked differences in spirometric values *(50,51)*. Both groups of transplant recipients exhibit

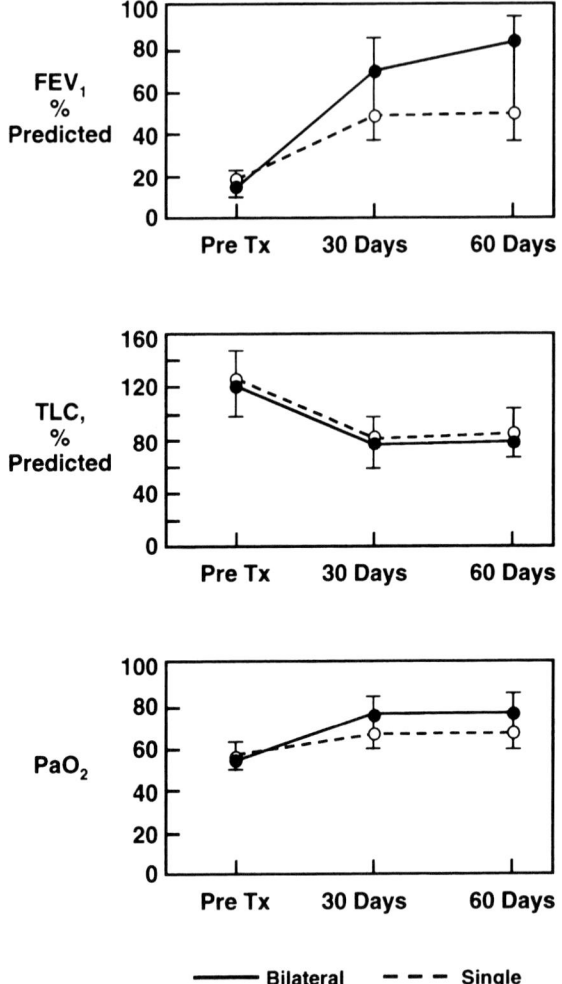

Fig. 3. Lung function before and early after single and bilateral lung transplantation for advanced pulmonary emphysema. Adapted from: (*30*) with permission.

the same degree of reduction in leg power and leg work capacity, reconfirming that it is peripheral skeletal muscle dysfunction that limits exercise performance in both groups *(50)*.

There are no studies directly comparing results of lung transplantation and LVRS. Comparison of published results of each procedure is complicated by whether patients underwent unilateral vs bilateral lung transplantation or unilateral vs bilateral LVRS. In one series, 33 patients who underwent bilateral LVRS via median sternotomy (mean age 57 yr) were compared with 39 patients who underwent single-lung transplantation (mean age 55 yr) and 27 patients who underwent bilateral lung transplantation (mean age 49 yr) *(52)*. At 6 mo after surgery, mean FEV_1 rose by 79% for LVRS, 231% for single-lung transplants, and 498% for bilateral lung transplants *(52)*. 6-minute walk distance increased by 28% for LVRS, 47% for single-lung transplants, and 79% for bilateral lung transplants *(52)*. Mean PaO_2 on room air was 72 mmHg for LVRS, 78 mmHg for single-lung transplants, and 92 mmHg for bilateral lung transplants.

Other centers have reported comparable results for LVRS *(53–56)*. In most studies, mean FEV_1 only improved by 30–80%, yet functional and exercise capacity improved to a greater extent *(53–56)*. In one study *(53)*, this was attributed to reduction of TLC (from 144% to 122%) and increased lung static elastic recoil pressure (from 11.3 to 16.3 cm H_2O), and in another report *(57)*, to improved diaphragmatic muscle pressures (from 41 to 65 cm H_2O) and increased diaphragm length in the area of apposition with the rib cage (2.1 to 3.0 cm) *(57)*. Finally, investigators have demonstrated improvements in exercise performance after LVRS, with higher levels of work (from 40 to 48 W) and O_2 consumption (from 0.73 to 0.76 L/min) than before LVRS, but these works levels remained far below those of normal subjects *(56)*.

A major concern regarding LVRS has been durability of results *(58,59)*. Although some centers have reported minimal loss in pulmonary function over time *(26,60)*, other centers have noted progressive decline in pulmonary function after 6 mo *(58,59)*. In one study, mean FEV_1 declined by 255 mL/yr after bilateral LVRS, and those patients who experienced the greatest short-term incremental response after LVRS also had the most rapid deterioration in FEV_1 *(58)*. Other investigators have raised concerns regarding marked variability in individual patient response, minimal beneficial effects on gas exchange, and the potential for raising pulmonary arterial pressures *(61–63)*.

UTILIZATION OF RESOURCES AFTER LUNG TRANSPLANTATION AND LVRS

Aside from improvement in pulmonary function, a strong argument in favor of LVRS is the limited supply of suitable donor lungs which restricts the option of lung transplantation to a small number of eligible patients. In 1998, 1067 lung transplant procedures (63% single lung, 37% bilateral lung) were recorded by the registry of the International Society for Heart and Lung Transplantation *(64)*. This number of lung transplant procedures represented a decline of 15% compared to the previous 3 yr, and occurred despite the use of increasingly older donors

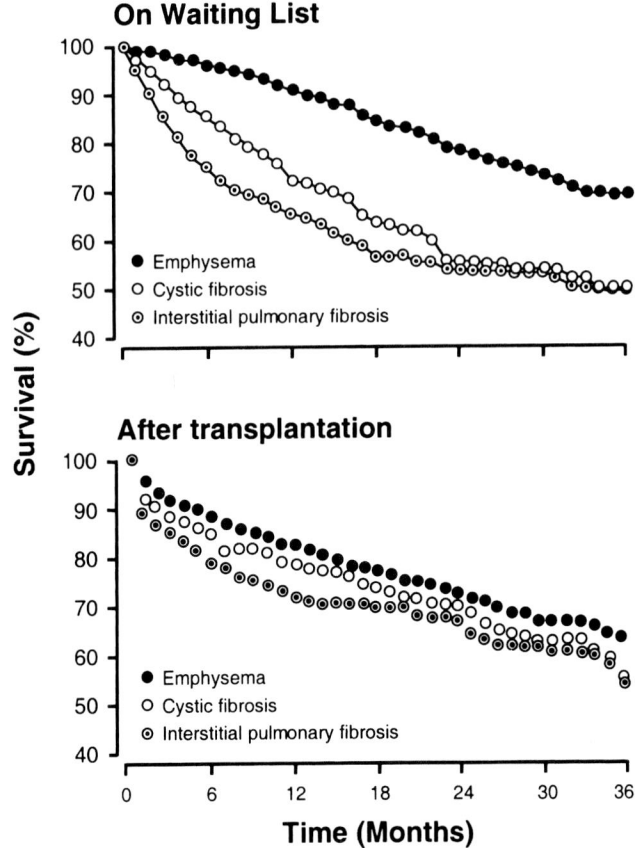

Fig. 4. Survival curves by diagnosis for patients waiting for lung transplantation (censored at time of transplantation) and after transplantation. Adapted *(63a)* with permission.

(64). Patients with advanced pulmonary emphysema constituted 45% of single-lung transplant procedures and 19% of bilateral-lung transplant procedures *(64)*. Patients with α-1 antitrypsin deficiency constituted an additional 11% of single-lung transplant procedures and 11% of bilateral lung transplant procedures *(64)*.

The number of transplant procedures performed for advanced pulmonary emphysema stands in contrast to the 2672 patients in 1998 who were awaiting lung transplantation *(65)*. This represents an increase of 64% in the number of patients awaiting lung transplantation compared to the previous 3 yr *(65)*. The number of transplant procedures for pulmonary emphysema also stands in contrast to the estimated 2000 LVRS procedures performed in the U.S. between 1994–1995, and to the estimated 1.7 million Americans who suffer disability from pulmonary emphysema *(66)*. It has been predicted that the greater availability of LVRS may be used to reduce the number of patients with pulmonary emphysema on transplant waiting lists *(67)*.

Along the same lines, costs associated with LVRS are far lower than those of lung transplantation *(66,68,69)*. Average hospital costs associated with LVRS have been estimated at $31000 *(66,68)*. In contrast, hospital costs associated with lung transplantation have been estimated at $108000 *(69)*. Furthermore, considerable costs remain after transplantation including greater than $1000 per month in medication costs *(69)*. By comparison, medication usage is often reduced after LVRS *(70)*.

MORTALITY AFTER LUNG TRANSPLANTATION AND LVRS

A second argument in favor of LVRS over lung transplantation is the high perioperative and later postoperative mortality associated with lung transplantation. Early postoperative mortality for all lung transplant recipients is 7–10% and 1-yr survival is approx 75% *(64)*. The average survival after lung transplantation is 3.8 yr *(64)*. Remarkably, patients with pulmonary emphysema fare better after lung transplantation than other diagnostic groups *(64)*. In one multivariate logistic regression analysis, the diagnosis of pulmonary emphysema reduced the risk ratio of 1-yr mortality after lung transplantation by 52% *(64)*. One-yr survival rates as high as 90–92% have been reported after single- and bilateral-lung transplantation for pulmonary emphysema *(52)*. Other centers have reported better survival results after bilateral lung transplantation (1-yr survival 90%) than after single-lung transplantation (1-yr survival 71%) *(71)*. Two-yr survival rates after lung transplantation for pulmonary emphysema decline to 82–90% for bilateral lung transplant recipients and 63–84% for single-lung transplant recipients *(71,72)*. Five-yr survival drops as low as 41–53% *(72)*. There have been no major changes in survival rates in the past few years *(64)*.

In view of the perioperative and later postoperative mortality risks for lung transplantation, some investigators have questioned whether there is a survival benefit associated with lung transplantation in the treatment of advanced pulmonary emphysema *(73)*. Hosenpud et al. utilized UNOS data to compare survival curves for patients waiting for lung transplantation and for those who received transplants (*see* Fig. 4) *(73)*. Since, strictly speaking, these survival curves cannot be compared statistically, the authors generated a model to estimate relative risk of death after lung transplantation relative to the risk of continued waiting on the transplant waiting list (*see* Fig. 5) *(73)*. For all diagnoses, the relative risk was high immediately after transplantation, reflecting

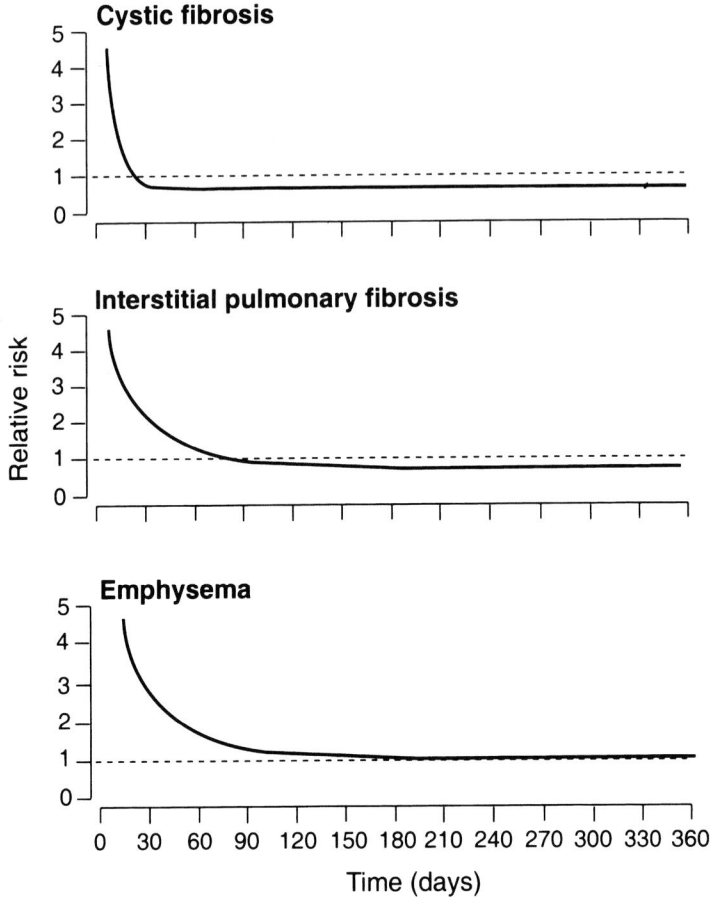

Fig. 5. Relative (transplantation/continued waiting) risk of death according to diagnosis. Adapted from: (*63a*) with permission.

perioperative mortality associated with transplant surgery (*73*). For patients with cystic fibrosis and idiopathic pulmonary fibrosis, the relative risk of transplant soon dropped below the risk of waiting, reflecting high mortality associated with continued waiting on the transplant waiting list. However, for patients with pulmonary emphysema, the relative risk of transplant never dropped below the risk of waiting, reflecting stable mortality rates associated with continued waiting on the transplant waiting list.

These data raise serious concerns regarding survival benefits of lung transplantation in the treatment of advanced pulmonary emphysema. The data, however, are based on a false premise. The analysis assumed that all patients with pulmonary emphysema listed for lung transplant were sick enough to need transplant surgery at the time of listing. Given the long waiting time for lung transplantation *(65)*, many centers may "list" a patient for transplant in anticipation of need at the end of the long waiting time. This unofficial policy biases results in favor of waiting list survival.

Another limitation of the analysis of Hosenpud et al. was that the data assessed only duration of survival, not quality of life. After successful lung transplantation, there are dramatic improvements in health status and quality of life *(74)*. One study of transplant recipients reported higher levels of happiness, more satisfaction with life and health, better function on the Karnofsky index and higher levels in every MOS 20 dimension except pain *(74)*. Furthermore, health-related quality of life remained stable 3 yr after transplantation, although there was some decline over time in patients who developed chronic rejection *(74)*. Between 85–90% of lung transplant recipients reported no activity limitation at 1 and 2 yr after transplant *(64)*.

These considerations highlight a major dilemma faced by transplant physicians and surgeons. On the one hand, guidelines for the referral of patients with pulmonary emphysema facilitate the identification of patients at risk for death in subsequent years *(6,75–78)*. However, the natural history of pulmonary emphysema is so variable that the exact timing of transplant surgery is difficult to define. Accordingly, transplant centers and the referring physicians rely on additional clinical criteria to determine optimal timing for lung transplantation. Such criteria include rapid decline in pulmonary function, frequent exacerbations, and deteriorating gas exchange *(79,80)*. If one waits too long before proceeding with transplantation, the patients may lose their suitability for transplantation by developing worsening debility or respiratory failure.

Despite the superior results of lung transplantation for pulmonary emphysema as compared to patients with other diagnoses, short-term mortality rates of lung transplantation exceed those reported for LVRS *(26,52,67,70,81)*. Operative mortality associated with LVRS has ranged from 3%–7.5%, but has also been reported to be as high as 13.8% *(26,52,67,70,81)*. Operative mortality from LVRS declines with surgical experience *(70)*.

One- and two-yr survival rates as high as 93 and 92% have been reported after LVRS, although other centers have noted slow continued decline in survival postoperatively *(26,70,81)*. In one study, 1-yr survival was 83–85%, and 2-yr survival 76–81% *(81)*. The continued decline in survival presumably reflects progression of the underlying emphysematous process, as well as morbidity related to the advanced lung disease itself. Indeed, survival was highest in patients who were

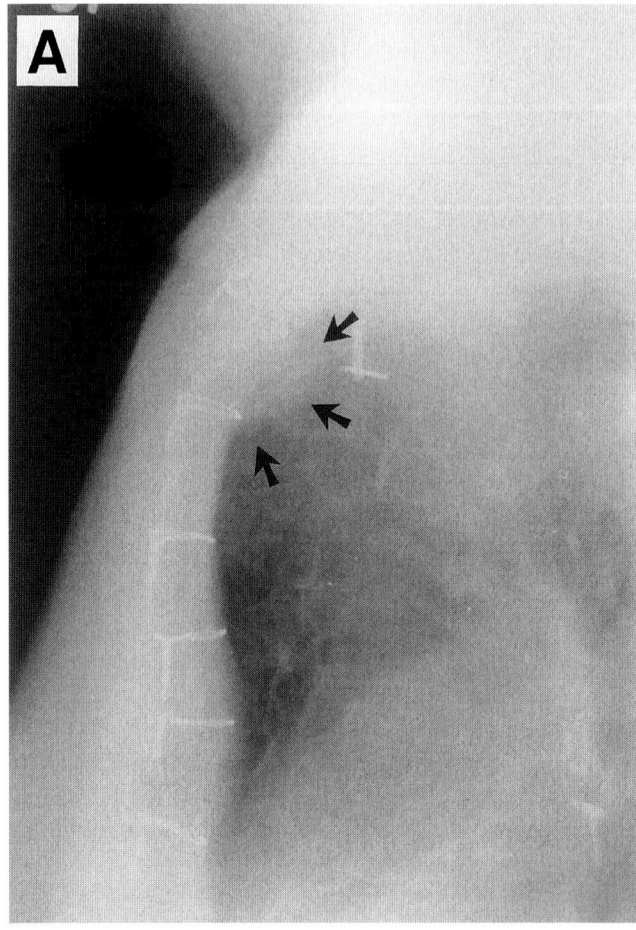

Fig. 6. *(this and opposite page)* A. Squamous cell carcinoma as a subtle irregular nodular opacity (arrows) adjacent to the left anterior chest wall, evident only in retrospect, on lateral chest radiograph of a 59-yr-old woman 11 mo after right single-lung transplantation for emphysema. B. Four months later, the carcinoma (arrows) has enlarged to a 4.5-cm mass.

younger, had higher baseline FEV_1, higher baseline PaO_2, and had the greatest short-term improvement in FEV_1 after LVRS *(81)*.

Just as in the analysis of lung transplantation and survival, some investigators have questioned whether there is a survival benefit associated with LVRS in the treatment of advanced pulmonary emphysema *(25,81)* (see Chapter 14). In this regard, issues concerning resources and optimal patient selection have also been raised *(25)*. To clarify these questions prospectively, the Health Care Financing Administration

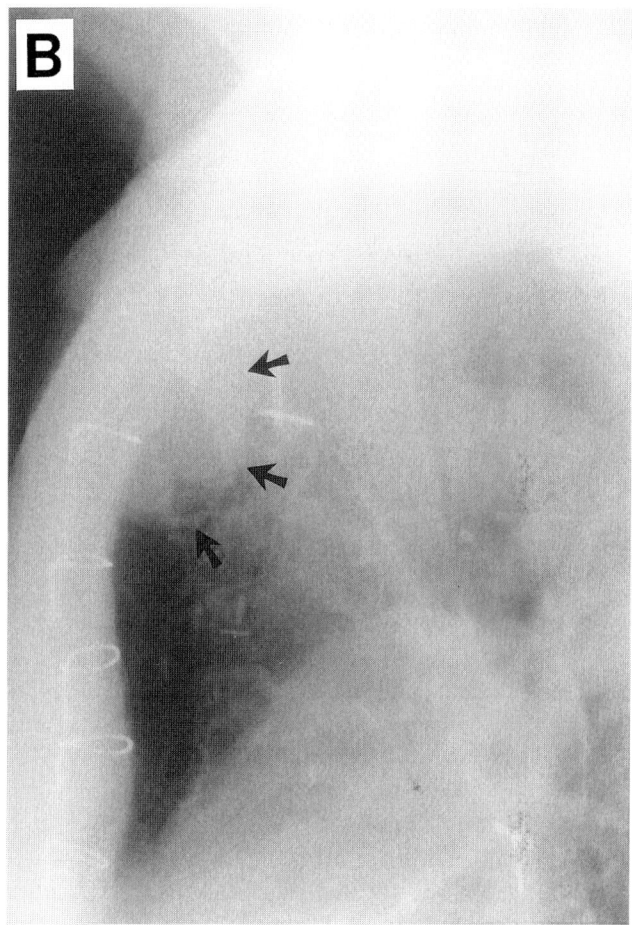

Fig. 6. (B)

(HCFA) is currently funding a randomized study designated as the National Emphysema Treatment Trial (NETT).

Morbidity after lung transplantation and LVRS

Despite improved pulmonary function and quality of life, transplant recipients face the risk of numerous postoperative complications *(7,8)*. One-half of transplant recipients require repeat hospitalization during the first yr after transplantation *(64)*. Postoperative morbidity may be conveniently divided into respiratory and nonrespiratory categories (see Table 2). In the perioperative period, respiratory complications include ischemia-reperfusion injury *(82–85)*, bronchial anastomotic complications (ischemia, dehiscence, stenosis) *(86–88)*, pulmonary vein thrombosis *(89,90)*, and pneumonia *(82,83)*. A complication that is unique to single-lung transplantation for pulmonary emphysema is acute mediastinal shift with hypoxemia and hypotension (*see* Fig. 2A) *(38)*. This is best managed with independent lung ventilation to deliberately underventilate the native, emphysematous lung, while maintaining normal ventilation parameters to the transplant lung *(38)*.

Later postoperative respiratory complications include acute rejection, opportunistic infection, and chronic rejection *(82,91–98)*. In lung transplant recipients, there appears to be a higher incidence of acute and chronic rejection than that observed with other solid organ allografts *(82,92)*. Acute allograft rejection, characterized by perivascular lymphocytic inflammation, is common, rarely fatal, and tends to respond favorably to augmented immunosuppression. In contrast, obliterative bronchiolitis (OB), which is generally considered to represent chronic allograft rejection, is characterized by fibrous obliteration of small airways, responds poorly to augmented immunosuppression, and is the major cause of long-term morbidity and mortality after lung transplantation *(94–96)*. A number of studies have identified multiple and high grade acute rejection episodes as the major risk factors for OB, yet the pathogenetic mechanisms linking acute perivascular rejection to chronic airway obliteration remain undefined *(94–96)*. These complications occur at similar rates for patients transplanted for pulmonary emphysema as compared to patients transplanted for other diagnoses.

Unique to single-lung transplantation for pulmonary emphysema is native lung hyperinflation with compression and atelectasis of the allograft. This issue will be addressed in more detail in the section discussing LVRS after transplantation. Other problems fairly specific to single lung transplantation for pulmonary emphysema are diseases related to the native lung *(99–101)*. These include pneumothorax, bronchogenic carcinoma (*see* Fig. 6), reactivation of dormant tuberculous and nontuberculous mycobacterial infections in the native lung *(101–103)*, and contamination of the transplant lung with pathogens colonizing the native lung such as gram negative bacteria and Aspergillus *(99,100)*.

Nonrespiratory complications after lung transplantation are numerous and include systemic hypertension, renal insufficiency, diabetes mellitus, hyperlipidemia, seizures, osteoporosis, gastroparesis, and post-transplant lymphoproliferative disorders *(7,8,22,23,104–107)*. Most nonrespiratory complications are related directly, or indirectly, to adverse effects of transplant medications. For example, it has been previously noted that the mean bone density of patients with emphysema is already in the osteoporotic range before transplantation (*see* Fig. 1) *(22)*. After transplant, Shane et al.

observed a further decline in bone density associated with effects of gluco-corticoids and cyclosporine *(24)*. The highest rate of fracture after transplant occurred in patients with the lowest bone density before transplant and with greatest duration of pretransplant glucocorticoid therapy. Patients with pulmonary emphysema were at highest risk for fractures after transplant, despite adequate antiresoprtive therapy.

A nonrespiratory complication seemingly unrelated to transplant medications is gastroparesis *(105,106)*. Gastroparesis is of special relevance to lung transplant recipients because by promoting bacterial overgrowth and enabling gastroesophageal reflux, gastroparesis may predispose to microaspiration, respiratory infection, and rejection *(105,106)*. The mechanism of gastroparesis is suspected to relate to operative vagal injury, and may be particularly important in patients with pulmonary emphysema who have a high incidence of reflux and peptic disease even before transplantation.

Postoperative complications after LVRS are far fewer than with lung transplantation. Early postoperative complications include prolonged air leak, sternal wound infection, and gastrointestinal complications *(26,70)*. Later postoperative complications relate predominately to the underlying obstructive lung disease (*see* Chapter 13 for a more detailed discussion of LVRS complications). The main difference compared to lung transplantation is absence of a requirement for immunosuppressive drug treatment.

Finally, both lung transplantation and LVRS have led to improvements in quality of life *(74,108)*. At present, there are no data to directly compare quality of life after lung transplantation and LVRS.

LVRS as a "Bridge" to Lung Transplantation

Patients who are suitable candidates for lung transplant and LVRS could be offered the opportunity for LVRS while being simultaneously listed for lung transplantation. Those with satisfactory results after LVRS could be deactivated from the waiting list. Those patients with unsatisfactory results after LVRS or those patients whose pulmonary function deteriorated after initial improvement could proceed with transplantation. Lung volume reduction via sternotomy or clamshell incision does not preclude successful subsequent lung transplantation. Preliminary experience in one center indicated that 23% of patients had an unsuccessful response to LVRS, and an additional 17% had significant deterioration during follow-up after LVRS requiring lung transplantation *(67)*. Widespread adoption of this approach could reduce the percentage of patients with pulmonary emphysema requiring lung transplantation, and could potentially reduce waiting times for all transplant candidates *(67)*.

Simultaneous LVRS and Single-Lung Transplantation

In an attempt to improve lung function after single-lung transplant, one center has reported preliminary experience with simultaneous single-lung transplantation and contralateral LVRS *(109)*. This approach may prevent problematic native lung hyperinflation after single-lung transplant and may yield levels of pulmonary function similar to those achieved after bilateral transplant.

LVRS after Single-Lung Transplantation to Reduce Native Lung Hyperinflation

Published reports from several lung transplant centers have indicated that LVRS may be beneficial after single-lung transplantation in selected instances where the native emphysematous lung undergoes hyperinflation, compressing and causing extrinsic dysfunction of a structurally normal allograft lung *(110–113)*. In these reports, surgical reduction of native emphysematous lung hyperinflation permitted improved expansion and function of the allograft lung. Ventilation and perfusion of the allograft increased, and the volume of the allograft lung increased *(113)*. Other centers have reported improved allograft function after native lung bullectomy, native lung lobectomy, or native lung pneumonectomy *(114–116)*.

LVRS after Single-Lung Transplantation to Salvage Chronic Allograft Rejection

Our transplant center reported data examining the utility of native LVRS in salvaging respiratory function for patients who had previously undergone single-lung transplantation for emphysema and who were disabled by severe obliterative bronchiolitis *(117)*. In contrast to reports cited earlier, the seven patients described in this series had severe intrinsic disease of the allograft lung. Under these circumstances, surgical reduction of native lung hyperinflation did not increase the volume of the allograft lung, and ventilation and perfusion of the allograft were further decreased *(117)*.

Nevertheless, mean FEV_1 rose from 0.68 ± 0.16 L before LVRS to 0.95 ± 0.22 L at 3 mo after LVRS, an increment of 40% ($p = 0.002$). In addition, mean 6-min walk increased from 781 ± 526 ft to 887 ± 539 ft ($p = 0.031$), and mean dyspnea index declined from 3.1 ± 1.1 to 1.6 ± 0.5 ($p = 0.010$). The LVRS procedure itself was notably safe with no mortality, minimal complications, and acceptable length of hospital stay. These clinical features were remarkable in view of the high surgical risk of this patient population who were maintained on chronic corticosteroids and chronic immunosuppression. In addition, these patients had a very low preoperative FEV_1 and all had had previous thoracic surgery.

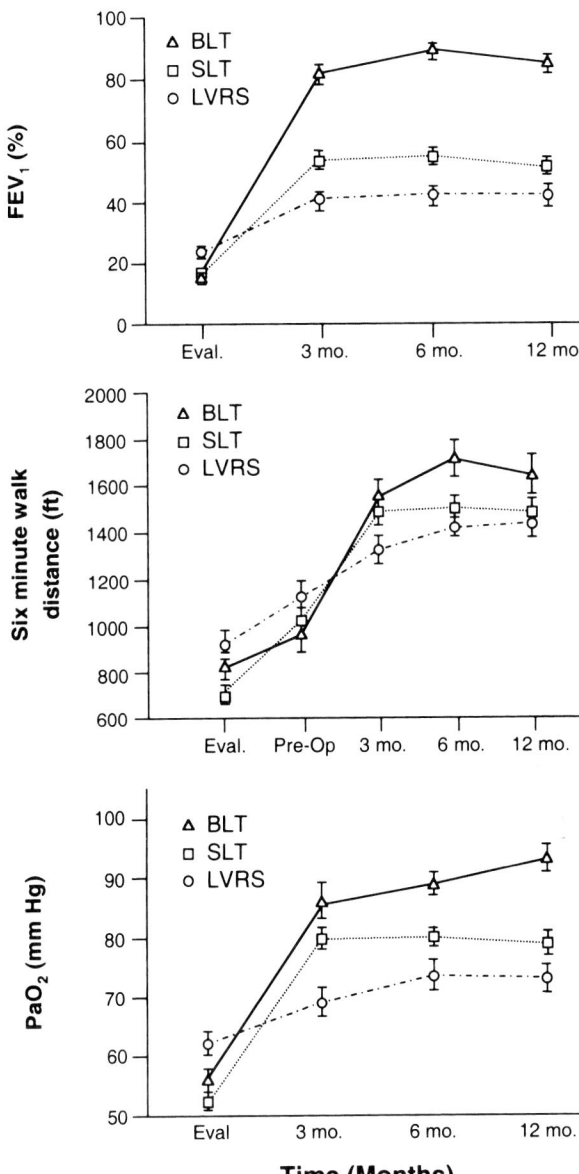

Fig. 7. Lung function before and after LVRS, single-lung transplantation (SLT), and bilateral-lung transplantation (BLT) for advanced pulmonary emphysema. Adapted from: *(52)* with permission.

The benefits, however, of LVRS in salvaging respiratory function appeared to be limited in magnitude and duration *(117)*. The degree of improvement in spirometry and other parameters of respiratory function were smaller than improvements noted in many series of unilateral LVRS for emphysema *(70)*. During follow-up, three of seven patients died within 1 yr after LVRS as a result of respiratory failure. Even survivors began to show deterioration in spirometry by 6 mo postoperatively. These limitations were most likely related to the severity of the underlying allograft dysfunction. The slow deterioration in FEV_1 seen in the 1-yr survivors after LVRS presumably reflected both progressive airflow obstruction in the allograft, as well as continued loss of elastic recoil in the native emphysematous lung. LVRS was able to salvage respiratory function in chronic allograft rejection in emphysema by reducing native lung hyperinflation, but the benefits were limited in magnitude and duration by the severity of the underlying allograft dysfunction *(117)*.

CONCLUSION

Lung transplantation and LVRS are becoming progressively interrelated in the approach to the treatment of advanced pulmonary emphysema. As clinical experiences with each procedure increases, optimal selection and utilization of these procedures will improve therapeutic options for patients. Further progress is needed in minimizing perioperative complications and optimizing postoperative management, especially in lung transplant recipients.

REFERENCES

1. Cooper JD (1997) The history of surgical procedures for emphysema. *Ann Thorac Surg* 63:312–319.
2. Nash ES, Briscoe WA, Cournand A (1965) The relationship between clinical and physiological findings in chronic obstructive disease of the lungs. *Med Thorac* 22:305–327.
3. Schulman LL, Lennon PP, Wood JA, Enson Y (1994) Pulmonary vascular resistance in emphysema. *Chest* 105:798–805.
4. Keller CA, Ohar J, Ruppel G, Wittry MD, Goodgold HM (1995) Right ventricular function in patients with severe COPD evaluated for lung transplantation. *Chest* 107:1510–1516.
5. Enson Y, Giuntini C, Lewis ML, Morris TQ, Ferrer MI, Harvey RM (1964) The influence of hydrogen ion concentration and hypoxia on the pulmonary circulation. *J Clin Invest* 43:1146–1162.
6. Joint statement of the American Society for Transplant Physicians, American Thoracic Society, European Respiratory Society, and International Society for Heart and Lung Transplantation (1998) International guidelines for the selection of lung transplant candidates. *Am J Respir Crit Care Med* 158:335–339.
7. Trulock EP (1997) Lung transplantation. *Am J Respir Crit Care Med* 155:789–818.

8. Arcasoy SM, Kotloff RM (1999) Lung transplantation. *N Engl J Med* 340: 1081–1091.
9. Kadikar A, Maurer J, Kesten S (1997) The six-minute walk test: a guide to assessment for lung transplantation. *J Heart Lung Transplant* 16:313–319.
10. Ries AL, Kaplan RM, Limberg TM, Prewitt LM (1995) Effect of pulmonary rehabilitation on physiologic and psychosocial outcomes in patients with chronic obstructive pulmonary disease. *Ann Intern Med* 122:823–832.
11. Shapiro PA, Williams DL, Foray AT, Gelman IS, Wukich N, Sciacca R (1995) Psychosocial evaluation and prediction of compliance problems and morbidity after heart transplantation. *Transplantation* 60:1462–1466.
12. Leibowitz, DW, Caputo AL, Shapiro GC, et al. (1994) Coronary angiography in smokers undergoing evaluation for lung transplantation: is routine use justified? *J Heart Lung Transplant* 33:701–703.
13. Snell GJ, Richardson M, Griffiths AP, Williams TJ. Esmore DS (1999) Coronary artery disease in potential lung transplant recipients > 50 years old: the role of coronary interventions. *Chest* 116:874–879.
14. Low DE, Trulock EP, Kaiser LR, et al. (1992) Lung transplantation of ventilator-dependent patients. *Chest* 101:8–11.
15. Flume PA, Egan TM, Westerman JH, et al. (1994) Lung transplantation for mechanically ventilated patients. *J Heart Lung Transplant* 13:15–21.
16. Dusmet M, Winton TL, Kesten S, Maurer J (1996) Previous intrapleural procedures do not adversely affect lung transplantation. *J Heart Lung Transplant* 15:249–254.
17. Detterbeck FC, Egan TM, Mill MR (1995) Lung transplantation after previous thoracic surgical procedures. *Ann Thorac Surg* 60:139–143.
18. Etienne B, Bertocchi M, Gamondes JP, Wiesendanger T, Brune J, Mornex JF (1997) Successful double-lung transplantation for bronchioalveolar carcinoma. *Chest* 112:1423–1424.
19. Garver RI, Zorn GL, Wu X, McGiffin DC, Young KR, Pinkard NB (1999) Recurrence of bronchioloalveolar carcinoma in transplanted lungs. *N Engl J Med* 340:1071–1074.
20. Schols AMWJ, Soeters PB, Mostert R, Pluymers RJ, Wouters EFM (1995) Physiologic effects of nutritional support and anabolic steroids in patients with chronic obstructive pulmonary disease. *Am J Respir Crit Care Med* 152: 1268–1274.
21. Schols AMWJ, Slangen J, Volovics L, Wouters EFM (1998) Weight loss is a reversible factor in the prognosis of chronic obstructive pulmonary disease. *Am J Respir Crit Care Med* 157: 1791–1797.
22. Shane E, Silverberg SJ, Donovan D, et al. (1996) Osteoporosis in lung transplantation candidates with end-stage pulmonary disease. *Am J Med* 101:262–269.
23. Aris RM, Neuringer IP, Weiner MA, Egan TM, Ontjes D (1996) Severe osteoporosis before and after lung transplantation. *Chest* 109:1176–1183.
24. Shane E, Papadopoulos A, Staron RB, et al. (1999) Bone loss and fracture after lung transplantation. *Transplantation* 68:220–227.
25. American Thoracic Society (1996) Lung volume reduction surgery. *Am J Respir Crit Care Med* 154:1151–1152.
26. Cooper JD, Patterson GA, Sundaresan RS, et al. (1996) Results of 150 consecutive bilateral lung volume reduction procedures in patients with severe emphysema. *J Thorac Cardiovasc Surg* 112:1319–1330.
27. Schulman LL (1998) Physiology of the transplanted lung. In: Norman and Suki, Eds., *Primer on Transplantation* Chelsea MI: Slack, pp. 519–526.
28. Martinez JA, Paradis IL, Dauber JH, et al. (1997) Spirometry values in stable lung transplant recipients. *Am J Respir Crit Care Med* 155:285–290.

29. Williams TJ, Patterson GA, McClean PA, Zamel N, Maurer JR (1992) Maximal exercise testing in single and double lung transplant recipients. *Am Rev Respir Dis* 145:101–105.
30. Low DE, Trulock EP, Kaiser LR, et al. (1992) Morbidity, mortality, and early results of single versus bilateral lung transplantation for emphysema. *J Thorac Cardiovasc Surg* 103:1119–1126.
31. Arens R, McDonough JM, Zhao H, Blumenthal NP, Kotloff RM, Grunstein MM (1998) Altered lung mechanics after double-lung transplantation. *Am J Respir Crit Care Med* 158:1403–1409.
32. Tamm M, Higenbottam TW, Dennis CM, Sharples LD, Wallwork J (1994) Donor and recipient predicted lung volume and lung size after heart-lung transplantation. *Am J Respir Crit Care Med* 150: 403–407.
33. Frost AE, Zamel N, McClean PA, Patterson GA, Maurer JR (1992) Hypercapnic ventilatory response in recipients of double-lung transplants. *Am Rev Respir Dis* 146:1610–1612.
34. Van Muylem A, Antoine M, Yernault JC, Paiva M, Estenne M (1995) Inert gas single-breath washout after heart-lung transplantation. *Am J Respir Crit Care Med* 152:947–952.
35. Chacon RA, Corris PA, Dark JH, Gibson GJ (1997) Respiratory mechanics after heart-lung and bilateral lung transplantation. *Thorax* 52:718–722.
36. Globits S, Burghuber C, Koller J, et al. (1994) Effect of lung transplantation on right and left ventricular volumes and function measured by magnetic resonance imaging. *Am J Respir Crit Care Med* 149:1000–1004.
37. Schulman LL, Leibowitz DW, Anadarangam T, et al. (1996) Variability of right ventricular functional recovery after lung transplantation. *Transplantation* 62:622–625.
38. Smiley RM, Navedo AT, Kirby T, Schulman LL (1991) Postoperative independent lung ventilation in a single-lung transplant recipient. *Anesthesiology* 74:1144–1148.
39. Cheriyan AF, Garrity ER, Pifarre R, Fahey PJ, Walsh JM (1995) Reduced transplant lung volumes after single lung transplantation for chronic obstructive pulmonary disease. *Am J Respir Crit Care Med* 151:851–853.
40. Kaiser LR, Cooper JD, Trulock EP, et al. (1991) The evolution of single lung transplantation for emphysema. *J Thorac Cardiovasc Surg* 102:333–341.
41. Mal H, Sleiman C, Jebrak G, et al. (1994) Functional results of single-lung transplantation for chronic obstructive lung disease. *Am J Respir Crit Care Med* 149:1476–1481.
42. Levine SM, Anzueto A, Peters JI, et al. (1994) Medium term functional results of single-lung transplantation for endstage obstructive lung disease. *Am J Respir Crit Care Med* 150:398–402.
43. Herlihy JP, Venegas JG, Systrom DM, et al. (1994) Expiratory flow pattern following single-lung transplantation in emphysema. *Am J Respir Crit Care Med* 150:1684–1689.
44. Estenne M, Cassart M, Poncelet P, Gevenois PA (1999) Volume of graft and native lung after single-lung transplantation for emphysema. *Am J Respir Crit Care Med* 159:641–645.
45a. Smiley RM (1991) Postoperative independent lung ventilation in a single-lung transplant recipient. *Anesthesiology* 74:1144–1148.
45. Cassart M, Verbandt Y, de Francquen P, Gevenois PA, Estenne M (1999) Diaphragm dimensions after single-lung transplantation for emphysema. *Am J Respir Crit Care Med* 159:1992–1997.
46. Pellegrino R, Rodarte JR, Frost AE, Reid MB (1998) Breathing by double lung recipients during exercise: response to expiratory threshold loading. *Am J Respir Crit Care Med* 157:106–110.

47. Evans AB, Al-Himyary AJ, Hrovat MI, et al. (1997) Abnormal skeletal muscle oxidative capacity after lung transplantation by ^{31}P-MRS. *Am J Respir Crit Care Med* 155:615–621.

48. Hall MJ, Snell GI, Side EA, Esmore DS, Walters EH, Williams TJ (1994) Exercise, potassium, and muscle deconditioning post-thoracic organ transplantation. *J Appl Physiol* 77:2784–2790.

49. Stiebellehner L, Quittan M, End A, et al. (1998) Aerobic endurance training program improves exercise performance in lung transplant recipients. *Chest* 113:906–912.

50. Orens JB, Becker FS, Lynch JP 3rd, Christensen PJ, Deeb GM, Martinez FJ (1995) Cardiopulmonary exercise testing following allogeneic lung transplantation for different underlying disease states. *Chest* 107:144–149.

51. Lands LC, Smountas AA, Mesiano G, et al. (1999) Maximal exercise capacity and peripheral skeletal muscle function following lung transplantation. *J Heart Lung Transplant* 18:113–120.

52. Gaissert HA, Trulock EP, Cooper JD, Sundaresan RS, Patterson GA (1996) Comparison of early functional results after volume reduction or lung transplantation for chronic obstructive pulmonary disease. *J Thorac Cardiovasc Surg* 111:296–307.

53. Gelb AF, Brenner M, McKenna RJ Jr, Fischel R, Zamel N, Schein MJ (1998) Serial lung function and elastic recoil 2 years after lung volume reduction surgery for emphysema. *Chest* 113:1497–1506.

54. Sciurba FC, Rogers RM, Keenan RJ, et al. (1996) Improvement in pulmonary function and elastic recoil after lung-reduction surgery for diffuse emphysema. *N Engl J Med* 334:1095–1099.

55. Argenziano M, Moazami N, Thomashow B, et al. (1996) Extended indications for lung volume reduction surgery in advanced emphysema. *Ann Thorac Surg* 62:1588–1597.

56. Ferguson GT, Fernandez E, Zamora MR, Pomerantz M, Buchholz J, Make BJ (1998) Improved exercise performance following lung volume reduction surgery for emphysema. *Am J Respir Crit Care Med* 157:1195–203.

57. Lando Y, Boiselle PM, Shade D, et al. (1999) Effect of lung volume reduction surgery on diaphragm length in severe chronic obstructive pulmonary disease. *Am J Respir Crit Care Med* 159:796–805.

58. Brenner M, McKenna RJ Jr, Gelb AF, Fischel RJ, Wilson AF (1998) Rate of FEV_1 change following lung volume reduction surgery. *Chest* 113:652–659.

59. Kesten S, Elpern E, Warren W, Szidon P (1999) Loss of pulmonary function gains after lung volume reduction surgery. *J Heart Lung Transplant* 18:266–268.

60. Cordova F, O'Brien G, Furukawa S, Kuzma AM, Travaline J, Criner GJ (1997) Stability of improvements in exercise performance and quality of life following bilateral lung volume reduction surgery in severe COPD. *Chest* 112:907–915.

61. Scharf SM, Rossoff L, McKeon K, Graver LM, Graham C, Steinberg HN (1998) Changes in pulmonary mechanics after lung volume reduction surgery. *Lung* 176:191–204.

62. Albert RK, Benditt JO, Hildebrandt J, Wood DE, Hlastala MP (1998) Lung volume reduction surgery has variable effects on blood gases in patients with emphysema. *Am J Respir Crit Care Med* 158:71–76.

63. Weg IL, Rossoff L, McKeon K, Michael Graver L, Scharf SM (1999) Development of pulmonary hypertension after lung volume reduction surgery. *Am J Respir Crit Care Med* 159:552–556.

63a. Hosenpud JD (1998) Effect of a diagnosis on survival benefit of lung transplantation for end-stage lung disease. *Lancet* 351:24–27.

64. Hosenpud JD, Bennett LE, Keck BM, Fiol B, Boucek MM, Novick RJ (1999) The registry of the International Society for Heart and Lung Transplantation: sixteenth official report. *J Heart Lung Transplant* 18:611–626.

65. 1998 annual report of the US scientific registry for transplant recipients and the organ procurement and transplantation network-transplant data 1988–1997. UNOS, Richmond, VA, and Div Transplantation, Bur Health Resources Develop, Health Resources Serv Admin, US Dept Health and Human Serv, Rockville, MD.
66. Huizenga HF, Ramsey SD, Albert RK (1998) Estimated growth of lung volume reduction surgery among Medicare enrollees: 1994 to 1996. *Chest* 114:1583–1587.
67. Bavaria JE, Pochettino A, Kotloff RM, et al. (1998) Effect of volume reduction on lung transplant timing and selection for chronic obstructive pulmonary disease. *J Thorac Cardiovasc Surg* 115:9–17.
68. Elpern EH, Behner KG, Klontz B, Warren WH, Szidon JP, Kesten S (1998) Lung volume reduction surgery: an analysis of hospital costs. *Chest* 113:896–899.
69. Ramsey SD, Patrick DL, Albert RK, Larson EB, Wood DE, Raghu G (1995) The cost-effectiveness of lung transplantation: a pilot study. *Chest* 108:1594–1601.
70. Argenziano M, Thomashow B, Jellen PA, Rose EA, Steinglass KM, Ginsburg ME, Gorenstein LA (1997) Functional comparison of unilateral versus bilateral lung volume reduction surgery. *Ann Thorac Surg* 64:321–326.
71. Bavaria JE, Kotloff R, Palevsky H, et al. (1997) Bilateral versus single lung transplantation for chronic obstructive pulmonary disease. *J Thorac Cardiovasc Surg* 113:520–528.
72. Sundaresan RS, Shiraishi Y, Trulock EP, et al. (1996) Single or bilateral lung transplantation for emphysema? *J Thorac Cardiovasc Surg* 112:1485–1495.
73. Hosenpud JD, Bennett LE, Keck BM, Edwards EB, Novick RJ (1998) Effect of diagnosis on survival benefit of lung transplantation for end-stage lung disease. *Lancet* 351:24–27.
74. Gross CR, Savik K, Bolman RM, Hertz MI (1995) Long-term health status and quality of life outcomes of lung transplant recipients. *Chest* 108:1587–1593.
75. The Alpha-1-Antitrypsin Deficiency Registry Study Group (1995) Survival and FEV_1 decline in individuals with severe deficiency of a1-antitrypsin. *Am J Respir Crit Care Med* 151:369–373.
76. Seersholm N, Kok-Jensen A (1998) Survival in relation to lung function and smoking cessation in patients with severe hereditary alpha1-antitrypsin deficiency. *Am J Respir Crit Care Med* 158:49–59.
77. Anthonisen NR (1989) Prognosis in chronic obstructive pulmonary disease: results from multicenter clinical trials. *Am Rev Respir Dis* 140:S95–S99.
78. Burrows B, Bloom JW, Traver JA, Cline MG (1987) The course and prognosis of different forms of chronic airways obstruction in a sample from the general population. *N Engl J Med* 317:1309–1314.
79. Gray-Donald K, Gibbons L, Shapiro SH, Macklem PT, Martin JG (1996) Nutritional status and mortality in chronic obstructive pulmonary disease. *Am J Respir Crit Care Med* 153:961–966.
80. Connors AF, Dawson NV, Thomas C, et al. (1996) Outcomes following acute exacerbations of severe chronic obstructive lung disease. *Am J Respir Crit Care Med* 154:959–967.
81. Brenner M, McKenna RJ Jr, Chen JC, Osann K, Powell L, Gelb AF, Fischel RJ, Wilson AF (1999) Survival following bilateral staple lung volume reduction surgery for emphysema. *Chest* 115:390–396.
82. Bando K, Paradis IL, Komatsu K, et al. (1995) Analysis of time-dependent risks for infection, rejection and deaths after pulmonary transplantation. *J Thorac Cardiovasc Surg* 109:49–59.
83. Christie JD, Bavaria JE, Palevsky HI, et al. (1998) Primary graft failure following lung transplantation. *Chest* 114: 51–60.
84. Anderson DC, Glazer HS, Semenkovich JW, et al. (1995) Lung transplant edema: chest radiography after lung transplantation the first 10 days. *Radiology* 195: 275–281.

85. Date H, Triantafillou AN, Trulock EP, Pohl MS, Cooper JD, Patterson GA (1996) Inhaled nitric oxides reduces human allograft dysfunction. *J Thorac Cardiovasc Surg* 111: 913–919.
86. Anderson MB, Kriett JM, Harrell J, et al. (1995) Techniques for bronchial anastomosis. *J Heart Lung Transplant* 14: 1090–1094.
87. Date H, Trulock EP, Arcidi JM, Sundaresan S, Cooper JD, Patterson GA (1995) Improved airway healing after lung transplantation. *J Thorac Cardiovasc Surg* 110: 1424–1433.
88. Griffiths BP, Magee MJ, Gonzalez IF, et al. (1994) Anastomotic pitfalls in lung transplantation. *J Thorac Cardiovasc Surg* 107:743–754.
89. Hausmann D, Daniel WG, Mugge A, et al. (1992) Imaging of pulmonary artery and vein anastomoses by transesophageal echocardiography after lung transplantation. *Circulation* 86(suppl II): II-251–II-258.
90. Leibowitz DW, Smith CR, Michler RE, et al. (1994) Incidence of pulmonary vein complications after lung transplantation: a prospective transesophageal echocardiographic study. *J Am Coll Cardiology* 24:671–675.
91. Yousem SA, Berry GJ, Cagle PT, et al. (1996) Revision of the 1990 working formulation for the classification of pulmonary allograft rejection: Lung rejection study group. *J Heart Lung Transplant* 15:1–15.
92. Schulman LL, Weinberg AD, McGregor C, Galantowicz ME, Suciu-Foca N, Itescu S (1998) Mismatches at HLA-DR and HLA-B loci are risk factors for acute rejection after lung transplantation. *Am J Respir Crit Care Med* 158: 1833–1837.
93. Cooper JD, Billingham M, Egan T, et al. (1993) A working formulation for the standardization of nomenclature and for clinical staging of chronic dysfunction in lung allografts. *J Heart Lung Transplant* 12:713–716.
94. Bando K, Paradis IL, Similo S, et al. (1995) Obliterative bronchiolitis after lung and heart-lung transplantation: an analysis of risk factors and management. *J Thorac Cardiovasc Surg* 110: 4–14.
95. Girgis RE, Tu I, Berry GJ, et al. (1996) Risk factors for the development of obliterative bronchiolitis after lung transplantation. *J Heart Lung Transplant* 15:1200–1208.
96. Sharples LD, Tamm M, McNeil K, Higenbottam TW, Stewart, Wallwork J (1996) Development of bronchiolitis obliterans syndrome in recipients of heart-lung transplantation: early risk factors. *Transplantation* 61:560–566.
97. Shreeniwas R, Schulman LL, Berkmen Y, McGregor C, Austin JHM (1996) Opportunistic bronchopulmonary infections after lung transplantation: clinical and radiologic findings. *Radiology* 200: 349–356.
98. Kramer MR, Denning DW, Marshall SE, et al. (1991) Ulcerative tracheobronchitis after lung transplantation: a new form of invasive Aspergillosis. *Am Rev Respir Dis* 144: 552–556.
99. Frost AE, Keller CA, Noon GP, Short HD, Cagle PT (1995) Outcome of the native lung after single lung transplant. *Chest* 107:981–984.
100. Horvath J, Dummer S, Loyd J, Walker B, Merril WH, Frist WH (1993) Infection in the transplanted and native lung after single lung transplantation. *Chest* 104: 681–685.
101. Schulman LL, Htun T, Staniloae C, McGregor C, Austin JHM (1999) Pulmonary nodules and masses after lung transplantation. *Am J Respir Crit Care Med* 159:A537.
102. Egan TM, Westerman JH, Lambert CJ, et al. (1992) Isolated lung transplantation for end-stage lung disease: a viable therapy. *Ann Thorac Surg* 53: 590–596.
103. Kesten S, Chaparro C (1999) Mycobacterial infections in lung transplant recipients. *Chest* 115:741–745.
104. Kesten S, Mayne L, Scavuzzo M, Maurer J (1997) Lack of left ventricular dysfunction associated with sustained exposure to hyperlipidemia following lung transplantation. *Chest* 112:931–936.

105. Reid KR, McKenzie FN, Menkis AH, et al. (1990) Importance of chronic aspiration in recipients of heart-lung transplants. *Lancet* 336:206–208.
106. Berkowitz N, Schulman LL, McGregor, C, Markowitz D (1995) Gastroparesis after lung transplantation: potential role in postoperative respiratory complications. *Chest* 108:1602–1607.
107. Aris RM, Maia DM, Neuringer IP, et al. (1996) Post-transplantation lymphoproliferative disorder in the Epstein-Barr virus-naive lung transplant recipient. *Am J Respir Crit Care Med* 154:1712–1717.
108. Moy ML, Ingenito EP, Mentzer SJ, Evans RB, Reilly JJ Jr (1999) Health-related quality of life improves following pulmonary rehabilitation and lung volume reduction surgery. *Chest* 115:383–389.
109. Todd TRJ, Perron J, Winton TL, Keshavjee SH (1997) Simultaneous single-lung transplantation and lung volume reduction. *Ann Thorac Surg* 63:1468–1470.
110. Yonan NA, el-Gamel A, Egan J, Kakadellis J, Rahman A, Deiraniya AK. Single lung transplantation for emphysema: predictors for native lung hyperinflation. J Heart Lung Transplant 1998;17:192-201.
111. Kapelanski DP, Anderson MB, Kriet JM, Colt HG, Smith CM, Mateos M, Jamieson SW (1996) Volume reduction of the native lung after single-lung transplantation for emphysema. *J Thorac Cardiovasc Surg* 111:898–899.
112. Kroshus TJ, Bolman RM, Kshettry VR (1996) Unilateral volume reduction after single-lung transplantation for emphysema. *Ann Thorac Surg* 62:363–368.
113. Anderson MB, Kriet JM, Kapelanski DP, Perricone A, Smith CM, Jamieson SW (1997) Volume reduction surgery in the native lung after single lung transplantation for emphysema. *J Heart Lung Transplant* 16:752–757.
114. Kuno R, Kanter KR, Torres WE, Lawrence EC (1996) Single lung transplantation followed by contralateral bullectomy for emphysema. *J Heart Lung Transplant* 15:389–394.
115. Le Pimpec-Barthes F, Debrosse D, Cuenod CA, Gandjbakheh I, Riquet M (1996) Late contralateral lobectomy after single lung transplantation for emphysema. *Ann Thorac Surg* 61:231–234.
116. Novick RJ, Menkis AH, Sandler D, Garg A, Ahmad D, Williams S, McKenzie FN (1991) Contralateral pneumectomy after single lung transplantation for emphysema. *Ann Thorac Surg* 52:1317–1319.
117. Schulman LL, O'Hair DP, Cantu E, McGregor C, Ginsberg ME (1999) Salvage by volume reduction of chronic allograft rejection in emphysema. *J Heart Lung Transplant* 18:107–112.

Index